Disaster Medicine

Editors: Lee Wallis and Wayne Smith

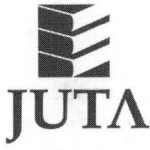

JUTA

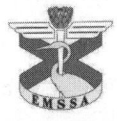

Emergency Medicine Society of South Africa

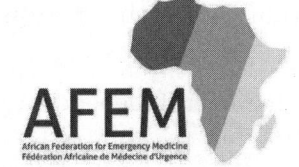

Disaster Medicine

First published 2011

Juta & Co Ltd
First Floor
Sunclare Building
21 Dreyer Street
Claremont
7708

PO Box 14373, Lansdowne, 7779, Cape Town, South Africa
© 2011 Juta & Company Ltd

ISBN 978-0-70218-670-7

Project Manager: Debbie Henry
Editor: Alfred LeMaitre
Proofreader: Glenda Younge
Typesetter: ANdtp Services
Cover designer: Marius Roux
Illustrations (pg 213 & 214): Carol Lochner

Printed in South Africa by Academic Press

The authors and the publisher have made every effort to obtain permission for and to acknowledge the use of copyright material. Should any infringement of copyright have occurred, please contact the publisher, and every effort will be made to rectify omissions or errors in the event of a reprint or new edition.

This book has been independently peer-reviewed by academics who are experts in the field.

Contents

About the Authors

Editors

Lee A Wallis
MBChB, MD, DIMC Dip Sport Med, FRCSEd(A&E), FCEM FCEM(SA)
Professor and Head: Division of Emergency Medicine
University of Cape Town and Stellenbosch University

Wayne P Smith
MBChB, EMDM, FCEM(SA)
Head: Disaster Medicine
A Division of Emergency Medicine
University of Cape Town and Stellenbosch University

Associate editors

Theo J Ligthelm
Colonel
MPA, B Soc Sc (Hon), Dip Adv Nurse, Dip H Ed, Cert AEA, Cert Aviation Nursing
Senior Staff Officer Strategy and Planning
Office of the Surgeon General
South African Military Health Service

Petra Brysiewicz
PhD, M Curationis, B Arts, B Soc Sc
Senior Lecturer and Nurse Educator
School of Nursing
University of KwaZulu-Natal

Timothy C Hardcastle
MBChB, MMed, FCS(SA)
Head of Clinical Unit: Trauma Surgery
Inkosi Albert Luthuli Central Hospital Durban

Contributors

Karen I Barnes
MBChB, MMed
Professor: Division of Clinical Pharmacology
Department of Medicine
University of Cape Town

Kathryn Chu
MD, MPH
Surgical Advisor
Médicins Sans Frontières
Cape Town

Nathan Ford
DHA, MPH, PhD
Head of Medical Unit
Médicins Sans Frontières
Cape Town

Daniël J van Hoving
MBChB, Dip PEC, MMed
Division of Emergency Medicine
University of Cape Town and Stellenbosch University

Melanie Stander
MBChB, MMed
Division of Emergency Medicine
University of Cape Town and Stellenbosch University

William Lubinga
MBChB, MFamMed, FCEM(SA)
Head: Emergency Medicine
University of Limpopo

Basil Bonner
MBBCh, DA
Manager Specialised Medical Projects, Medi-Clinic
Honarary Senior Lecturer: Joint Division of Emergency Medicine
University of Cape Town and Stellenbosch University

Ben Steyn
MBChB, MMed
Colonel
Chemical and Biological Defence Advisor to the Surgeon General
South African National Defence Force

Andrew C Argent
MBBCh, MMed, DCH(SA), FCPaeds(SA), FRCPCH(UK)
Professor: School of Child and Adolescent Health
University of Cape Town

N Kissoon
MD, FRCP(C), FAAP, FCCM, FACPE
Vice President: Medical Affairs
Associate Head: Department of Pediatrics
Professor: Pediatric and Surgery (EM)
BC Children's Hospital
University of British Columbia

Helena J Ras
Brigadier
Section Head: Technology Management
Criminal Record & Forensic Science Services
South African Police Service

Jean E Augustyn
MA, B.Cur, Dip Nursing Education
Nurse Educator: Emergency Nursing
Medi-Clinic Learning Centre

Jacques Goosen
MBChB, FCS(SA), Cert Trauma Surgery
Professor
Head: Charlotte Maxeke Johannesburg Academic Hospital Trauma Unit
University of the Witwatersrand

Susan P Hattingh
D Litt et Phil, MA Cur, BCur (Hons), BCur IetA, Dipl Gen Nurse, Dipl Midwifery,
Dipl Theatre, Dipl Psych
Professor and Associate Dean: College of Nursing
National Guard Al Ahsa
Saudi Arabia

Mande J Toubkin
Dip Gen Nurse, Dip Midwifery, Dip Paediatrics, Dip Medical and Surgical Nursing
Trauma, Dip Medical and Surgical Nursing Critical Care
General Manager: Emergency, Trauma, Disaster Management and Transplant
Netcare

Samuel J Stratton
MD, MPH
Professor: UCLA School of Public Health
Centre for Public Health and Disasters

John Frean
MB BCh, MMed, DTM&H, MSc, FACTM, FFTMRCPSG
Head: Special Bacterial Pathogens Reference Unit
Parasitology Reference Unit, Microbiology Division
National Institute for Communicable Diseases

Lucille Blumberg
MBBCh, M Med, Cert ID, FFTMRCPS, DOH, DTM&H, DCH
Professor: Epidemiology Division and Special Pathogens Unit
National Institute for Communicable Diseases

Robert Swanepoel
BVSc, DTVM, PhD, MRCVS
Professor: Viral Haemorrhagic Diseases Section
National Institute for Communicable Diseases

Marc Mendelson
BSc, MBBS, PhD, FRCP(UK), DTM&H
Associate Professor and Head: Division of Infectious Diseases and HIV Medicine
University of Cape Town

Vernon Wessels
MBChB, Dip PEC
Deputy Director: Emergency Medical Services
Gauteng Department of Health and Social Services

Preface

Whether due to global warming, better reporting, or other causes, disasters are on the increase across the globe. Almost every day, news channels report on natural disasters causing untold devastation and human suffering. Luckily, our region has been spared the worst of these recent disasters. On a smaller scale, however, 'major incidents' are an everyday part of our lives, from taxi collisions and multi-car pile ups, to stampedes at sports events – the list is endless. Between them, disasters and major incidents exact a disproportionate load on developing countries, which are less prepared and less able to deal with the after effects.

While facing major incidents almost weekly in South Africa, we are fortunate to have some of the best legislation in the world on the subject. The Disaster Management Act of 2002 makes it clear that preparedness and response to such events is everybody's business, but health services are critical participants in dealing with these incidents. Healthcare professionals, however, often feel unprepared for the role that they have to play in such events – whether responding to the aftermath of an earthquake overseas, or dealing with yet another overturned taxi on the side of the freeway. This text is intended to help these people – you – to be better equipped and better prepared to achieve what needs to be done at such times; in other words, to do the most for the most number of people.

Lee Wallis and Wayne Smith

Chapter 8 is dedicated to the memory of the late Professor Barney de Villiers, Department of Community Health, Stellenbosch University.

Introduction to Disaster Medicine

W Smith and L Wallis

1. Introduction

The intent of this manual is by no means to educate the reader in all facets of disaster medicine. What is important to understand is that disaster medicine is a line function operating within the guidelines of disaster management. It is thus necessary to understand the phases of a disaster, as well as the definitions and terminology used in this discipline.

2. Definitions

Note that more formal definitions are provided in Chapter 1.

Disaster management

For our purposes, disasters can be said to have occurred when normal community and organisational arrangements are overwhelmed by an event, and extraordinary responses are needed.

Disaster medicine

Disaster medicine is the study and collaborative application of various health disciplines to the prevention, preparedness, response to and recovery from the health problem arising from a disaster. This must be achieved in cooperation with agencies and disciplines involved in comprehensive disaster management.

Types of disasters

Natural disasters

These include earthquakes, tsunamis, volcanoes, floods, avalanches, thunderstorms and lightning strikes, tornadoes, hurricanes, pandemics, wild fires, famine, droughts and other severe weather extremes. These natural events result in a multiplicity of secondary effects, including loss of human life, significant damage to property and the environment, and economic and social losses.

Man-made disasters

These include wars, terrorist activities, nuclear and industrial accidents, travel and transportation accidents, explosions and bombs, fires/arson and epidemics. They are virtually all preventable, and are within the control of administrative authorities. Man-made disasters invariably require a formal investigation to determine causation, accountability and, where necessary, measures to avert similar incidents in the future.

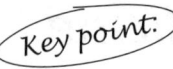 Both natural and man-made disasters can have devastating effects on the community. This effect can be reduced by adequate mitigation plans.

Phases of a disaster

The Disaster Management Act, 2002 (No 57 of 2002) describes the following phases of a disaster:

Table 1: The phases of disaster

Pre-disaster risk reduction	Post-disaster recovery
* Prevention	* Response
* Mitigation	* Recovery
* Preparedness	* Rehabilitation
* Early warning	* Reconstruction

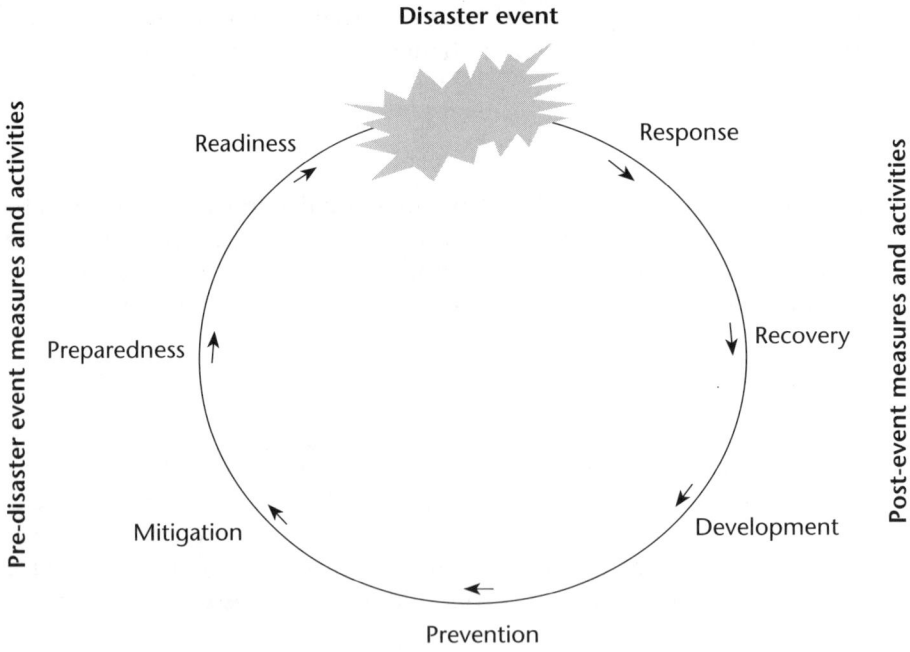

Figure 1: Pre- and post-disaster measures and activities

Pre-disaster phases

The pre-disaster phases of prevention, mitigation and preparedness are defined in Chapter 1.

Here, the emphasis is on being able to provide a rapid response plan, and includes aspects such as hospital disaster plans and regular multi-disciplinary exercises.

Mitigation and preparedness are often considered one and the same.

Early warning can be defined as the collection and analysis of information for the purpose of:

- anticipating the escalation of life threatening situations;
- the development of strategic responses to these situation;
- presentation of options to the relevant decision-makers.

The primary aim of early warning is a timely response to threats.

Disaster occurrence

The disaster phase is the period during which extraordinary measures have to be taken in order to save lives, protect property and secure livelihoods.

A disaster phase may be quite extensive (as in the case of a slow-onset disaster, such as the outbreak of a haemorrhagic fever). It can also be relatively short-lived (for example, an earthquake or aircraft accident).

Post-disaster phases

The response phase is really the relief and rescue phase. It is during this time that survivors need to be found, be given emergency treatment and then transported to hospitals. The activity at the hospital during this time is also part of the response phase, as extra resources are utilised to save life and time.

The recovery and rehabilitation phases refer to that time following a disaster during which the aim is to restore the community to former conditions (restoring normality). The two go hand in hand in this process, with 'recovery' referring more to processes and infrastructure and 'rehabilitation' referring to the human element, with specific reference to mental and physical health.

RISK AND EMERGENCY MANAGEMENT

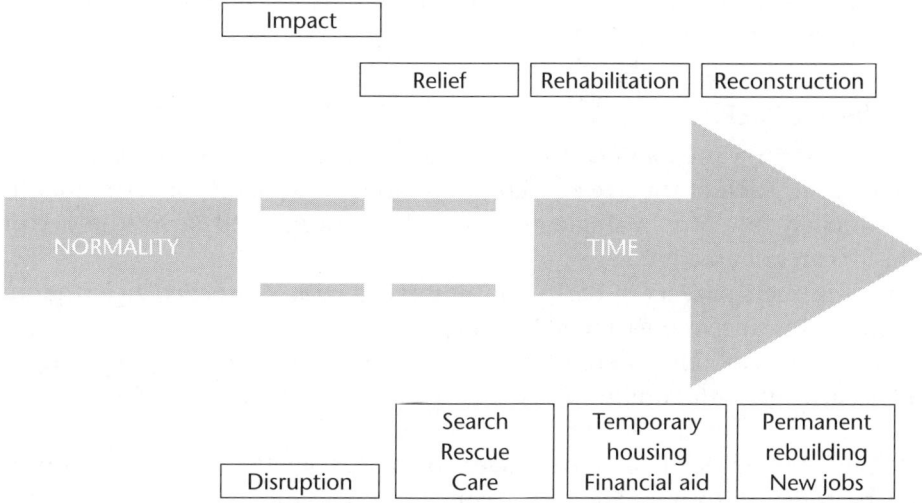

Figure 2: Post-disaster phases

Reconstruction is the phase during which attempts are made to re-establish a community. Attempts should be made not only to re-establish the community to the pre-disaster state but to aim at developing resilience in the community, the hope being that the community will be in a better state to withstand a similar disaster in the future. For health and emergency services, this represents the time of review and debriefing. Disaster plans are revamped according to lessons learnt.

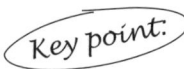 **The phases of a disaster highlight the importance of planning in an integrated manner**

3. Case study

This case study deals with the Sarin gas attack on the Tokyo subway, which occurred in March 1995. This incident is an ideal case study in that many lessons were learnt both by disaster management authorities as well as the medical fraternity. These will be reviewed later in terms of the phases of a disaster.

Background

The attack came at the peak of the Monday morning rush hour on one of the world's busiest commuter transport systems. On 20 March 1995, members of the doomsday cult Aum Shinrikyo released the deadly Sarin gas and liquid on several lines of the Tokyo subway. Prior to this attack there were many other incidents when gas was released or canisters found containing gas. In most of these cases, links could be made to the Aum Shinrikyo: the most deadly incident was a Sarin gas leak at the Aum Shinrikyo compound in Matsumoto in June 1994, in which seven people were killed and about 200 injured.

The cult played down the incident, claiming that the chemical precursors were being used for industrial purposes and that no one in the cult had the knowledge to produce Sarin. They claimed that the whole episode was part op a United States-led campaign against the group.

The subway attack

The liquid Sarin was contained in plastic bags which cult members had wrapped in newspaper. Each of the five perpetrators carried two packets of Sarin, totalling approximately one litre. A single drop of 100% concentrated Sarin (the size of a pinhead) can kill an adult.

Carrying their packets of Sarin and umbrellas with sharpened tips, the men boarded trains at five prearranged stations. At predetermined times and places, the sharpened umbrellas were used to pierce the packets, thereby releasing the deadly Sarin gas. Maximum effect was achieved in that five individual lines became contaminated.

Despite many reports of ill passengers being taken off trains throughout the network, some trains were allowed to continue operating for as long as one hour and 40 minutes following the Sarin release.

The injured

Television footage showed subway entrances that resembled battlefields. In many cases, the injured simply lay on the ground, many unable to breathe. Incredibly, several of those affected by Sarin went to work, despite their symptoms, thereby contaminating others in the workplace.

Several of those affected were exposed to Sarin only by helping passengers from the trains (these included passengers on other trains, subway workers and health care workers).

The signs and symptoms were similar in most of those affected, and included:

- Bleeding from nose and mouth;
- Coma;
- Convulsions;
- Choking;
- Shortness of breath;
- Extreme sensitivity to light;
- Foaming at the mouth;
- Tremors.

Many passengers presenting with similar signs and symptoms should have been an early indication of a chemical contamination. Unfortunately, this was not the case.

Emergency services

Emergency services, including police, fire and ambulance, were criticised for their handling of the attack. The Subway Authority was also criticised in that they failed to halt trains despite reports of several passengers being taken ill.

Health services, including hospitals and staff, were ill-prepared, and many health workers themselves became infected.

Secondary contamination at hospitals

There was secondary contamination of hospital personnel who had treated passengers. Since the information that the incident was caused by a poison gas was not available in the first few hours, decontamination and personal protection procedures were not instituted. As a result, 245 of the 5 500 victims were hospital and emergency service personnel. The final casualty toll was 5 500 people injured, and 11 deaths.

Current activities

Shortly after the attack, Aum Shinrikyo lost its status as a religious organisation, and its assets were seized. However, the government rejected a request from security officials to outlaw the sect outright, because the officials could not prove that it posed an immediate danger to Japan, despite ten of its members being convicted for the subway attack. The cult reportedly still exists under the name Aleph, has 2 100 members and owns numerous businesses throughout Japan.

Lessons learnt

The attack resulted in many changes to the way disaster management is structured in Japan, including the way hospitals practise disaster medicine. The attack can be reviewed in terms of the phases of a disaster as outlined below.

Pre-disaster

Prevention

- Tighten security protocol;
- Mapping of dangerous substances;
- Ongoing risk analysis (Aum Shinrikyo).

Mitigation

- Adequate ventilation in subways;
- Pre-determined mass communication policies.

Preparedness

- Emergency services – disaster management plan;
- Hospital – mass casualty plan;
- Strategic resource stockpile (Atropine);
- Personal protection protocol;
- Mass decontamination protocols and exercises;
- Subway disaster planning.

Early warning

- Previous attempt (Matsumoto 1994);
- Political climate;
- Recent terrorist trends as regards mass casualties.

Post-disaster

Response

- Activation of pre-hospital mass casualty plan;
- Implementation of decontamination protocol;
- Incident management system;
- Early activation of hospitals;
- Hospitals activate mass casualty plan;
- Personal protection;
- Additional Atropine and ventilators;
- Constant communication.

Recovery and rehabilitation

- Cleaning of the subway;
- Hospital loads redistributed;
- Prolonged medical treatment;

- Dealing with mass hysteria;
- Dealing with a large number of fatalities – including colleagues;
- Early intervention of psychological support.

Reconstruction

- Re-opening of the subway;
- Hospitals back to pre-disaster loads;
- Re-examine disaster plans;
- Re-look at personal protection;
- Re-look at Atropine availability.

The Tokyo subway attack highlights the importance of adequate planning among all disciplines. Identifying and understanding the phases of a disaster assists practitioners to describe disaster-related needs, inclusive of adequate planning.

The pre-disaster risk-reduction phase enjoys huge emphasis within the South African environment: the primary focus of the Disaster Management Act of 2002 is to prevent and mitigate. Review of previous incidents and experience in dealing with such incidents is critical in the whole process. It gives the option to associate probability (what might happen) with experience (what did happen).

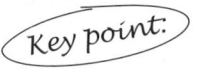 **There are always valuable lessons to be learnt from previous incidents and disasters. This highlights the importance of being prepared to share the lessons learnt, as well as documenting them.**

4. Historical overview of disaster management in South Africa

Until June 1994, South Africa did not have a holistic approach to dealing with disasters. South Africa had until then followed the traditional trend, viewing disasters resulting from 'acts of nature' as rare, inevitable events that could not be predicted or avoided. Because of this belief, the approach to dealing with such disasters was focused solely on measures that were reactive – in other words, the focus was only on *post*-disaster measures designed to deal with the consequences or adverse effects of a disaster.

In the years after the Second World War, following the German air raids on London, the concept of establishing civil defence organisations was introduced in South Africa. The purpose of these organisations was to develop contingency plans designed to respond to the impact of man-made disasters, and to introduce measures to provide for the safety of people and property *during* such catastrophes.

The South African government became concerned that a similar attack on South Africa would have severe consequences. South Africa would not have been able to protect its citizens against such actions. Although almost stillborn from its inception, the fact that South Africa never experienced any bombing raids in the Second World War led to the civil defence services being dismantled shortly after the war.

In 1959, a Council for Civil Defence Services was established but was disbanded in 1962 to make way for the Directorate for Emergency Planning. In 1963, this Directorate made way for the Directorate of Civil Defence! It became apparent that the government of the day had no idea what to do with the orphan called civil defence/protection. It was only in 1966 that a piece of legislation governing civil defence was promulgated by Parliament: the Civil Defence Act 39 of 1966. This act focused mainly on establishing civil defence as a function of national government, and accordingly many local and provincial authorities refrained from rendering civil defence services. In 1977, the Civil Defence Act 39 of 1966 was revoked and replaced by the Civil Defence Act 67 of 1977, which provided for the promotion of civil defence at all tiers of government.

Civil defence in South Africa coexisted with many of the other functions within the civil service. In many instances, local authorities were not quite sure what to do with this 'newly adopted child'. Accordingly, the function of civil defence was shuffled between numerous line functions and departments, with no one really sure where it should fit into their hierarchy.

Internationally, however, while the traditional perceptions remained, there was growing realisation that the focus had to broaden to include not only man-made disasters, but also major catastrophes resulting from natural hazards such as floods, tornadoes and earthquakes. Furthermore, by introducing preparedness programmes (prevention and mitigation), the effects of a disaster could be minimised. As a result, an increasing emphasis on community disaster preparedness programmes began to emerge. The term 'civil defence' was disposed of in many countries and was replaced by the more appropriate term, 'civil protection'. In South Africa, the Civil Defence Act was amended (Civil Defence Amendment Act No 82 of 1990) whereby all references to 'civil defence' were amended to read 'civil protection'.

Civil Protection services were rendered under the Civil Protection Act 67 of 1977 (as amended) and the Fundraising Act 107 of 1978. The first Act provided for the operations of civil protection, while the Fundraising Act provided mechanisms for the funding of disaster rehabilitation and reconstruction.

In 1989, a general session of the United Nations declared the coming ten years the International Decade for Natural Disaster Reduction (IDNDR). This declaration was a clear international call to all member countries to revisit their approach to dealing with disasters, in order to ensure disaster prevention, mitigation, relief and preparedness. This newly found interest in the field of disaster management slowly but surely brought on the paradigm shift from the civil defence/protection approach to more holistic disaster management as we know it today.

The devastating floods which occurred in the Cape Flats in June 1994, together with the emergence of our new democracy, were the catalysts that heralded the paradigm shift in South Africa. As a result of the extreme hardship suffered by the poorest of the poor when events of this nature occurred, government decided to take a firm stand on the matter. This resulted in a Cabinet resolution to follow international trends and take a new look at the whole concept of civil protection. In 1997, government established an Inter-Ministerial Committee for Disaster Management (IMC). This not only showed government's commitment to disaster reduction, but also, in line with our new Constitution, its commitment to making South Africa a safer place for all.

For the first time in South Africa, a process of wide consultation on the whole approach to the management of disasters followed, culminating in February 1998 with the publication of the Green Paper on Disaster Management. The Green Paper, which highlighted the need for a holistic mechanism for the management of disasters in South Africa, was followed in the ensuing year by the White Paper process, and in January 1999, South Africa had its first-ever national policy on the management of disasters.

In early 2000, the Disaster Management Bill was published for public discussion. Public hearings on the Bill took place in 2001, and the Disaster Management Act was promulgated by Parliament in 2002.

5. Disaster management structures in South Africa

The primary responsibility for disaster management in South Africa rests with government. In terms of Section 41(1)(b) of the Constitution of the Republic of South Africa, Act No 108 of 1996, all spheres of government are required to 'secure the well-being of the people of the Republic'. According to Part A, Schedule 4, disaster management is a functional area of concurrent national and provincial legislative competence. However, Section 156(4) of the Constitution provides for the assignment and, by agreement and subject to any conditions, the administration of any matter listed in Part A, Schedule 4, which necessarily related to local government, if that matter would most effectively be administered locally and if the municipality has the capacity to administer it.

Apart from the fact that local government is required under Schedules 4 and 5 of Part B of the Constitution to provide for functions which are closely allied to disaster management, Section 152(1)(d) also requires that local government 'ensure a safe and healthy environment'.

The Disaster Management Act provides for an integrated and coordinated disaster management policy that focuses on preventing or reducing the risk of disasters, mitigating the severity of disasters, emergency preparedness, rapid and effective response to disasters and post-disaster recovery, the establishment of national, provincial and municipal disaster management centres, disaster management volunteers and matters incidental thereto.

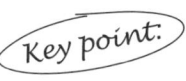 **The Disaster Management Act focuses on risk reduction and highlights the fact that disaster management is everyone's business.**

6. Major incidents

This book, as in many disaster medicine texts, will use the terms 'disaster' and 'major incident' interchangeably. Traditionally, a disaster has been taken as a natural event (flood, earthquake, etc), while man-made events have been termed 'major incidents'. More formal definitions are presented in Chapter 1.

CSCATTT

The principles of scene management will introduce concepts that are not unique to disaster medicine. The priorities for effective management, summed up by the mnemonic CSCATTT, are as follows:

- Command and control;
- Safety;
- Communication;
- Assessment;
- Triage;
- Treatment;
- Transport.

METHANE

A second useful mnemonic, METHANE, is used to pass disaster messages:

- My call sign/major incident (declared or standby);
- Exact location (grid reference);
- Type of incident;
- Hazards;
- Access routes;
- Number of casualties;
- Emergency services (on scene and required).

1

Background

P Brysiewicz, S Stratton, W Smith and L Wallis

Objectives

By the end of this chapter, the reader will:

- have an understanding of the common terminology used in major incidents and disasters;
- understand the legal framework in which health services respond;
- know the four ethical principles governing medical ethics;
- have an overview of various ethical challenges faced during a disaster situation;
- have an overview of the various research methodologies used in disaster research.

1.1 Terminology

In communicating between the many disciplines involved in disaster medicine, it is essential that a common understanding of terminology be established. The World Association for Disaster and Emergency Medicine (WADEM) has formulated a research template for disaster medicine research, and clarified key definitions to enhance commonality. These are discussed in the following sections.

Hazard

A *hazard* is anything, natural, man-made or a combination thereof that may pose a danger to adversely affect human health, property, activity and/or the environment. The specific hazard varies in space and time and differs between populations. Only when a hazard is converted to an *event* can it potentially become a *major incident* or *disaster*. Examples of *hazards* include floods, fire, explosions etc. Hazards are classified as natural (for example, a wind storm), man-made (caused by human actions; for example, a transport hazard) or mixed (where natural and man-made hazards combine; for example, a fire). The identification of a new flu virus could be classified as a natural hazard.

Risk

A *risk* refers to something negative happening. It refers to the probability that a *hazard* may become an *event* – the probability that the hazard '*may happen*'. A risk only applies to one specific hazard. *Risk factors* refer to measures taken to modify the hazard. Risk markers are an attribute of the hazard, indicating that an *event* may occur. Falling pressure in a gas pipeline is a risk marker that a leak may have occurred and that the hazard (the gas) may explode (the event).

Prevention

This is what is done to prevent the *event* from happening. Prevention is thus the aggregate of approaches and measures to ensure that the *hazard* does not cause an event. It does not refer to decreasing the intensity or scale of the *event*. Removing all sources of ignition from the area of the gas leak or vaccinating against the new virus are examples of prevention.

Modification

This refers to the approaches and measures taken to modify the intensity or scale of the event. Opening the windows to ensure that some gas from a gas leak is blown away by the wind modifies the scale of the event should the gas (*hazard*) explode (the *event*). Prohibiting public gatherings of large groups in small areas are measures to modify the scale of the outbreak of a disease (the *event*).

Event

The *event* refers to the occurrence that has the potential to negatively affect living beings and/or their environment. Events may have a sudden, gradual or delayed *onset* – for example, an explosion versus a famine. The *duration* of an event may be short or prolonged. It is also possible to distinguish between *primary events*, responsible for initiating the damage, and *secondary events*, occurring as a result of the impact of the primary event. The hurricane may be the primary event, with mudslides caused by the rain as secondary events. The term *incident* is used in some literature as being synonymous to *event*.

Impact

This refers to the influence of the *event* on society or the environment. The impact is the precipitating cause of the *damage* that may result from an *event*.

Mitigation

This is the process that is undertaken to reduce the immediate *damage* by the impact on society. Isolating victims with a new strain of flu is an example of mitigating measures.

Preparedness

This is the aggregate of all measures and policies taken *before* the event occurs, and which reduce the *damage* that would have been caused by the *event*. For example, stockpiling of specific treatment drugs will reduce the damage caused by the new disease.

Damage

Damage refers to the *negative* result of the *impact* of an *event*. The number of patients is an example of damage.

Absorbing capacity

This is defined as the ability of the affected society to absorb the *impact* of the *event* without sustaining a loss of essential functions. This refers to those goods and services that are available on a day-to-day basis within a society, and which can be consumed before there is a negative effect on essential functioning of the society. Absorbing capacity is often part of preparedness, and includes actions such as stockpiling, training and protective equipment.

Buffering capacity

Buffering capacity refers to the ability of society to minimise the change of essential functions. This differs from society to society; and greater the buffering capacity, the less likely a disaster will result from the impact of an event.

Major incident

In the health services, a *major incident* is defined as any *event* (incident) in which the location, number, severity or type of live casualties requires extraordinary resources. It is therefore an event in which the impact causes damage (casualties) that could not be absorbed within the buffering capacity of the society, and extraordinary resources are required to mitigate the damage on society.

Simple/compound major incidents

In a *simple incident* (event), the infrastructure, such as communication lines and roads, remains intact; in a *compound incident* (*event*), the impact results in damage to the infrastructure, making it more difficult to respond to, or manage, the situation.

Compensated/uncompensated major incidents

Compensated incidents refer to a situation where the casualties can be managed by utilising the preparedness and buffering capacity of the society. The extraordinary resources that are activated can deal with the casualties – the load is less than the capacity. An *uncompensated incident* refers to a situation where the impact of the event causes so much damage (including number of casualties) that, in mobilising all the available resources, using all the preparedness measures and taking buffering capacity into account, the society (or health care facility) will not be able to cope with the number of casualties – the load exceeds the capacity.

Disaster

The World Health Organization (WHO) defines a *disaster* as 'the result of a vast ecological breakdown in the relationship between man and his environment, a serious and sudden disruption of such a scale that the stricken community needs extraordinary efforts to cope with it, often with outside help or international aid'. If this definition is broken down into the elements discussed earlier it is clear that a hazard caused an event in which the impact resulted in damage that exceeded the *mitigation* and *preparedness* of the community. The community does not have the ability to absorb the damage and the extraordinary resources that the community could mobilise are not adequate to compensate for the damage. It is therefore an *uncompensated major incident*. Disasters are often also compound in nature, as damage is caused by the impact to infrastructure, making recovery more difficult.

Recovery

Recovery occurs when all of the damage from an event has been repaired or replaced. All responses to the damage are aimed at achieving recovery. A new balance is established within society.

   Note: For the purposes of this text, we shall use the term 'major incident' as the preferred term. It should be considered largely interchangeable with the term 'disaster' for the majority of concepts presented in this book. Where the text refers to disasters, it is in the context of larger incidents (uncompensated major incidents).

1.2   Legal framework

The appropriate management of a disaster requires international strategies and collaborations with many organisations to ensure disaster preparedness and disaster reduction. This collaboration needs to occur at international, national and regional levels.

International organisations

United Nations organisations

The United Nations International Strategy for Disaster Reduction (UN/ISDR) is an essential tool of the UN disaster system, which:

● Promotes, links and coordinates disaster-reduction activities;
● Supports policy integration;
● Produces international information on disaster reduction, develops awareness campaigns and produces articles, journals and other promotional materials related to disaster reduction.

The ISDR aims to establish disaster-resilient communities by ensuring communities are aware of the importance of disaster reduction and have the necessary information. The ISDR builds on partnerships and takes a global approach to disaster reduction, seeking to involve every individual and community towards achieving the common goals of reducing the loss of life, property and environmental damage caused by natural hazards.

   The ISDR has the following objectives:

● Increase public awareness regarding disaster risk and ways to reduce these risks;
● Obtain the commitment from public authorities to implement disaster-reduction policies and actions;

- Stimulate interdisciplinary and intersectoral partnership to address disaster reduction;
- Improve scientific knowledge about disaster reduction.

The ISDR involves the Inter-Agency Task Force on Disaster Reduction (IATF/DR) as well as the Inter-Agency Secretariat of the ISDR (UN/ISDR) in order to attempt to meet these objectives. The IATF/DR is the principal body for the development of disaster-reduction policy, and is involved in discussing issues of common and global relevance to disaster reduction.

To address disaster risk reduction in Africa, UN/ISDR established a regional office in Nairobi in October 2002. UN/ISDR Africa's main areas of focus are:

- Supporting disaster policy and strategy development;
- Advocating and raising awareness in disaster risk reduction;
- Promoting information-sharing;
- Networking, partnership-building and coordination of disaster risk reduction.

African Union

African countries have various disaster risk-reduction policies. However, their effectiveness is limited, and there was a need for a more cohesive and strategic approach to disaster risk reduction. To address this, the African Union (AU)/New Partnership for Africa's Development (NEPAD), African Development Bank (ADB) and the UN/ISDR Africa have all been working together since the beginning of 2003.

The Hyogo Framework for Action (2005–2015) led to 24 countries submitting reports; seven of these were in sub-Saharan Africa. This allowed an initial mapping of the international partners of the ISDR system in this region, and a Status Report on Disaster Risk Reduction in Sub-Saharan Africa was produced in May 2009. The Member States of the African Union then demonstrated their commitment to disaster risk reduction (DRR) by adopting the Africa Regional Strategy for Disaster Risk Reduction (ARSDRR) at the tenth meeting of the Africa Ministerial Conference on the Environment (AMCEN) in 2004. The African Union Commission (AUC) then formulated and endorsed the Programme of Action for the Implementation of the Africa Strategy for DRR (2005–2010) at the First African Ministerial Conference on DRR in Addis Ababa in 2005. The Second Africa Regional Platform in Nairobi in May 2009 then amended these action plans and extended the timeframe to 2015, as well as aligning it with the HFA.

The ARSDRR is an African regional disaster risk-reduction framework for action. It has the following objectives:

- To reduce social, economic and environmental impacts of disasters on African people and economies;
- To increase understanding and knowledge of DRR;
- To increase capacity at sub-regional and national levels for implementing DRR (3).

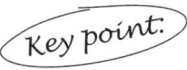 **The Member States of the AU adopted the Africa Regional Strategy for Disaster Risk Reduction (ARSDRR).**

Southern African Development Community (SADC)

The Southern African Development Community originates from the Southern African Development Coordination Conference (SADCC), which was formed by nine countries in 1980. In 1992, it became the Southern African Development Community (SADC), and was concerned with encouraging development, economic growth and poverty alleviation. SADC has engaged in disaster risk reduction since 1999; in 2001, SADC developed a new strategic framework, the Regional Indicative Strategic Development Plan (RISDP), to provide Member States with a development agenda on social and economic policies over fifteen years. Although it included a disaster management plan, this was oriented towards disaster response, and progress in disaster risk reduction led to a revision of this plan in 2006. The revised plan, the Disaster Risk Reduction Strategic Plan 2006–2010 set out the SADC strategic direction to achieve the following objectives:

● Strengthen governance, legal and institutional frameworks at all levels of disaster risk reduction;
● Facilitate the identification, assessment, and monitoring of disaster risks and enhance early warning systems;
● Promote the usage and management of information and knowledge, innovation and education to build a culture of safety and resilience;
● Ensure that disaster risk reduction is a national and local priority;
● Integrate preparedness and emergency response into disaster risk reduction interventions.

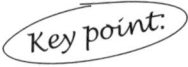 **SADC developed the Disaster Risk Reduction Strategic Plan 2006–2010 to guide Member States in disaster risk reduction.**

International, national and regional coordination

The need for the coordination of activities in times of disaster has long been recognised by the international community.

The United Nations Disaster Assessment and Coordination (UNDAC) team brings together disaster management professionals, who are nominated and funded by member governments, the Office for the Coordination of Humanitarian Affairs (OCHA), UN Development Programme (UNDP) and operational humanitarian United Nations agencies such as the World Food Programme (WFP), UN Children's Fund (UNICEF) and the World Health Organization (WHO). When requested, this team can be deployed within hours to carry out rapid assessment of priority needs and to support national authorities and the United Nations Resident Coordinator to coordinate international relief on site.

The UNDAC system is made up of four parts, namely:

● Specially trained and experienced staff;
● Predefined methods of information management, assessment and coordination necessary during the first phase of a disaster;
● The ability to mobilise and deploy an UNDAC team so that it can arrive within 24 hours at any disaster site anywhere in the world;
● The equipment necessary to be self-sufficient when deployed to a disaster.

SADC established the SADC Disaster Management Unit to work and coordinate with relevant individuals and institutions at regional and global levels. The national disaster management authorities in the individual SADC Member States therefore play an important coordinating role.

The South African government and a number of stakeholders developed the Disaster Management Act, 2002 (Act No 57 of 2002), which came into force on 15 January 2003. The Act provides for the following:

- An integrated and coordinated disaster risk management policy to reduce or prevent disasters;
- Effective response to disasters;
- The establishment of national, provincial and municipal disaster management centres;
- Disaster risk management volunteers.

The Act recognises that there are many ways to reduce or avoid disasters through the combined efforts of all spheres of government, civil society and the private sector, but there is also a need for uniformity in the approach taken. The national management framework is the legal instrument specified by the Act to ensure this consistency, by providing 'a coherent, transparent and inclusive policy on disaster management appropriate for the Republic as a whole' (Section 7(1)). The Disaster Management Act of 2002 dramatically reorganised disaster management structures, and introduced a culture of disaster preparedness.

International humanitarian law

International disaster response is indeed more effective and more efficiently coordinated through internationally agreed standards. However, the legal framework for international disaster response requires significant improvement in order to create genuinely favourable conditions for all efforts to enhance that response. Laws and regulations in a disaster situation should:

- Waive import, export and transit restrictions and duties for relief goods;
- Waive overflight and landing restrictions and duties;
- Grant landing rights and facilitate telecommunications in emergency situations;
- Waive visa and other immigration restrictions.

In addition, the regulations should provide for the right to exercise medical and other professional services, directly benefiting disaster victims. At the same time, in order to benefit from these measures, relief organisations and their personnel should be required to respect local laws and internationally agreed standards.

International humanitarian law is a set of rules which, for humanitarian reasons, limits the effects of armed conflict. It protects persons who are not, or are no longer, participating in the hostilities, and restricts the means and methods of warfare. International humanitarian law is also known as the law of war or the law of armed conflict.

Cooperation with non-governmental organisations (NGOs)

During a disaster situation non-governmental organisations (NGOs) play a very important role. NGOs are non-profit organisations or associations made up of private citizens with a common interest in providing humanitarian assistance activities during or after a disaster. The term 'NGO' can be applied to any non-profiting organisation which is independent from the government, and they may be international or local. Examples of NGOs involved in disaster and humanitarian crisis response are Oxfam, Red Cross and Gift of the Givers.

NGOs are typically value-based organisations which depend, in whole or in part, on charitable donations and voluntary service. Although the NGO sector has become increasingly professional over the last two decades, principles of altruism and voluntarism remain key defining characteristics. The role of NGOs is essential in building the resilience of local communities to disasters and supporting local-level implementation of the Hyogo Framework for Action.

The benefits of NGOs are as follows:

- Excellent advocacy or lobbying capacity;
- Can fill gaps – specialised skills/capacity;
- Mobilise quickly;
- Well connected at local level.

NGOs do have limitations, and it is essential to work together to try to maximise the impact of the limited resources available. NGOs potentially have a key role to play in disaster management, and they have been identified as an effective alternative means of achieving an efficient communication link between disaster management agencies and an affected community.

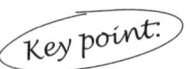 **NGOs have a very important role to play in a disaster situation.**

The South African disaster system

South Africa's National Disaster Management System (NDMS) has three levels: at national level is the National Disaster Management Centre (NDMC); at provincial level there are nine Provincial Disaster Management Centres (PDMCs); and at local level there are Municipal Disaster Management Centres (MDMCs).

The NDMS strives to successfully implement the Disaster Management Act by ensuring well-trained, well-resourced and committed people in order to maintain disaster preparedness and response. It attempts to do this in the following ways:

- *Integrated institutional capacity for disaster risk management* – ensuring all the necessary requirements are available to implement disaster risk management a national, provincial and municipal level;
- *Disaster risk assessment* – how to implement disaster risk and monitoring;
- *Disaster risk reduction* – plans, programmes and projects that reduce disaster risks;
- *Response and recovery* – ensuring all the roles and responsibilities of organisations concerned are clear during a disaster and in the post-disaster phase.

In order to be able to achieve this, it is important that there are effective information management and communication systems for disaster risk management. There needs to be education, training, public awareness and research on all aspects of disaster management.

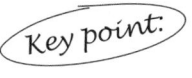 **The South African National Disaster Management System is made up of national, provincial and municipal disaster management centres.**

Integrated National Early Warning System (INEWS)

This system was developed to integrate all emergency warning into a single framework, including meteorological, hydrological, related health hazards, and geological hazards, in order to ensure disaster preparedness and disaster response. National and regional forecasting offices liaise directly with the relevant national, provincial and municipal disaster management centres before, during and after the disaster event.

South African National Fire Danger Index

During 1998, South Africa passed the National Veld and Forest Fire Act (Act 101 of 1998), which provided for the prevention of fires by using a National Fire Danger Rating System (NFDRS). The NFDRS allows for the prediction of potential conditions conducive to fires, thus allowing for preventive measures to be taken. The NFDRS should also be regarded as one of the early warning systems required by the National Disaster Management System (NDMS).

Flash Flood Guidance System (FFGS)

This system was designed to improve flash flood warnings in flood-prone regions.

Ensuring that a country is adequately prepared for a disaster requires a great deal of international, national and local collaboration and policy development. Additional legislation needs to be developed to guide this collaboration, and the practical application of the legislation must be made clear to all concerned parties so that there is a common understanding. South Africa has made a great deal of headway in this (thanks in part to the 2010 FIFA World Cup) although there is always room for improvement.

1.3 Ethics

Ethics can be defined as the study of standards of conduct or moral judgment, or as a system of a code of morals – concepts of right and wrong. Medical ethics are governed by the following four principles:

- *Beneficence* – doing the best for the patient in order to promote the most advantageous outcome; achieve the greatest amount of good.
- *Non-maleficence* – doing no harm; provide helpful treatment rather than inflict harm.

- *Autonomy* – respect for the individual patient's informed choice as it pertains to their own medical care.
- *Justice* – equitable distribution of medical resources among all patients; recommend actions that are fair to those involved.

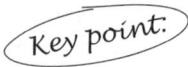 **Medical ethics are guided by the ethical principles of beneficence, non-maleficence, autonomy and justice.**

On a day-to-day basis, medical professionals are required to weigh up their actions according to these principles in the treatment of individual patients. In disaster medicine the same principles need to be taken into account, not only on an individual level, but on a collective ethical level as well. The unique challenges presented to the medical fraternity in disaster situations may seem to be in direct conflict with these principles. The overarching principle described in the Hippocratic Oath – that is, to assist in the relief of human suffering and the alleviation of pain – remains intact, however: the challenge is in the practical application.

Below are some ethical situations to be considered in the disaster situation. This is by no means a comprehensive list, but serves to highlight some of the more common challenges and their ethical complexity:

- *Duty to care:* The American Medical Association (AMA), in a 2004 policy document, states that 'Because of their commitment to care for the sick and injured, individual physicians have an obligation to provide urgent medical care during disasters. This ethical consideration holds even in the face of greater than usual risk to their own safety, health or life.' While there is no formal guidance regarding this from either the Nursing or Health Professions Council of South Africa, the ethical mandate is the same in our country provided the safety of the health care worker is observed prior to engaging with such care.
- *Triage:* The aim of triage in any situation is to prioritise patients in order to do the most good for the most number of patients. This embraces the principle of justice in that it requires that care and medical resources be distributed equally, without consideration of race, age, gender or creed. In the disaster situation, during which by definition there are inadequate resources to deal with the load, it is deemed unethical to concentrate resources (equipment or personnel) in an effort to save an individual life at the expense of others who may benefit from the scarce resources. In the same vein, patients who were not direct victims in the disaster, but are also under the care of the limited resources, will need to be triaged alongside the disaster victims.

  In cases of severe resource constraints, it may be necessary to invoke the 'expectant' category for those patients who are suffering from injuries so severe that survival is unlikely, and the level of care necessary is such that it compromises the care given to patients with a greater chance of survival. In such cases, the expectant patients would receive palliative care and would thus not be completely abandoned. The expectant triage code is unlikely to be used in civilian incidents, and more likely in the military environment.
- *Informed consent:* On a day-to-day basis, the principle of individual consent to medical care and treatment upholds the principle of autonomy. In a disaster

situation, the balance must necessarily shift to doing the most for the most; thus there may not be time/opportunity to gain informed consent.

- *Sustainability:* Specifically in the case of the response of outside medical agencies, consideration needs to be given as to whether, if started, medications and treatment can be sustained in the long term once these parties withdraw. The appropriate time of withdrawal of medical professionals also needs to be considered.
- *Humanitarian assistance:* In the context of civil war, humanitarian groups are often commandeered by one or other warring faction to take care of their sick and wounded, and thus their presence may serve to prolong the conflict. The withholding of humanitarian assistance may, however, lead to the continued severe suffering of innocent victims.
- *Armed conflict:* The World Medical Association (WMA) advises that medical ethics in a time of armed conflict should be exactly the same as during peacetime. The medical professional's primary obligation is to perform his or her medical duty and, in so doing, have their conscience as their supreme guide.
- *Media:* The media have a responsibility to inform the world of the occurrence and development of disaster situations. Prudent, timely reporting of accurate information may serve to direct attention and subsequent support to the disaster area. Medical professionals need to be aware of the important role that the media can play, while at the same time ensuring that patient dignity and confidentiality are protected. Specifically, control must be effected in order to ensure that photographs or footage of patients are not taken without their express permission.
- *Disaster research:* Research in disaster situations is extremely important if geared toward learning for future, similar events. The timing, however, must be appropriate, considering that, by definition, resources are scarce. Thus, in the acute phase particularly, it would not be ethical for researchers to stand by and record proceedings when all available hands are needed to assist with victims. Therefore research conducted in the latter phases of a prolonged incident may be more plausible.

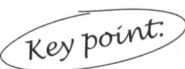 **There are many unique challenges faced by the medical fraternity in disaster situations, and these may appear to be in direct conflict with ethical principles.**

Much of the controversy surrounding ethics in the disaster setting can be obviated if these dilemmas are taken into account and addressed in the planning stages of disaster preparedness. The ethical codes for disasters should be dealt with in a manner that is transparent and inclusive so that all role-players are comfortable and conversant with them and are willing and able to apply them in the event of a disaster.

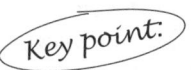 **Ethical principles should be taken into account during disaster preparedness in order to address these ethical challenges.**

Children in disasters

Essentially, it is likely that in most countries of the world there would be limited capacity within the health systems to deal with a significant surge in demand for acute services for children. In most developing countries, there is simply no capacity at present to deal with the current demand, and in both situations we will have to work out how to provide the best possible care to the affected children.

While some general principles appear to be recognised for the triage of adult patients, there is very little published material on the allocation of scarce resources for children in the context of mass casualties or disasters. The tenets of the accountability for reasonableness may be useful in working through this process. As it is simply not tenable for clinicians involved in disaster care to make these decisions on their own, there is an urgent need for communities across the world to consider and discuss the possible approaches to allocation of scarce clinical resources in disasters in their region. This may be relatively straightforward within countries, but it becomes extremely problematic in the context of disasters in countries where foreign healthcare workers are brought in as part of the response to the emergency.

Summary

Ethical principles are an essential guide for health personnel when dealing with the numerous challenging ethical issues found within the disaster situation, although many of these unique challenges may appear to be in direct conflict with these principles. Dealing with children in a disaster is an example of one of these specific challenges. It is, however, essential that health personnel are aware of these dilemmas and actively attempt to address them in the planning stages of disaster preparedness.

1.4   Research in disaster medicine

Disaster medicine research is in the early phases of development in comparison to that of other areas of medicine. Research in disaster medicine is challenging because the variables that affect an outcome of a disaster event are often uncontrollable and cannot be predicted. In contrast, areas of medicine that have developed over a far longer time, such as the study of infectious disease, have established methods to define and control variables such that comparative studies can be conducted. While it is a challenge to design controlled disaster medical studies, the study of disaster medical problems does not require extensive statistics or complicated methodological approaches. This section provides an overview of medical research techniques that apply to the study of disaster medicine. In presenting the material, the intent is not to provide an exhaustive or detailed discussion of methodology or statistics.

Disaster medical research is different from classic disease-based research, in that comparing disaster events and outcomes is difficult. Disease states are identified by case definition and predictable outcomes and variables. Disasters vary from event to event. To aid researchers in reporting outcomes and variables tested in disaster medical research, a multinational group of experts have developed a set of guidelines, which are set out in *Health Disaster Management: Guidelines for Evaluation and Research in the Utstein Style*. These guidelines provide a standardised vocabulary and event reporting structure that allow for comparison of different disaster research and reports.

Field disaster research is usually descriptive in design. The survey method is a common type of disaster medical research. Also common in disaster medical research are field reports and cross-sectional studies. Field reports and cross-sectional methods are descriptive in nature, as opposed to another form of research called observational analytical studies. Experimental studies, including randomised controlled trials, are considered the most valid forms of clinical research and the only type of study that can establish causal relationships. A causal relationship is one in which the investigator can state that a tested variable causes an outcome: for example, with exposure or presence of variable X, outcome Y is caused in a predictable amount of the time. Randomised trials rarely fit into disaster research projects because they require strict control of study variables and the ability to randomly assign individuals to a test and control (unexposed) group.

Randomised controlled disaster medical trials can be designed if variables that apply to an entire population are defined and controlled and study interventions can be measured reliably. The use of a randomised study is applicable to planned and well-controlled disaster exercises and computer modelling formats.

Recognising that almost all disaster medical studies are descriptive or observational due to the lack of ability to control variables in the disaster environment, the focus of this section is on descriptive reports and observational studies.

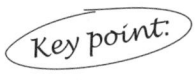 **Research in disaster medicine is challenging as the variables that affect an outcome of a disaster event are often uncontrollable and cannot be predicted.**

Initial steps of a medical disaster study

Development of a study objective

The initial step in developing disaster medical research is the formulation of a hypothesis or research objective. A hypothesis is a statement of the study question to be answered by the data that is included in a study. A research objective is similar to a hypothesis, but rather than asking a question to be proven, an objective states concisely what the study data or information is expected to show. For this section, the term 'study objective' will be used for descriptive studies, and 'hypothesis' used for comparative studies.

While seemingly a simple task, the development of a study objective is actually one of the most difficult aspects of designing a scientific study. Developing a focused, concise study objective allows for a directed and organised approach to the project. A tendency for descriptive researchers is to form an objective that lacks focus and is too broad to allow for an organised study.

A poorly defined hypothesis leads to a confused and hard-to-understand research experience. A strong research objective or hypothesis has the following characteristics:

1. It is clearly stated in one to two sentences;
2. It is focused, and contains one primary question;
3. It can be accomplished with the data available to the investigator;
4. It addresses an important issue;
5. The information derived by accomplishing the objective will add to the scientific knowledge base.

A study objective must be stated in a way that allows for study of an issue. A well-stated study objective generally includes an exposure, measurable variable(s) and outcome that can be derived by analysis of the measured variables.

Study population

A study population is that group of persons that are the subject of a study. For disaster research, defining the study population is important. There are various population dynamics that can affect who should be included in a study population, such as timeframes for exposure, location of exposure, economic status and environmental variation. For example, while the 1994 Northridge earthquake in southern California was believed to have had an effect on all residents of Los Angeles, the location of residence had a marked impact on how people were exposed to the effects of the quake. Those living in the Harbor area of Los Angeles suffered little impact from the event, while those living in the Valley area suffered major impacts. A study of the effects of the Northridge earthquake would be profoundly affected by how the study population is selected – for example, including all of those living in Los Angeles versus those living in the Valley region.

Prospective and retrospective data

Data used for research are obtained in either prospective or retrospective fashion. Prospective data are collected as a study occurs. For prospective data collection, the researcher must define the data elements to be collected, design a collection tool and arrange to collect the data while conducting the study. Stated in terms of disaster research, a prospective study would be one in which the data to be collected are determined prior to the disaster event or exercise and then collected using a standardised collection instrument (form) as the event or exercise occurs.

In a retrospective study, data is collected after the event or exercise has occurred. The terminology 'retrospective' and 'prospective' is often confused by researchers. In essence, both types of studies begin and end in the present, but a retrospective study is one that draws data from the past. Common types of retrospective studies are those in which data is collected from hospital records, field reports and established databases. Of the two types of data, prospective is preferred because the study data elements can be collected without as much risk for variation in definitions of terminology, loss of information from failure to record specific data and loss of records (cases).

Study bias

Different from the common meaning for bias or prejudice, bias in research relates to deviation from the true outcome in nature. There are many forms and causes for research bias. Bias stems from poor and invalid data, improper selection of those studied, poor case definition, bias in information obtained for study and, most important, the personal bias of investigators. All effort should be placed on avoiding bias in research. This is a difficult task, as there are many forms of bias; even in the most rigorous of studies, limitations occur which may bias both the study outcomes and its conclusions.

Triangulation in descriptive reports

With descriptive design, some types of data are uncontestable: for example, the number of death certificates issued in relation to a disaster. But often, data is potentially in error or contestable, such as the number of heart attacks related to an earthquake event. When contestable data is reported, triangulation is preferred to improve the report. A triangulated data element is one that has been determined using three independent data sources. Triangulation allows for determining if the phenomenon or case data found remains the same at other times, in other spaces, or from different independent data sources. An example of triangulation is the determination of eye injury during an earthquake using hospital records, emergency medical services field reports and insurance billing records. Triangulation is difficult, but should be a goal in descriptive study when data is 'soft' or has a high possibility for error.

Study design

Surveys

Surveys are a common method used for disaster medical research. A survey is a means of collecting information to describe knowledge, attitudes, experience and reported behaviour. For the purposes of this section, a survey is a means of providing quantitative descriptions of the opinions or experiences of a fraction of a study population. Survey data is generated by means of asking questions of a representative portion of a population of interest. The survey method is considered by some to be a descriptive form of research. Data for surveys can be collected using various methods, including telephone, internet, direct mailing, group distribution and interviews. In all cases, the basic structure of a survey is questions designed to elicit the information needed to answer a study objective. Surveys are prone to a number of forms of bias, and study questions must be presented and worded in such a way that prejudice and bias are minimised. Surveys are also prone to cultural and temporal bias, meaning that the same experience or information may be expressed in different cultural ways, and for the same person may vary with time. A common problem with the use of the survey method is poor response rates, which can lead to selection bias and lack of ability to validate the response data as representative of the population of interest.

Surveys can measure a variety of types of information, including the attitudes of the population being studied. Factual information, such as injury during a disaster event or loss of shelter, can be determined using the survey method. Surveys are ideal for measuring the perceived needs of a population in relation to a disaster event. Surveys designed as a knowledge testing tool can help determine the understanding and information held by a study population. Finally, surveys allow for measurement of perceptions of study subjects.

There are essential steps that should be taken when conducting survey research. The first is to define the survey study objective and the study population. It is important to define the information a survey will provide before developing the survey questions or tool. Lack of a focused study objective leads to a survey that is confusing and lengthy, decreasing the probability that an adequate number of persons will respond.

Establishing how a survey will be conducted is also an important first step. It is important to consider the potential need for ethics committee review of the research project if the survey will involve collection of personal identifiable information. Determination of a sampling system is necessary for survey research, including determination of the population to be studied, how many of that group will be surveyed and whether the survey sample represents the whole study population.

Development of a valid survey involves more than simply listing questions to be answered by respondents. Survey questions must be developed such that internal and external bias is minimised. Table 1.1 lists the essential elements for survey question development. Experienced survey researchers usually pre-test survey questions on a test group of the study population to determine the understandability, cultural competency and minimisation of external bias (prejudice caused by the survey or surveyors).

Table 1.1: Survey question development

1.	Survey questions should be directed at answering the study question
2.	Demographic survey questions should help to define who took the survey and how well they represent the study population
3.	Survey questions must be constructed in such a way that they do not cause bias
4.	Survey questions must be culturally correct for the persons being surveyed
5.	The study question should be explored by asking for research information in more than one way in more than one question
6.	The survey should have no more questions than those necessary to answer the research question and establish the characteristics of the group that participates in the survey

One advantage of the survey method is that data can be collected and measured quantitatively. Demographic data are helpful for comparison and validation of the response group to the study population and are usually collected in single-answer questions that allow for measures of frequency, means and medians. Questions structured to provide categorical answers, such as gender, allow for proportional analysis. Answers can be designed along an ordinal scale that will allow for comparison of ranges of answers and determination of the strength of the opinion of those surveyed. The most common ordinal scale used in survey research is the Likert Scale, which measures a response as between one to five or one to ten based on lowest-to-highest strength of the individual respondent's answer. Open-ended questions can also be used in survey research to allow for development of themes and give depth to quantitative answers. Finally, mixed methods can be used in a single question, or data can be developed for the same study objective using mixed methods of questioning.

When conducting a survey, one must determine how long to wait for replies or completion of interviews before reminding non-responders of the request to participate. Data should be collected into a database that will allow basic statistical analysis. It is considered most appropriate to analyse data only after all final responses to the survey have been received. The survey tool (questions) should not be altered during the conduct of the survey as this will change responses and result in data that is mixed in outcome with respect to a specific point or question. It is important to determine who will be surveyed and how many persons will be included in a survey.

Analysis of survey data should include information that reflects how those who took the survey represent the population that is the object of the study. This is usually done by comparing the demographic features of those who completed the survey with the demographics of the study population. Survey conclusions should be based only on the data collected. It is important to estimate the potential error in the survey analysis that occurred as a result of sample size and lack of responses.

Survey research is at risk for bias. Many high-level medical journals avoid considering publication of surveys because of the multiple areas of bias that must be considered. Table 1.2 lists common causes for bias in survey research. Even when surveys are conducted with strong efforts to avoid bias, uncontrolled factors, such as events occurring at the time of the survey (economic and social) and cultural interpretation of questions and appropriate answers, can affect the research conclusions.

Table 1.2: Potential sources of bias in survey research

1.	Personal or institutional bias imparted by an interviewer or researcher to the survey participant
2.	A motivation on the part of the survey participant to answer questions to please or argue with the researcher
3.	Poorly constructed questions that lead to lack of clear understanding of questions by those taking the survey
4.	External bias based on current news reports, community information or political concerns
5.	Risk that those participating in the survey do not represent the study population
6.	Survey fatigue, failure to honestly or thoughtfully answer questions later in the survey because the survey is too long
7.	Selection bias that may occur from poor selection of participants
8.	Situational bias caused by changing personal situations of participants and environment
9.	Recall decay from past time of the event
10.	Lack of adequate number of survey participants
11.	Data analysis poorly done or data not definitive to support an answer to the study objective; data collected such that the actual study objective is not possible to answer
12.	Failure to account for effect of non-responders in data analysis

Descriptive reports and observational studies

The terms 'descriptive' and 'observational' are often used interchangeably. But, there is a distinction between what is considered a descriptive and an observational study. Descriptive studies are structured reports of an event, often with a focus on a particular issue. Such studies can generate baseline and statistical data that help to define or illustrate an important issue. On the other hand, observational studies are those in which analysis of data allows for the development of an association between a variable and outcome. Descriptive and observational studies are described in more detail in the following sections. Descriptive studies are important at this point in the evolution of medical disaster research.

Descriptive reports

Descriptive reports are structured examinations of an event, population, location, or similar study subject. A descriptive report describes the existing distribution of variables during a defined period without regard to causes or hypotheses. Descriptive reports do not test a hypothesis; rather, they are used to generate hypotheses. They are also used to establish baseline demographics or characteristics of populations or other groupings. A descriptive study does not generally incorporate a comparison group. Of primary importance in the validity of descriptive studies is the careful collection of data to be reported in the study. Data reported in descriptive reports have a hierarchy of validity (see Table 1.3). Data with high validity are least biased and have the least risk of error.

Table 1.3: Potential sources of descriptive data, ordered from top to bottom by degree of validity

1.	Measurable numerical data that can be confirmed
2.	Measurable nominal data (for example, gender or death)
3.	Formal reports (for example, coroner's reports)
4.	Surveys designed to minimise bias
5.	Structured interviews
6.	Measurable indicators (for example, hospital visits as an indication of medical effect)
7.	Databases that are compiled using verification methods
8.	Newspaper accounts
9.	Legal court records

While descriptive reports are designed to systematically collect and analyse available data, there are a variety of types of descriptive studies. Some of these include:

- *Purely descriptive reports*
  1. Case reports – a detailed report of a single case or event.
  2. Case series – a detailed aggregate analysis of cases in one report
- *Prevalence studies*
  1. Cross-sectional studies – a prevalence study of a population; a description of study variables within a population at a specific point in time.
  2. Surveillance studies – the report and analysis of data generally gathered through traditional channels (disease reports, death certificates and others).

3. Correlation studies – the correlation between exposures and outcomes in a population.

Appropriate statistical measures in descriptive reports are measures of central tendency. Mean, median and mode are descriptive statistics to report for this form of disaster research. Data optimally should be dispersed in a near-normal manner (bell curve) to properly apply these statistical measures. Mean calculations are used to measure the central tendency for continuous data, while the median is used for ordinal or ordered data, such as that generated by use of the Likert Scale or Glasgow Coma Score. When measuring means (averages), confidence intervals, usually 95%, or standard deviation should also be reported to allow for determination of the central tendency or inherent strength of a reported mean to reflect the norm for the test population. When a mean cannot be calculated, the median and range with quartiles should be reported to allow for estimation of the dispersion of the data elements from the central measured median.

Cross-sectional studies are descriptive reports that can be used to calculate prevalence for a disease or event. Surveillance and correlation studies are considered sophisticated forms of descriptive reports. They can be used to calculate prevalence and incidence (these statistics are discussed below). In addition, the validity of surveillance data measured as sensitivity and positive predictive value can be calculated.

Two types of descriptive study are common in disaster research: the case series and cross-sectional study.

Case series

Case series are common in epidemiological disaster research. This method of research is more precise than a descriptive case report, with the focus being on known cases of an outcome. Generally, the cases are reviewed and described in detail with similarities identified. For example, if during an inhalational anthrax bioterrorism event, there were ten cases that occurred, a case series would be initiated to find any similarities in the cases, to determine the source and time of infections. As with any descriptive study, a case series helps to generate a hypothesis for further research, such as hypothesising that the anthrax was released at a public site at a specific time.

Cross-sectional studies

Cross-sectional studies are also common in disaster research. In a cross-sectional study, the investigator takes a study population and collects information about an outcome or variable of interest. If there has been a disaster occurrence that affected a population, a cross-sectional study can generate information that can be compared with the times before and after the disaster. In a cross-sectional study, subjects are entered (enrolled) into the study because they are members of the population at risk (were affected by a disaster event). Selected outcomes of interest are measured within the study population to determine the rate of occurrence of the study outcome within the population. Cross-sectional studies are well suited for calculations of comparative prevalence statistics within a population.

Often, cross-sectional studies are performed using a selected sample of an entire population. Sampling a population allows for quicker and less costly examination of a portion of the whole population, with the intent of extrapolating the sample results to make conclusions about the whole population. Proper sampling of a population can be difficult and complicated. A population sample must reflect all aspects of the whole population before the results generated by sampling can be considered representative of the entire population.

Prevalence and incidence

Prevalence and incidence are measures of occurrence of an event or variable within a population. Prevalence is an important statistical measure used in disaster research, and it is important to understand the difference between it and incidence measures. Often the terms 'incidence' and 'prevalence' are used interchangeably by mistake. Each term has a very specific meaning.

- *Prevalence* = existing cases/study population.
- *Prevalence* measures the proportion of study cases present in a population.

Stated another way, *prevalence* measures the frequency of existing disease or the study variable within the population. Technically, there are two types of prevalence – point prevalence and period prevalence. *Point prevalence* refers to the frequency of an event in a population at a single point in time. *Period prevalence* refers to the frequency of an event during a specified period of time.

Measures of prevalence are strong tools used in disaster research. The prevalence of a condition or event during a disaster can be compared to the prevalence for the same variable before or after a disaster event, and can be shown to increase or decrease in frequency. This allows one to form conclusions of association for variables and specific disaster events.

Incidence is defined as the occurrence of new cases that arise during a period of observation. When referring to incidence, it is very important to realise that it is *new cases* that are being measured. Prevalence, as described above, measures all cases within a population, both new and existing. Because of this, incidence is usually considered a more specific epidemiological measure because it gives a measure that helps predict forward development of a measured variable. In other words, it does not include old cases, and focuses on developing or new cases during a period of time.

- *Incidence* = new study cases / study population per time.
- *Incidence* measures the development of an outcome of interest within a population.

As with prevalence, incidence, when it can be measured, is a tool that allows a disaster researcher to make associations between a disaster and the development of an outcome, when the incidence of an occurrence during a disaster period is compared to incidence rates prior to or after recovery from an event.

To further emphasise, prevalence and incidence are powerful disaster research statistics. Prevalence measured in a study can be compared to known or baseline measures of the same statistic. For example, after the Northridge earthquake, the prevalence of coccidoidomycosis increased over the usual prevalence for the area. From this data, it was hypothesised that dust rose into the air as a result of the earthquake, increasing infection with coccidioidomycosis. Comparison of incidence and prevalence with baseline rates before a disaster help one make conclusions in a research effort.

Observational analytical studies

While descriptive reports include observation of subjects or variables as part of the process for conducting the study, the term 'observational study' is usually reserved for studies that include observations of comparison and control subgroups within a defined population. These types of studies are called analytical studies because the method allows for data analysis and statistical measures that show the degree of association between a variable and outcome. The difference between observational or analytical studies and descriptive studies is that an analytical study utilises controls to analyse the affected group.

Observational studies are used whenever possible in conducting disaster research to limit bias in data results and study conclusions. The ability to make associations between events and outcomes is a strong tool provided by observational methodology. While observational methodology does allow for stronger interpretation of appropriate data and the ability to analytically approach a research problem, there is still risk for study error and bias in results and conclusions (see Table 1.4). There are two primary types of observational analytical studies: the cohort and case-control study.

Table 1.4: Potential causes of bias in observational studies

1.	Lack of enough cases to make a valid conclusion (poor sample size) – generally the more cases included, the lower the risk for study error
2.	Poorly controlled data – data that is 'soft' and unreliable
3.	Error in the conduct of the study leading to bias in results:
	a. poor definition of exposure or outcome
	b. failure to include cases that reflect the study population
	c. failure to compare data or study groups to appropriate controls
4.	Confounding, defined as failure to recognise variables that affect the outcome of interest, and not including those variables in the study analysis
5.	Lack of appropriate selection of comparison groups
6.	Lack of accurate determination of exposure and/or outcome status

Cohort studies

In a cohort study, cases are entered into the study because they have been exposed to the event of interest. For example, if one wanted to determine if exposure to a disaster resulted in higher rates of gastroenteritis, the study subjects would be only those who were exposed to the disaster. A cohort study typically measures the effects of an exposure, with the subjects defined according to their exposure levels and followed for the disease occurrence. Cohort studies can be either prospective or retrospective, with the key aspect of the study being that cases are selected into the study group based on an exposure being studied.

Cohort studies allow for actual comparison of control groups, and therefore for an analytical approach. To develop an analytical cohort study, one must:

- Establish the exposure criteria for entering cases into the cohort study group;
- Define the outcome of interest and find people with that outcome;
- Identify a group comparable in all aspects with the cohort study group, except with respect to the exposure, to compare with the cohort group.

A classic example of a cohort study is the Framingham study of cardiovascular disease, which started in 1948 in the United States. This study sought to establish the association of smoking, obesity, elevated blood pressure, cholesterol levels and physical activity with coronary artery heart disease. The study focused on a defined population (those living in Framingham), and compared the development of coronary heart disease with the study variables. An important point is that the Framingham study allowed for the calculation of incidence rates for the population. The ability to calculate incidence rates is an advantage for the cohort study design.

Case-control study

For a case-control study, the investigator selects the study group based on their outcome status, regardless of the exposure of interest. The prior exposures are then determined. Stated in a different way, a case-control study examines the relation of a defined disease or occurrence to a certain exposure (disaster event). A group of individuals with the disease or occurrence (cases) are compared to a group of individuals without that disease or occurrence (controls) to determine what proportion of those with the disease or occurrence were exposed to a disaster event and what proportion were not.

For example, if post-disaster-event diarrhoea is the outcome of interest, and the investigator hypothesises that exposure to a specific water supply available during a disaster event may have an association with development of acute diarrhoea, the investigator would collect all those with diarrhoea within the study population and determine the rates of exposure to the water supply in question. In effect, a case-control study looks at an issue in the opposite way that a cohort study does.

Case-control studies allow for analysis using comparison groups. The following are essential to developing an analytical case-control study:

- Establish or define the outcome of interest;
- Define the exposure being tested for;
- Identify a group comparable in all aspects with the case-control study group except with respect to the outcome or interest to compare with the case-control group.

Data analysis methods used in observational studies

Cohort and case-control studies are appropriate methods for disaster research. These types of observational study allow for an analytical approach to specific hypotheses that apply to disaster events.

In cohort studies the prevalence (cases/population) and incidence (new cases/population) are the simplest measures that can be applied. 'Risk' and 'risk ratio' are also measures commonly used in cohort studies:

- *Risk* = number of cases or occurrences/number of people at risk (study population).
- *Risk ratio* = risk in exposed group/risk in non-exposed group.

For case-control studies, an odds ratio is calculated to measure the association between exposure and the outcome of interest. Odds are the number of times something occurs divided by the number of times something does not occur. Importantly, the case-control method does not allow for calculation of prevalence because the denominator of the prevalence equation or total population cannot be determined using this study method.

- *Odds* = number of cases or occurrences/number exposed or not exposed.
- *Odds ratio* = odds of occurrence exposed/odds of occurrence in non-exposed.

Because this section is a basic discussion on disaster research methodology, the reader who is considering the determination of risk ratios and odds ratios for a study should refer to basic statistical texts for more detail on these calculations.

Experimental studies

Experimental studies or trials use experimental methods derived from laboratory research methodology to control variables and compare two or more groups. Experimental studies are designed so that all variables but the one being tested are controlled and held constant within the total population tested. The population is then divided into groups and the variable being tested for cause or effect on an outcome is applied to a comparison or intervention group, while a control group does not have the study variable applied to them.

The grouping of those who receive an intervention and who are controls can occur naturally within a population (called a natural experiment) or can be accomplished by the researcher selecting who is assigned to either group. Most researchers use a method to randomly select those assigned to intervention and control groups, resulting in the form of experimental study referred to as a randomised trial. Randomised trials are felt by most researchers to be the only method that allows an investigator to show causal effect. Use of the term 'causal effect' implies that the cause for an outcome is directly related to a specific variable (intervention). In non-experimental studies, association for an effect by a variable is usually shown as opposed to the causal effect shown by experimental studies.

Active manipulation or control of study variables by the investigator is the hallmark of experimental studies called randomised controlled trials. Randomised controlled trials are considered to be the most rigorous, or highest level of clinical study method. Experimental studies of human populations during disaster events are extremely difficult to perform because of the lack of ability to control all variables within the study population. Because the investigator randomises and applies the study variable within the population that is being studied during a randomised controlled trial, this type of experimental study is prospective in design.

Randomised trials or experimental studies allow for application of robust statistical measures. The statistical test applied for an experimental study is determined by the type of data collected. There are multiple statistical tests that are appropriate and used in experimental studies. For the investigator, it is important to realise that, when designing an experimental study, one must determine the appropriate statistical analytical method for use in the study. Most often, the type of data collected determines the appropriate statistical test for the study. The following are example of tests that are commonly used in experimental studies:

- *Nominal data* (named categories – for example, lived/died)
  1. McNemars Test (when groups are matched).
  2. Chi-Square.
- *Ordinal data* (discrete categories – for example, GCS Scale)
  1. Wilcoxon Rank Sum Test.
  2. Wilcoxon Signed Rank Test (matched groups).
  3. Friedman 2-Way Anova (multiple matched groups).
  4. Kruskal-Wallis 1-Way Anova.
- *Continuous data* (numerical data – for example, age)
  1. T-Test (data normally distributed in a bell curve).
  2. Wilcoxon Rank Sum Test.
  3. Wilcoxon Signed Rank Test (matched groups).

While experimental study methods are considered the most rigorous of the types that can be done in medical research, there is potential for error in these types of studies. The most common types of error that can cause an experimental study to have a serious flaw include selection bias (inappropriate selection of subjects or variables) and poor sample size.

Comparison of study designs

Each study design has strengths and weaknesses; they should be considered carefully when choosing the right design for your study. A researcher should choose a design based on the study objective or hypothesis and the availability of study data. Most researchers will choose the highest level of study method possible to avoid risks of study bias and error.

As stated above, experimental studies are the highest form of clinical research and the only design that allows for making a causal inference. Experimental studies require control of all variables that may affect the outcome of interest for the study. For this reason, experimental studies are rarely considered in disaster research because, by the very nature of a disaster event, variables that can affect outcome are uncontrolled.

Descriptive and observational studies are appropriate methods for disaster medical research. The following list describes the major aspects of common descriptive and observation study methods, which can help determine the appropriateness of each in designing a study.

Strengths of descriptive and observational studies

1. *Cross-sectional study*
   a. Allows for descriptive analysis of a population with calculation of prevalence that can be compared to the same measures from different times.
   b. Allows for the generation of future study hypotheses.
2. *Case series*
   a. Allows for a case description for future study.
   b. Allows for the generation of future hypotheses.
3. *Cohort studies*
   a. Suited for examining effects of rare exposures.
   b. Can determine multiple outcomes from one exposure.
   c. Allows for analytical measurement of risk.
   d. Allows for measurement of prevalence and incidence.
4. *Case-control studies*
   a. Suited for study of rare outcomes.
   b. Shows relationship of multiple exposures to outcome of interest.
   c. Of all observational studies, this provides the best ability to determine differences between a group of interest and comparison group.

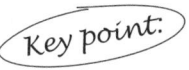 **Most disaster research makes use of descriptive or observation types of methods.**

Summary

Various established clinical research methods are used in disaster medical research. Most disaster research is done using descriptive or observation types of methods. This is because study groups exposed to disaster events are difficult to randomise, and disaster event variables are uncontrollable. Descriptive reports are helpful in generating hypotheses and providing an overview of the variables that are of interest in relation to a disaster event. Case series help one to understand the characteristics of subjects that have an outcome of interest. Cross-sectional studies allow for statistical measures of prevalence and measures of central tendency that can be used for comparison to similar data. Cohort and case-control studies are the more powerful of the observational study types, and allow for application of analytical methods (such as comparing a study group to a control group).

1.5   Resources

Hardcastle, T. (In press). 'The ethical and medico-legal issues of trauma care'. *South African Journal of Bioethics and Law*, 3(1).

Kramer, E. (2008). '"No one may be refused emergency medical treatment" – ethical dilemmas in South African emergency medicine'. *South African Journal of Bioethics and Law*, 1(2): 53–6.

United Nations: International Strategy for Disaster Reduction Africa – www.unisdr.org/africa/

International Committee of the Red Cross – www.icrc.org/eng

South African National Disaster Management Center – www.ndmc.gov.za/Home.aspx

1.6 References

1. Advanced Life Support Group. *Major incident medical management and support.* 2nd ed. London: BMJ Books; 2002.
2. United Nations. United Nations International Strategy for Disaster Reduction. Accessed July 2010. Available from: www.unisdr.org/#.
3. Disaster reduction in Africa. ISDR Informs. 2009 issue.
4. International Committee of the Red Cross. 2004. What is international humanitarian law? Advisory Service on International Humanitarian Law.
5. Sundres KO, Birnbaum ML (editors). Health disaster management guidelines for evaluation and research in the Utstein Style. *Prehospital and Disaster Medicine* 2003;17(supplement 3).
6. Aschengrau A, Seage GR. Epidemiologic approach to causation. In: *Essentials of epidemiology.* 2nd ed. Boston: Jones and Bartlett; 2008. pp. 382–409.
7. Turchin P. *Complex population dynamics: a theoretical/empirical synthesis.* Princeton, NJ: Princeton University Press; 2003.
8. Gehlbach SH. Prospective and retrospective. In: *Interpreting the medical literature.* 3rd edition. New York: McGraw-Hill; 1993. pp. 29–32.
9. Grimes DA, Schultz KF. Bias and causal associations in observational research. *Lancet* 2002;359:248–52.
10. Stake RE. Triangulation. In: *The art of case study research.* Thousand Oaks, CA: Sage Publications; 1995. pp. 107–20.
11. Groves RM, Fowler FJ, Couper MP, Lepkowski JM, Singer E, Tourangeau R. *Survey methodology.* New York: John Wiley and Sons; 2009.
12. Grimes DA, Schultz KF. Descriptive studies: what they can and cannot do. *Lancet* 2002;359:145–9.
13. Savage J. Ethnography and health care. *British Medical Journal* 2000;321:1400–02.
14. Aschengrau A, Seage GR. Measures of disease frequency. In: *Essentials of epidemiology.* 2nd edition. Boston: Jones and Bartlett; 2008. pp. 33–54.
15. Aschengrau A, Seage GR. Overview of epidemiologic study designs. In: *Essentials of epidemiology.* 2nd edition. Boston: Jones and Bartlett; 2008. pp. 139–67.
16. Schneider E, Hajjeh RA, Spiegel RA, *et al.* A coccidioidomycosis outbreak following the Northridge, California, earthquake. *Journal of the American Medical Association* 1997;227:904–08.
17. Gordis L. Case-control and cross-sectional studies. In: *Epidemiology.* 2nd edition. Philadelphia: WB Saunders; 2000. pp. 140–56.
18. Liao Y, McGee DL, Cooper RS, Sutkowski MB. How generalizable are coronary risk prediction models? Comparison of Framingham and two national cohorts. *American Heart Journal* 1999;137:837–45.

2

Major Incident Management in the Pre-Hospital Environment

T Ligthelm, T Hardcastle, M Stander, B Bonner, D van Hoving and V Wessels

Objectives

By the end of this chapter, the reader will:

- be able to adequately plan for a major incident;
- understand the different tiers of command;
- understand the Incident Command System (ICS);
- understand the need for an efficient message structure;
- understand the different methods of communication;
- understand the principles of radio communication;
- understand the all-hazards approach to scene safety;
- appreciate the various hazards that can confront the emergency care provider;
- know the key principles of search and rescue operations;
- be able to triage using the triage sieve and the triage sort;
- understand the dynamic nature of triage;
- be able to understand treatment priorities in a major incident;
- be aware of the importance of a coordinated transport strategy;
- understand the importance of PPE as well as incident-specific equipment;
- realise the importance of regular exercises and continual training.

2.1 Introduction

The pre-hospital environment is a challenging venue to manage a disaster or major incident. In many countries, implementation of formalised major incident management systems has been achieved. In South Africa, in addition to the obvious resource constraints under which we operate, major incident response is further complicated by the presence of different EMS service providers (communications, for instance, become challenging with three or four services, each of whom have their own radio channels and control centres). However, despite challenges there is no doubt that South Africa has a wealth of experience in dealing with major incidents, and this should be built on with formalised systems.

2.2 Planning

Effective response to a major incident is critically dependent on pre-event planning. All EMS services must have a Major Incident Plan in place.

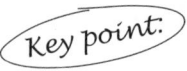 **Failing to plan is planning to fail!**

However, the plan is only as good as the personnel who are there to implement it; therefore it is vital that all role-players are consulted in the development of the plan, that it is circulated to all personnel who may be involved in managing the response, and that it is continually audited and updated as part of the post-response recovery process.

In addition to the plan being known to all key EMS role-players, it must also be shared with other pre-hospital service providers (police, fire, etc) and local hospitals.

2.3 Command and control

Command and control should be the first priority to establish when any major incident occurs. Time is critical; for every five minutes without command in place, it takes about 30 minutes longer to bring the incident under control. The overall control of the scene should be the responsibility of one of the emergency services. The specific service responsible for control differs between countries but it often falls under the auspices of the police.

Control entails one individual being responsible for horizontal communication and coordination between all the emergency services present (or needed) at the scene.

Command, on the other hand, refers to the authority within each emergency or support service. Each service has one individual who is in command (for example, the incident medical commander), who communicates through vertical channels within the service.

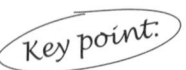 **Command and control must be established immediately on arrival at a major incident.**

Tiers of command

The different command tiers are recognised internationally.

- *Gold* command is the strategic backbone of the incident. It may involve local, provincial or national authority and is often remote from the scene.
- *Silver* command is confined by the outer cordon at the scene and is tasked with all the tactical aspects related to the incident. A silver commander is usually designated by each service (see later) to form a unified command team.

- *Bronze* command performs the operational tasks and is situated in the 'hot' zone, bounded by the inner cordon. Each service is also represented by a designated sector commander.

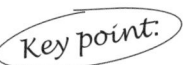 **The responsibility of control falls under the auspices of one service (often the police).**

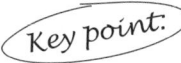 **Command entails authority and communication within each emergency service.**

Incident Command System

The beginning

The conception of the Incident Command System (ICS) is credited to the fire services in the aftermath of the devastating 1970 wild fires in California (FIRESCOPE). The ICS really refers to this modular structure, as developed in the United States of America. There are other systems, all with similar outcomes – that of ensuring rapid and efficient multi-disciplinary command and control of major incidents.

In South Africa, a simple structure has been put in place for incident command. This is available for free download from www.emssa.org.za.

The purpose of incident command

Incident command allows an effective response to any disaster by bringing together different agencies (e.g. fire, medical and police). The common language and familiar organisational structure simplifies communication. Major incidents without the establishment of an appropriate and integrated command structure will lack coordination, with potential catastrophic outcomes for the casualties.

The modular structure of the ICS

The ICS, as utilised in the United States of America, consists of five functions (modules) that can expand or collapse as the incident evolves (see Table 2.1). A single person can effectively run a small incident, covering all the functions. As the incident increases in magnitude, an individual is allocated to take responsibility for each function. Smaller sections can be added underneath, if need be.

The assignment of roles and tasks is made at the scene according to incoming resources. Typically, the first responding unit needs to establish incident command by using available resources. Incident command is the only functional position that must always be filled. When needed, the underlying functions should be dedicated to different individuals that report directly to the incident commander. The ICS system works best if roles are filled only to the required extent. The allocation of roles should take into account the experience of the individual. It is best to allocate duties to individuals who perform similar duties on a day-to-day basis. To maintain reliability, the assignment (and re-assignment) of personnel to different positions should be made in relation to any situational change. The allocated individuals should wear marked vests in order for other providers to identify them.

Unity of command specifies that each person reports to only one person; with the command structure supervising three to seven persons. If this clear line of supervision is violated, it may result in delays in decision-making and increased confusion if supervisors give conflicting instructions.

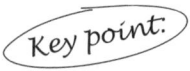 **The ICS allows for a multi-organisational all-hazard approach.**

Individual roles within the ICS

The incident medical commander (IMC) is the highest-ranking position in the ICS. The initial tasks of the IMC include:

- An assessment of the situation;
- Identification of any contingencies;
- The development of objectives;
- Establishing the resources needed;
- Generating an initial action plan.

The IMC should also allow lower-ranked personnel to make decisions if they are better qualified or more experienced in the relevant field. This should be viewed as utilising available resources and not as giving over command. A balance should be maintained between a centralised, explicit organisational structure versus a more diffuse, improvisational approach.

Unified command

Unified command represents a management system that involves all participating services. Each emergency service is represented by its respective commander. This team of commanders functions on equal par and is responsible for their specific service. This unified command (*silver command*) is ultimately responsible for the overall management of the major incident. The development and implementation of strategic decisions, as well as the order and release of required resources, falls under their jurisdiction.

The other building blocks of the ICS consist of:

- *Operations:* Responsible for the development of tactical operations to achieve the primary objectives.
- *Planning:* Involves the development of an action plan to accomplish the objectives.
- *Logistics:* Supports the ICS by providing services and resources required to manage the incident.
- *Finance/administration:* Handles all costs related to the incident.
- *Information:* Supplies information to the media and other relevant organisations.
- *Safety:* Ultimately responsible for the safety on the scene, survivors and personnel.
- *Liaison:* The dedicated contact point for assisting agencies.

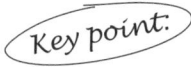 **The ICS consists of functional modules that can be extended or contracted according to situational demands.**

Key roles and action cards for roles, as adapted for the South African environment, are available at www.emssa.org.za.

Key position identification

The above-mentioned key positions should ideally be allocated prior to the occurrence of a major incident. To ensure that a major incident plan can be declared at any given time, it is better to identify and train a group of persons to fill each position, so that the initial incident command can be replaced by a predetermined and trained individual, once they arrive at the incident site. Transfer of command, when deemed necessary, should occur only once, to the most experienced and qualified person and not necessarily to the highest-ranking individual. The transferring of command must be very explicit, face-to-face and must include a full up-to-date report.

Situational awareness

The cognitive and perceptional requirements of the tasks are extremely demanding, and personnel may struggle to maintain awareness of the surrounding system (situational awareness). Traditionally, this has been performed by means of paper or radio, but new technology can provide a real-time view of the situation.

Why the ICS might fail

Various authors have established why the ICS works so well for emergency responders. On the flip side, it may be less successful for law enforcement, public health and public works, probably because these organisations are not formal first responders and hence not that familiar with the system.

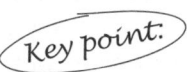 **Unified command organises various autonomous emergency services into one combined command.**

Summary of ICS

The ICS is a highly formalised system with extensive rules, procedures, policies and instructions that focuses on operations, planning and logistics. Its most attractive qualities are flexibility, adaptability and reliability. These qualities are needed to achieve specific objectives by coordinating diverse resources under turbulent, time-constrained and even hazardous conditions. Table 2.1 lists six key principles pertinent to the ICS that allows the system to be applied to any type or size of disaster.

Table 2.1: Key principles of the Incident Command System (ICS)

1.	Modular organisational structure
2.	Consistent basic structure
3.	Functional hierarchy
4.	Key position identification
5.	Early implementation
6.	All-hazard approach

International command

The ICS might also fail during international disasters. Because multinational organisations respond to these disasters, responders include volunteers and non-governmental organisations who might not be involved regularly with major incidents. The lack of technical knowledge and confidence, together with minimal interpersonal trust, might lead to failure. On the international scene, working under the auspices of global organisations, such as the United Nations (UN) or the World Health Organization (WHO), becomes critical.

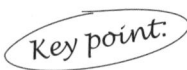 **Global organisations such as the UN should take command during international disasters.**

Summary

Command and control are the most important aspects of major incident management. Effective command requires strict discipline and excellent communication between responding services. The ICS provides an approach to any major incident, regardless of type and size. It ensures common ground between different services (and even different nationalities) when responding to a major incident. International command requires responding agencies to work under the auspices of global organisations such as the UN or the WHO.

2.4 Communication

Communication is essential to human existence. Without the ability to communicate, humans cannot relate feelings, emotions and facts. In major incidents, this is even more important as the lack of efficient communications leads to the failure of effective command, control and scene safety. Indeed, the failure of services to work together effectively at major incidents in the past has been blamed squarely on ineffective communication.

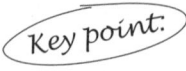 **Efficient communication is the pivot point around which major incident management stands or falls.**

Efficient message structure

The METHANE system is a mnemonic used in the MIMMS system (Major Incident Medical Management and Support) to convey an efficient message regarding a major incident within, and between, emergency services.

METHANE is an acronym for the following components of an emergency message:

- *M*ajor incident: My call sign, whether a 'standby' call, a declared incident or an update. A stand-down will be given when the incident is completed.
- *E*xact location: with GPS coordinates if possible.
- *T*ype of incident.
- *H*azards present and potential.
- *A*ccess and egress routes, including a vehicle staging area location, if appropriate.
- *N*umber of casualties on scene (actual or estimate).
- *E*mergency services: those present and those required; also for the hospitals: is a 'go' team required?

Another acronym, MIST, is a useful brief patient handover between the various levels of emergency medical care providers during the extrication and evacuation at a major incident:

- *M*echanism of injury;
- *I*njuries identified;
- *S*ymptoms and signs identified;
- *T*reatment given.

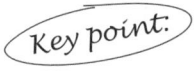 **Any emergency message must be complete in structure and yet brief enough for effective onward transmission. METHANE is one such system.**

Methods of communication

Telephone (land line) is the most common method for the initial alerting of the emergency services of a major incident by members of the public. Dedicated emergency lines and easy, short emergency numbers linked to multi-service call centres with trained emergency dispatchers allow for optimal call assimilation. The challenge is that land lines can only take a single call at one time (except for conference call services, which are limited) and are likely to become 'jammed' in an emergency. In South Africa, the challenge is made worse by the fact that the universal 107 and 112 systems are not available in all parts of the country; neither do all the services subscribe to the universal number, with many private ambulance services and local fire services having their own emergency numbers.

Cellular networks are the other single-user system, where calls can be directed to other cellular devices or to land lines. The problem with cellular networks is that they rely on a system of 'available cells', and the likelihood is great that during major incidents the first system of communication to be lost is the cellular network.

Radio networks are the most common method of communication for emergency services within South Africa. These require the use of either 'base stations', usually of around 25-watt signal strength, or handheld devices of about 5-watt strength that are linked via either simplex (line of sight, often on HF or VHF) or repeater stations to boost the signal (often VHF systems). Radio networks have several advantages, namely, that the other responding vehicles can receive simultaneous updates from the scene, get ongoing directions to staging areas and, through dedicated emergency channels, allow day-to-day calls to be attended to without disruption of their communications. Trunking systems allow multiple talk-groups through complex computer controlled linking, thus allowing better use of frequencies and some degree of privacy.

Written messages sent by runners are often useful at the incident scene or within control rooms, both to maintain records and to pass on sensitive information.

Hand signals are often of value at the bronze/hot zone, when the noise and other distractions make radio or cellular communication difficult to hear. These may vary from service to service so one must check the system used in one's local area.

Whistle signals have been used for many years by the fire and rescue services to pass instructions and signal the need for rapid evacuation. A single long blast on a whistle should stimulate rapid evacuation of all staff due to impending danger.

Personal interaction is most likely to occur at the strategic (silver or 'cool' zone) command centre between the responsible members of various services and at the bronze/hot zone between operation personnel as they work to free trapped individuals and tend to injured patients. A face-to-face meeting is often the most opportune method to resolve differences of opinion and heated emotions, and to gain perspective and direction. Personal communication by loud-hailer may also enable instructions to be provided to multiple providers at one time.

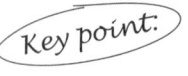

There are many forms of acceptable communication – utilise them timeously and appropriately. Know the warning signals for evacuation.

International rules for radio communication

The international laws governing radio communications, to which the Independent Communications Authority of South Africa (ICASA) is a signatory, require the use of English as the only acceptable official language for emergency communications. Radios must be licensed and regularly checked and tested. Bandwidth must be used sparingly and profanity is not allowed. In South Africa, all radio communication is subject to the Telecommunications Act 13 of 2000.

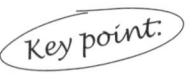

Radio communication is subject to international law.

Practical principles of radio communication

Radio airtime is valuable, and therefore brief, clear and unambiguous messages should be transmitted. For efficient radio communication the voice procedure should be as follows: smooth controlled normal speech of mid-range pitch, at normal volume (no shouting), should be used. Wait for free airtime and then proceed to call the intended responder using their call sign, with your call sign to follow. Await a response and then transmit your message. At the end of every message, say 'over' and await response. Keep messages to about 30 seconds, with a warning issued for long messages – rather break these up into segments. For spelling and numbers, use the universal NATO phonetic alphabet. In this system, the letters of the alphabet are given names (for example, A = Alpha, B = Beta, O = Oscar, P = Papa, etc.). Ideally, the recipient will respond with an acknowledgement (roger/ wilco/message received) and repeat the details of your message. The controller will be the one to end the call with 'out'. Do not use profanity or shouting on the air and avoid 'radio gibberish' such as 'over and out'.

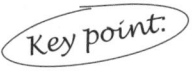 **Radio procedure is standardised, and all operators of radio equipment must adhere to the procedures to optimise airtime usage.**

Summary

Communication is essential for effective major incident management – without it, the command and control and safety structure would collapse. No effective patient care will result without good information flow. There are numerous methods of communication, yet radio networks offer the best method of emergency communication currently available.

Standardisation of international practice leads to efficient message delivery.

2.5   Safety

The scene of a major incident is a potentially dangerous place. Without implementation of a robust command system, such as that taught in the Major Incident Medical Management and Support course, needless additional casualties may result from heroic staff members attempting hazardous rescues in an unstable bronze (hot) zone with inadequate personal protective equipment (PPE) and without listening to the wisdom of other services with more expertise in a particular field.

Safety is the first intervention step after an incident is declared and a command and control structure has been initiated, using a multi-service Incident Command System approach.

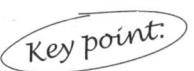 **Safety must always come first – there is no point in going from hero to zero!**

Aspects of scene safety

Safety at the scene incorporates everything from the initial safety assessment to the determination of the potential and actual hazards present on the scene and the need for special equipment. A safety officer should be appointed by each service, or the decision can be taken to devolve this responsibility to one coordinator for all services on the scene, most often the fire service safety personnel.

Some of the aspects to assess from a safety perspective are the following:

- Is the bronze/hot zone safe to access for extrication and evacuation?
- Is there any actual hazard present on the scene (e.g. fire, electrical live wires, chemical spill, secondary device, etc.)?
- Is there a potential hazard on the scene that should be mitigated prior to accessing the scene (e.g. flammable liquids or gases, structural instability, oncoming traffic, violent, distressed family members, etc.)?
- Is there the need for special personal protective gear, specifically chemical, biological PPE, or will standard protective gear be adequate?
- Can hazardous materials be adequately identified by known signs and markings?
- If staff are working in standard rescue attire ('bunker gear'), are there ambient climatic conditions that could affect the safe work duration and need for on-site rehabilitation services? What is the wind direction and temperature on the scene?
- Is there a need to call in specialists from other disciplines (e.g. medical physicists or hospital 'go' teams) to the scene to provide specific expertise?

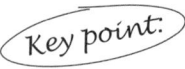 **Appoint a safety officer, who must assess all possible and present hazards.**

Specific safety issues on the scene

'It's management, not just equipment, that keeps first responders safe at large-scale incidents.' So said David Bates, the former editor of *Homeland Security Today* magazine. In order to be properly prepared to be safe on a scene, responders must be aware of some of the specific threats they may face.

Biohazards

A biohazard can be in the form of any body fluid contaminant at the scene, bioterrorism or even a biohazardous load in transit. Suspicion is the watchword and the use of at least basic 'standard precautions' should apply when engaging in the treatment of any casualty with a potential biohazard.

Chemical or radiation hazard

Many incidents will involve chemical spills and potential contamination of victims. It is essential, for safe management of the incident, that the chemical is identified, the risks associated with the chemical are proclaimed to all staff and appropriate steps are taken to contain and neutralise hazardous or flammable chemicals (if required).

Staff exhaustion/rehabilitation

One of the greatest challenges with major incidents is the desire of staff to go the extra mile and then exert themselves beyond safe physiological limits, thus endangering themselves and their co-workers. The safety officer has the responsibility to check not only the PPE of personnel going into a scene, but also their physiological and psychological state of mind. There are good studies that have shown that the ideal time to rotate staff in full PPE in a warm environment is around 20–30 minutes.

Secondary devices

With terrorism, the aim is to kill and maim, as well as cause confusion and anarchy. When a team responds to an explosion or other suspected terrorism event, the risk of a secondary device is high and must feature on the agenda of the safety officer.

Structural stability

While every effort is taken to ensure a safe environment for self, scene and patient, it is often the obvious that is overlooked. Part of the provision of a safe scene is through engaging support services to provide shoring and chocking devices to ensure structural stability to prevent collapses, or to provide support during trench rescue situations.

Adequate visibility

One common error in major incident management, and of particular relevance in protracted or night operations, is the lack of adequate lighting units to aid accessibility and visibility. This includes the use of special lighting devices such as infrared cameras, endoscopic search devices and personal headlamps.

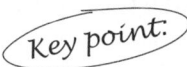 **Safety is dependent upon good visibility on scene, appreciation of staff physiology and addressing all risks.**

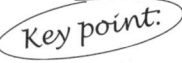 **No staff member should enter the bronze/hot zone without appropriate equipment and until the safety officer has declared the site safe for evacuation.**

Personal protective equipment (PPE)

The US Environmental Protection Agency (EPA) classifies PPE according to four levels, depending on the level of protection offered against hazardous chemicals and fire. Level A should be worn when the highest level of respiratory, skin, eye and mucous membrane protection is needed. This includes positive-pressure enclosed breathing apparatus within an encapsulating suit, with chemical double gloves and boots. A hard hat and inclusive non-sparking radio communications device are optional if required. Level B provides for less eye and skin protection, with the same level of chemical protection for hands and feet. Level C is for known chemicals with moderate risk, and the standard firefighter bunker gear is equivalent to this level of protection. Finally, level D is a work uniform, such as a flight suit or overalls, which is for use with 'nuisance contamination' only. Safety boots and medical gloves should still be utilised.

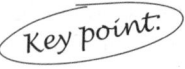 Appropriate PPE is essential – bunker gear is usually the minimum required at the scene unless specific hazards are identified and have to be mitigated.

Summary

Safety at the scene of a major incident is a multifactorial consideration, combining personnel aspects, incident aspects and the safety (or decreased additional risk) of the victims. A safety officer should make the final decision as to when it is safe to enter the bronze/hot zone and also for how long it is safe to utilise a staff member in a particular area before relief is provided. The safety officer must also ensure the safe use of all equipment and the appropriate level of PPE.

2.6 Search and rescue (SAR)

The fundamental goal of emergency medical response in disaster is to save lives and reduce injury and permanent disability. Urban search and rescue operations are an integral part of the response to major incidents and disasters. In virtually all major incidents there is some attempt to rescue victims presumed lost and trapped. This desire is inherent in all societies, and is a logical response to any disastrous situation. Typically, in initial stages, this response is provided by the lay public closest to the incident.

Deployment challenges

There are a number of models for the deployment of search and rescue services, but the vast majority of deployments are for people trapped under rubble. Clearly, the nature of the incident dictates the techniques and equipment required, as well as the level of expertise and experience needed. Equally important is that the rescue of trapped individuals by untrained and unsupervised lay public may be just as detrimental to the outcomes of both patient and rescuer. It is therefore imperative that rescuers and potential rescuers (in areas where the likelihood of collapses is high) be trained and equipped accordingly. The teams should have a basic knowledge of rescue, as well as an understanding of the principles of effective life-supporting first aid and advanced trauma life support (ATLS) principles at the scene.

Urgent medical care of victims trapped under rubble cannot be provided unless the victims have been extricated and removed to treatment facilities, or are accessible to field rescue and medical teams. Indeed, the most significant improvements in response over the last three decades have been the advances in the recovery of victims trapped for prolonged periods. The emergence of the science of confined space medicine – medical care rendered to those trapped in confined spaces – has lent additional credibility to search and rescue medicine.

Major incidents, irrespective of whether man-made or natural, present extreme challenges to emergency services. In most incidents, once command and control has been established, the principle of doing the greatest good for the greatest number is then put to use by determining the area of search and rescue within the inner cordon (bronze area). Within the search and rescue area, a coordinated response is then established by the designated team or teams. The team(s) need to be adequately briefed and equipped with both PPE and appropriate rescue equipment. Communication systems must be implemented and tested before teams are deployed. All SAR efforts at the scene should be controlled and integrated, often in parallel to overall command and control, and should be done as rapidly and safely as possible taking care to ensure that rescuers do not become victims.

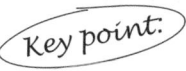 **All SAR operations must be properly coordinated as part of the command and control of the incident.**

Search and rescue typically occurs after the initial stage of chaos, followed by the organisational period, and coincides with the period during which site-clearing and evacuation occurs. Initial treatment of victims identified by the SAR team may need to be done at the scene, before the casualty clearing station is even established. This may require skilled treatment teams to be operational even before the actual medical treatment hierarchy is properly established. This important process must be with the knowledge and tacit approval of the overall incident command and control.

Outcomes

The search and rescue effort is designed to achieve a number of specific outcomes. These include:

1. A detailed description of the incident site;
2. Identification of the potential and actual hazards;
3. Determination of the terrain and challenges;
4. Allowance for the update of the operational plan;
5. Communication of the need for additional resources, both personnel and logistical. This will often allow for more details to be added to the initial METHANE report, particularly as far as casualty numbers and resources are concerned.

Stages of urban search and rescue

There are five recognised stages to an urban search and rescue operation:

1. Reconnaissance;
2. Assessment of survivors/victims;
   (These two stages are surface operations only, and are designed to give knowledge and allow for planning of the rubble penetration that follows in the next three stages. Initial reconnaissance is vital to ensure that the most appropriate resources are deployed to the scene.)
3. Detailed search of the area for potential victims;
4. Guided small-scale debris removal;
5. Large-scale debris removal.

During the first two stages, logistics and safety planning are paramount, and all information about the buildings/rubble pile or incident site are gathered as rapidly as possible to determine rescue needs and potential treatment volumes. The initial search of the area is only a probe, without dogs or other sophisticated equipment, and will only identify those victims closest to the edge.

A more detailed search commences as soon as the team and equipment arrive. This is much like peeling an onion, layer by layer, taking care not to topple further structures. This part of the search is guided by the information gained earlier, and often focuses on specific areas. It commences with manual debris removal, and machinery is only allowed into the area once all casualties are removed, or at least identified for removal. Further structural collapse and injury to victims and rescue personnel is avoided at all cost.

Medical management

As victims are located, a rapid triage will be done, and an assessment of their medical needs will be made, the degree of entrapment established and the presence of other survivors determined. Treatment may be started before or during the extrication, especially if the entrapment has been prolonged, or the extrication complicated and delayed. This is particularly important in trapped victims with possible crush injuries and dehydration. Other injury patterns are also typical in confined-space rescue depending on the cause of the building collapse. Where structural integrity is the cause of collapse, the injuries are typically those of crush and entrapment, as well as falling debris. When an explosion is the cause of building implosion, blast injuries become significant and important. There are four types of blast injury – primary to quaternary – where the pressure wave ruptures hollow organs; flying debris inflicts shrapnel-type injury; the victims are thrown around into solid or penetrating structures; and, finally, building collapse with the associated injury. The search and rescue teams need to be aware of these aspects in order to assist with the treatment determinations.

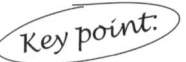 **Injuries can be predicted by the mechanism of the incident.**

Where entrapment has been prolonged, attention must always be paid to the degree of exposure, the level of starvation and dehydration, and the possibility of concomitant infection. These syndromes may need to be addressed at the scene, once access is achieved, even if release from entrapment is likely to still be delayed a while.

Summary

The greatest risk to a good outcome for victims of a major incident lies in the failure of search and rescue teams to prepare adequately.

2.7 Triage

Triage is essential if the major incident response is to fulfil the aim of 'doing the most for the most'. The word 'triage' is derived from the French word, *trier* (to sort). Baron Dominique Jean Larrey has been credited as the originator of modern triage: during the Napoleonic wars, he developed and implemented a system whereby soldiers requiring the most urgent medical care were attended to, and treated first, regardless of rank. The aim was to get as many men back into fighting-fit condition as quickly as possible. Casualty outcomes during times of conflict, including the two world wars, the Korean War and the Vietnam conflict, have continued to improve and mortality rates have decreased because of the implementation of triage and the decrease in time to definitive treatment.

Recently, South African emergency centres and EMS systems have both been utilising the South African Triage Score (SATS) on a day-to-day basis to prioritise patients; numerous other systems are available and are in use in other African settings. Such systems balance accuracy against speed in their measurements; the faster a tool triages a patient, the less accurate it will be. On a day-to-day basis, there are usually enough resources to spend time on individual patients in this regard. In a major incident, however, local resources are inadequate to deal with the casualty load; triage becomes critical for the effective and efficient use of limited on-scene resources, but these very same restrictions mean that dedicating staff for triage is difficult. A simple, easy-to-learn and fast triage tool is essential to facilitate this process.

One of the key early role allocations in the incident command structure is the triage officer; this person is in charge of the overall triage process and may have teams working under their command, depending on the size of the major incident. The triage officer's job is only to assign the casualty to the correct triage category, not to institute treatment. Any suitably trained health worker can perform effective triage. Triage is a dynamic process and needs to be repeated; at a minimum, this should be in the bronze area, and at the casualty clearing station.

Triage systems

There are numerous triage systems in use internationally, confirming that there is currently no gold-standard system. One of the reasons is due to the lack of robust research into triage systems and the difficulty of performing randomised control studies during major incidents. It is also unclear as to which system results in the best utilisation of available resources or which system results in the optimum outcome. Most international triage methods are based on consensus opinion. Currently, no specific recommendation based on strong evidence can be made to support any one triage system over another.

Despite the numerous systems in use, they all have similar outcomes – they all attempt to designate patients into colour categories depending on certain criteria. Almost all systems initially separate the walking wounded from the rest of the casualty cohort. These patients are typically designated the colour *green* (*Priority 3*). *Yellow* patients, also referred to as *Priority 2*, are considered urgent and need treatment within 2–4 hours. *Red* patients (*Priority 1*) represent the group of patients that have a direct threat to life which must be immediately corrected. Dead patients are triaged as dead and dealt with appropriately. A final category, which may be used in extreme circumstances, is the 'expectant' category (*Priority 4*); these patients are not expected to survive, even if they are the only patients injured. In a major incident, dedicating resources to their care may compromise the care of others who have a higher likelihood of survival. The abbreviations P1, P2, P3 and P4 are used to denote these treatment categories.

The most common triage system followed in South Africa is the Triage Sieve/Sort system, as taught in the MIMMS course. The Triage Sieve is used as the primary triage tool on the scene. It was developed to be rapid and reproducible, and has been shown to be easy to use and reasonably accurate.

TRIAGE SIEVE

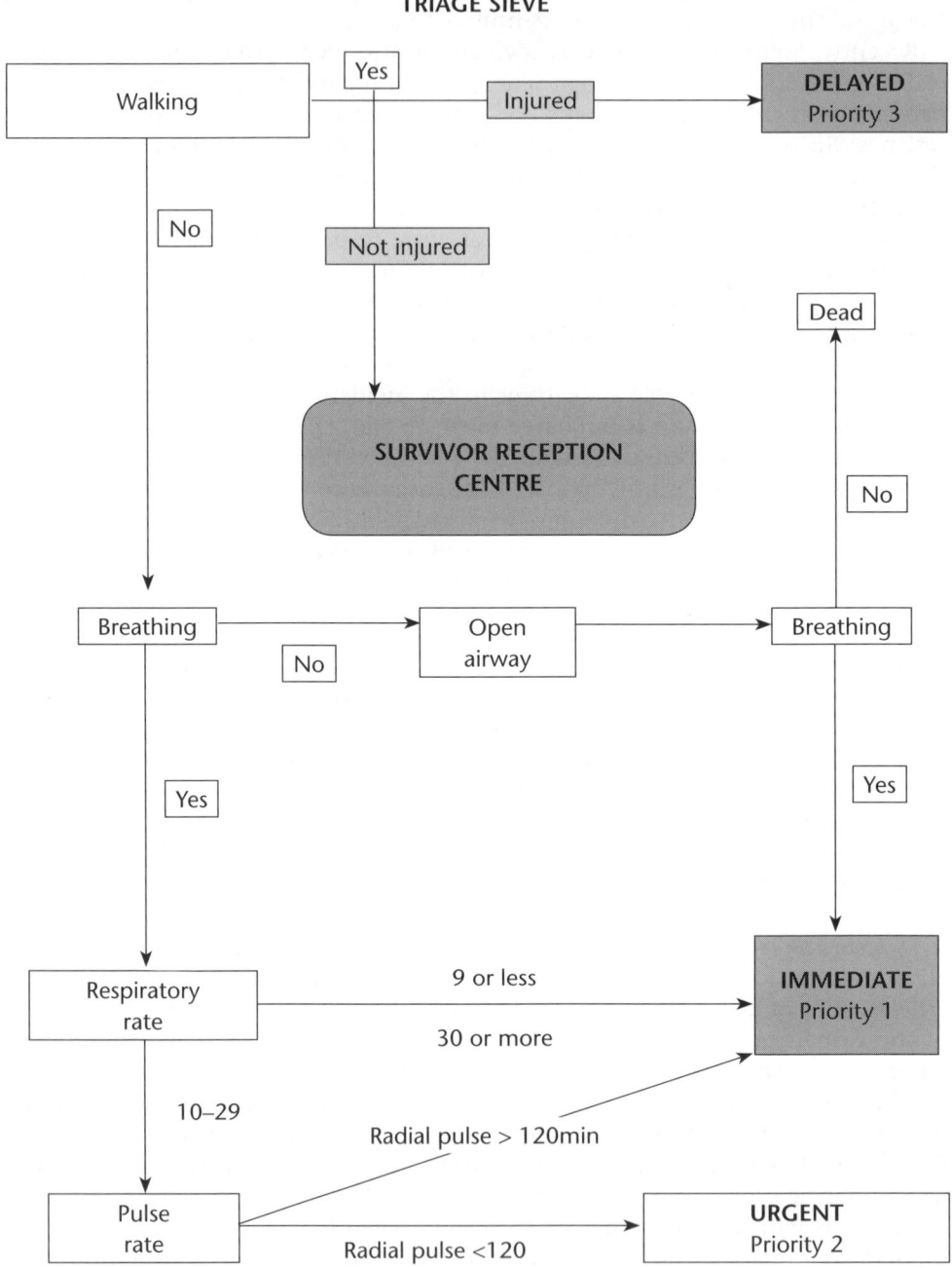

Capillary refill test (CRT) is an alternative to pulse rate, but is unreliable in the cold or dark: if it is used, a CRT of > 2 seconds indicates **PRIORITY 1**.

Figure 2.1: Triage Sieve

The Triage Sieve system uses adult parameters, and if applied to children can result in over-triage of these patients. The Paediatric Triage Tape was developed using different values for these parameter algorithms for children aged 1–10 years. This tape is laid out next to the child; where the child's heel touches the tape will be the corresponding algorithm for that child. If the child is walking (or the infant is alert and moving all four limbs), the child is considered to be Priority 3.

Other primary triage tools include JumpSTART (a physiological triage system for use on children below 8 years based on the START system) and Careflight (also based on physiology).

Secondary triage occurs at the casualty clearing station. As a complement to the Triage Sieve, the Triage Sort is in use in South Africa. It is based on the physiologic components of the Triage Revised Trauma Score (TRTS), and adds anatomical information to upgrade the triage category as needed. The parameters needed to calculate this score include the Glasgow Coma Scale, systolic blood pressure and respiratory rate.

STEP 1: Calculate the GLASGOW COMA SCORE (GCS)

1. Eye opening:		2. Verbal response:		3. Motor response:	
Spontaneous	4	Orientated	5	Obeys commands	6
To voice	3	Confused	4	Localises	5
To pain	2	Inappropriate	3	Pain withdraws	4
None	1	Incomprehensible	2	Pain flexes	3
		No response	1	Pain extends	2
				No response	1

GCS = A + B + C

STEP 2: Calculate the TRIAGE SORT SCORE

X GCS			Y Respiratory rate			Z Systolic BP	
13–15	4		10–29	4		≥ 90	4
9–12	3		≥ 30	3		76–89	3
6–8	2	+	6–9	2	+	50–75	2
4–5	1		1–5	1		1–49	1
3	0		0	0		0	0

TRIAGE SORT SCORE = X + Y + Z

STEP 3: Assign a triage PRIORITY

12	=	**PRIORITY 3**
11	=	**PRIORITY 2**
≤10	=	**PRIORITY 1**

STEP 4: Upgrade PRIORITY at discretion of senior clinician, dependent on the anatomical injury/working diagnosis.

Figure 2.2: Triage Sort

If using START/JumpSTART, secondary triage may be done with the Secondary Assessment of Victim Endpoint (SAVE) triage system. Careflight is a system that can be used for both primary and secondary triage.

Triage labelling

There are certain concepts about triage labelling that are important. These include: the label must be highly visible under most conditions; the different triage categories must be displayed (including colours, letters and words); the label must be securely attached to the patient; and the label must allow for a change of triage category if the patient's condition changes. The material used for the label must be durable and waterproof and ideally should have a space for clinical notes, and each label should have a unique number.

Triage training

Training must emphasise the assessment and methodology of the triage system, as well as provide practical application of the information. Each provider should be taught to implement the triage system in a real-life situation, as this will ensure a successful mass-casualty management system. Training should also be provided to any individuals who may interact with fire and EMS personnel while managing the mass-casualty incident. Police and traffic officers, dispatchers, nurses, doctors, forensic pathologists and others who may interact with the scene, as well as the first responders should have a basic understanding of the triage system. This ensures effective communication and interaction among all individuals involved in the mitigation of the incident.

Summary

Triage remains one of the fundamental steps in the coordinated response to a major incident, and if performed correctly will result in a decreased overall morbidity and mortality. Regardless of the type of major incident, triage can be difficult to perform due to prevailing conditions (terrain, environment or type of casualties – for example, major incidents involving a large number of children) but it also has a significant emotive and ethical component which must not be underestimated.

2.8 Treatment

Treatment of victims involved in any major incident remains a significant, immediate and important priority. This is often the single most important outcome factor, and usually provides and determines the most important 'value' placed on the incident outcome. The loss of life and injury statistics are regarded, and reported, as defining outcome parameters, and are often more important than the damage to the buildings or, indeed, the costs thereof. Although the outcome is affected by many other equally important parameters, medical treatment remains the most important determinant of favourable patient outcome.

Initially, the scene of any incident will be chaotic. This is inevitable, but should progress through a number of defined phases, with increasing organisation and intensity. This approach will allow the aim of doing the most for the most. There are always factors such as human emotion, medico-legal issues and moral and ethical challenges to be considered as the phases of medical care unfold.

Medical treatment is best considered in a number of clearly determined, planned phases. These phases are outined in the following sections.

Early spontaneous treatment

The early rendering of care in any major incident situation will be done by others in the same situation, either less severely injured or coincidentally medically experienced. Bystanders who are caught up in the incident, but not involved or injured, often provide early attention and care in the form of first aid and possibly basic life support, as do the early search and rescue teams. Information about the need for treatment is also obtained in this early phase. The arrival of the search and rescue teams heralds the next phase of care.

Early coordinated contact and treatment

This early treatment phase, while significant, addresses the needs of very few, and is mainly important in terms of information gathering from the scene. It can provide valuable planning insight for the medical component of command and control structures in determining early needs. This information will help to modify the early METHANE report relayed to emergency services, emergency centres and hospitals. This action allows for better planning of medical needs in terms of resources and service requirements, and facilitates appropriate treatment and care plans.

Among the first responders will be fire and police officers, who, if trained in the basics of medical care provision, are often in a forward position and able to do Triage Sieve, basic evaluation and life-saving first-aid interventions required on the scene. Although the intention of sieve is not to treat, but to determine who needs treatment, some basic care will always be rendered (even if deferred). This defines the beginning of the emergency treatment phase, and is best considered as early (on scene) and late (in the casualty clearing station, or CCS).

The emergency treatment phase

The ambulance service has the overall responsibility to treat, but will only be allowed on the scene once it has been declared safe. Their responsibility is to organise the order of treatment by conducting triage, ensuring life-saving basic life support, and coordinating the orderly, safe evacuation of the victims to the designated treatment area (casualty clearing station) that has been established, beyond the bronze area cordon (inner cordon). Occasionally, where there is entrapment of survivors, or more immediate and specific specialist type care is required on scene (e.g. amputation is required to free a victim and general anaesthetic is needed), highly skilled teams may be required in this early phase, but this is exceptional.

The late emergency treatment phase

The casualty clearing station usually performs the late emergency treatment phase which is characterised by the stabilisation and treatment of patients by detailed assessment and the commencement of definitive care procedures in preparation for safe evacuation. The establishment of the casualty clearing station is a responsibility requiring careful planning. It must be set up out of harm's way, but close enough to the scene to allow ready access, and it needs to be close to access and egress routes for ambulances and other transport vehicles, to allow for orderly and organised loading and transport of the injured to hospitals for definitive care.

In the casualty clearing station, treatment priorities are determined, and victims are exposed to specific advanced life support interventions or appropriate treatment interventions, by specially tasked and trained emergency medicine providers – doctors, nurses and paramedics. The clearing station requires a great deal of organisation and communication, in preparation for the next phase of care – transport to the nearest, most appropriate facility for definitive care.

The medical staff in the CCS comprises an officer in charge, a secondary triage officer (or two) and a number of treatment teams with specific designation instructions – P1 or P2, and P3. It may not be feasible or desirable to have the P3 survivors in the same general area, unless there is a large amount of space or enough personnel to address everyone's needs. In many instances, it might be more logical to bypass the CCS with the P3 victims, and arrange transport directly to the nearest appropriate P3 treatment facility. Where the remoteness of the incident means that there are scarce resources and facilities, it might be an option to get the P3 patients to the hospital, and have them cleared and sorted before the P1s and P2s arrive for more demanding care. All these decisions need to be taken in consultation with the medical command and control structures.

Priorities in the Red or P1 zone would include advanced airway protection and stabilisation, intubation and chest decompression, pain control and volume resuscitation. Splinting of fractures and the stabilisation of the cervical spine (and the rest of the spine) would be done in order to allow for safe transport to the hospital, where X-rays and definitive care and admission will be carried out. Environmental exposure issues would be addressed here too, prior to transport.

The layout of the casualty clearing station should delineate areas where priority cases are dealt with accordingly, and these areas need appropriate resource supply. Logistics back-up is therefore essential, and these needs are communicated back to the command centre (silver command). Logistics resupply in remote areas may be a significant challenge, and delays may even be seen to be affecting care and therefore outcome. Decisions would need to be made by command structures regarding these issues.

The duration of the incident will also require that the staff are able to be relieved for comfort and nutrition/rehydration breaks. This again requires coordination and resources, and in remote areas the local populace will often provide valuable assistance in this regard.

Early information that is reliable and appropriate will allow the major incident to be declared, and hospital planning can then proceed to ensure that resources both medical – staff, beds, theatres and supplies – and non-medical are made available. In order to ensure that the best outcomes are achieved, it is imperative that there is a seamless step-up in the level of care as the patient passes from one phase of treatment to the next – from the scene to the casualty clearing station to the hospital.

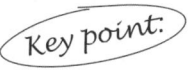 **Treatment provided at scene will vary from life-saving first aid to advanced medical interventions, depending upon the resources available at scene.**

2.9 Transport

Transportation is the final major component of medical support in a major incident. It is a critical component, and poses major challenges for the medical command, especially when the incident is of a large nature or is in a remote area far from hospital back-up and support. Furthermore, triage and treatment decisions play a significant role in determining appropriate transport. Hence, a transport officer should be appointed to assist both silver command and the casualty clearing station with the function of organising and coordinating transport.

The location and maturity of the service also plays a role in determining what resources are available, but, generally speaking, most medical transportation vehicles will be able to be upgraded to provide advanced life support (ALS) type care fairly easily – whether by placing appropriate personnel with equipment on the vehicles, or by supplying the basics needed for safe transportation – under prevailing circumstances.

Transport is best considered in two stages: that which moves patients from the incident zone to the CCS, and that which moves the patient to definitive care.

Transportation at the scene is usually done by manual stretcher-bearers, as the terrain may not allow for transport vehicles of any substantial size. However, golf cart-sized response vehicles might be able to be used very effectively to transport severely injured patients from the scene to the casualty clearing station. The recruitment of stretcher-bearers requires a great deal of cooperation between the services, and traditionally, once the scene safety issues and contamination have been resolved, the fire services personnel and some of the police and traffic personnel might be well placed to assist with the manual ferrying of the triaged cases to the casualty clearing station. This is usually arranged through the command and control structures where all services are represented, and where such decisions can be made and enforced centrally and jointly.

Transport from the scene, however, requires a great deal of forethought and planning, and must be carefully coordinated in order to achieve the goal of getting the correct-priority patient, with the correct category of transport, in the appropriate time, to the appropriate treatment destination.

The scene of a major incident is usually congested, and in many instances the roads to and from the scene are blocked by curious onlookers or concerned bystanders and families. The traffic department needs to be cognisant of this and ensure that the outer cordon is effective and promotes a clear unidirectional flow of emergency vehicles into and out of the cordon. The movement of vehicles into the area should ensure that the vehicles are parked and manned, ready to be loaded and despatched according to need. Ideally these vehicles should be 'recycled' (cleaned and rapidly restocked) at the receiving facility, and returned to the queue of waiting transport vehicles ready to receive load instructions. It is also possible then for these available crews to be allowed to refresh before being tasked again with another load.

In major incidents, it is critical for best outcome to ensure that appropriate levels of care are upheld, once P1 patients are identified and stabilised. This implies that the transport vehicle and crew need to be designated appropriately, and hence the sooner the triage assessments are done, the sooner the command can determine the number and type of vehicles to be made available. It is therefore crucial that all patients and their triage codes are relayed to a central command and control point, in order that resources are appropriately utilised.

There may be a number of voluntary or private ambulances available, and many such organisations may have a number of medically intended patient-transporter-type vehicles.

In addition, bus companies are often able to assist by loading a large number of walking wounded survivors, and this mode can be used very efficiently and safely by placing a trained medical person on the vehicle for the duration of the trip to the receiving facility. This option requires a great deal of coordination and pre-planning, as the resources may not be readily available on standby unless specifically arranged.

Receiving facilities must be warned, and must be prepared to receive a large number of patients all at once to avoid moving chaos and congestion from the scene to the hospital or receiving facility. If there is an outpatient-type facility, this will cater more appropriately for the load, while a single-entrance emergency centre with a few stretchers would not cope well.

It is the responsibility of the health services command to determine which facilities are to be used as receiving hospitals, and how many patients of each triage category can be accommodated at these facilities. Patients requiring specialist care services like neurosurgery, and burn cases, can be sent, after arrangement, to super-specialised facilities straight from the CCS.

The determination of the destination facility for the respective triage-category patients is the final aspect of transportation decision-making that needs to be considered. While triage and treatment needs are important, the preparation for transport needs to be complete. Non-critical treatment should not delay transport, but, equally so, all patients transported must be packaged and prepared correctly.

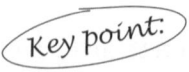 **Transport logistics, both at the scene and from the scene, require extensive coordination and prior planning.**

2.10 Equipment

Major incidents can affect communities in many ways, from destruction of transport and communication infrastructure to loss of personal property and protection, and may even overwhelm the capacity of the medical and health systems to provide assistance and support.

The type and amount of medical equipment and pharmaceuticals required for any major incident response will be determined by the nature, type, location and size of the incident itself. As an example, the medical supplies and equipment used to address incidents involving military forces would differ from those needed to respond to a natural disaster, although many crossover synergies exist.

Incidents can be classified in many different ways as either natural or man-made, and can be considered in terms of size. Pre-planning with scenario training creates awareness and insight into major incidents, and assists with preparation in order to be able to respond effectively. Equipment pre-planning is paramount to effective response in the time of major incident need.

During the planning phase for any major incident, recognition should be given to the fact that in natural disasters (flooding etc.) it takes considerable time to mobilise resources and move them from stores and depots to the scene. This might be from several hours to a day or so, whereas international aid, when required, could take several days.

Equipment and supplies that are essential to response capacity can be divided into several categories:

- Direction, command and control;
- Communications;
- Mass care survival;
- Health and medical supplies;
- Medical logistics and occupational health supplies – which includes *personal equipment*, with the emphasis on safety (PPE) and operational efficiency, and *medical supplies*, with the focus on medications, medical equipment and supplies that are necessary for direct patient care. This should include provisions for maintaining primary care services, including pharmaceutical needs.

Determining the quantity of supplies and equipment needed will depend on a number of factors:

- The specific threat or disaster – for example, war versus radiation contamination;
- Availability of medical services and medical assets in the community/region/ country;
- Extent of disruption of the health services (and the stature of thoses services to begin with);
- Number and severity of live patients;
- Time to recovery phase of the incident.

There are multiple sources for clinical recommendations with regard to treatment of casualties of events involving CBRN (chemical, biological, radiation and nuclear). Recommendations regarding PPE support the use of level C personal protection (splash suits, gloves, boots and masks). Pre-hospital-care clothing must provide safety, with comfort and durability, and should be functional in all climates and terrains. While it is possible to have different clothing needs on a single scene – rain-resistant in the bronze zone, while indoors in the CCS there might be no need to have rainproof suits – there will always be a standard that must be upheld to ensure the protection of self, and scene, then survivors.

All staff despatched to a scene should therefore check in with the designated safety officer before being deployed in the field. An 'all hazards' approach is the safest option, and therefore all vulnerable body areas need a protective clothing solution – from jackets and hard hats to ear/eye protection and gloves and boots. All of these issues can be provided well in advance in any system planning for major incidents. Allowing for appropriate staff to take personal responsibility for their PPE ensures that response and activation times will be kept to a minimum. Once basic protection is provided, over-vests can be used to designate role and responsibility, a feature needed for proper command and control. Additional items are added to the list as part of PPE during major incidents; these include appropriate personal and professional identification, communication and reporting equipment, and loose change for necessary sustenance until organisation prevails and logistics are available on scene.

Incident command will require equipment for the effective running and management of the scene. This includes radios, phones, maps, triage cards and note pads. A source of electricity generation and a light source are essential, too. Mostly this equipment is kept together in an incident response vehicle or trailer, and should be serviced and checked regularly to prevent breakdown at critical times. Since the practised *modus operandi* in a major incident is to have an established CCS, some form of portable makeshift protective structure should be part of the equipment armamentarium. The size of the structure will determine the expectation of treatment volumes, and may assist with patient flow, until a more suitable structure is available – such as a school hall or similar.

Medical equipment is crucial right from the initial response to a major incident, and should be organised in advance in preparation. It is best considered in a functional, logical and organised way: from the initial response, through primary triage, and BLS (basic life support), with scene removal, to secondary triage and CCS stabilisation and ALS treatment, on to early definitive care. This equipment should be stored securely and accessibly, with a detailed legacy of use and an inventory for resupply – item for item, together with source knowledge. It is important that the scene and local hospital supply are not one and the same, as the simultaneous use of this equipment is usually the norm rather than the exception. Most trained providers will have their own appropriate level-response bags, with the necessary BLS and ALS equipment, but may only be able to treat a few patients from one bag. This essential replenishment therefore is required early on in the incident, at the scene, and should be ready as the need arises. Clearly it would do no good to identify P1 cases and then fail to treat them appropriately because of a lack of equipment and resources. This requires careful preparation and planning, and can be practised in regular exercises.

The set-up and supply of the CCS is akin to the field hospital/emergency centre, and should be set up as such. Thus, it will contain all the ALS equipment, beds, lights and 'light' surgical instruments, as well as a comprehensive pharmaceutical supply for resuscitation, essential emergency drugs and appropriate associated equipment (such as ECG monitors).

The transport of patients to hospitals sees them leaving with essential equipment items, particularly immobilisation and stabilisation items, and hence equipment resupply here is also required timeously to ensure that undesirable time delays do not occur.

Incidents, particularly those in remote areas or akin to disasters, may be protracted, and providers will not only need to look after the needs of the victims, but tend to the needs of the community too. This is part of a much larger consideration, but will include a pharmaceutical supply that covers vaccines and emergency antibiotics, and should include primary-health-type medications for symptom management as well as chronic disease control. A reliable source for medical and pharmaceutical needs is the WHO's 'New Emergency Health Kit'.

It is of critical importance that in-depth review takes place throughout the incident to reassess the true needs as the incident unfolds. This will enable resources to be forthcoming as they are required, and in the appropriate incremental amounts.

Resources are required that most immediately address critical medical needs of the affected victims. Water, food, shelter and equipment are needed next. Effective resource management requires several basic actions:

- Determining specific resources and amounts;
- Procuring the resources;
- Preparing and securing a storage facility for the resources;
- Preparing to receive the medical and operational equipment;
- Identifying a means to transport and distribute the resources where and when they are needed;
- Finding locations from which, and personnel, to dispense medication and medical equipment.

2.11   Training

Major incidents pose a very real threat to every individual. One way to mitigate the threat of disaster is through preparedness. This was a lesson learned the hard way in the 9/11 disaster, and is repeated time after time when major incidents strike.

Preparedness involves individuals, groups, systems and communities. The community in general often bears the brunt of any incident, and relies on the emergency services at large to be prepared and to have a plan.

Despite having an overarching plan, many operatives rarely get the chance to use the plan, and often lose interest in the challenge of planning. This can be averted by a focus on training and practical exercises around aspects of the plan.

Why do we need to train and exercise?

The reasons for training and exercises, and appreciation of the real benefits of being prepared, are best summarised as follows:

- Reduction of fear, anxiety, panic and losses that often accompany major incidents. Knowing what to do when faced with incidents, with regard to basic medical and survival needs and shelter, goes a long way towards improving overall outcome.
- Improved risk awareness and knowledge of how to reduce the impact of a major incident.

It is vital however, that major incident planning remains a priority, and that interest and commitment is maintained through regular planning exercises, taking numerous forms, and involving different groups of people.

It is just as important to focus on the community who are exposed, or at risk, as it is to reflect on the issues that face the operations team. Functional exercises represent an important link between disaster planning and disaster response. Exercises need to be performed, but must be evaluated in order to make them meaningful.

In the pre-hospital environment, the daily routine keeps the professional and the planner focused on the practical tasks at hand, and prepares the emergency services for more of the same controlled volume and circumstance. However, this practice never really tests the responses of individuals, communities or systems to overwhelming volume or circumstance. As simulated exercises are expensive and time-consuming to run, with dubious long- or short-term benefit, it is important to provide a parallel training medium to test parts of the readiness under differing circumstances.

Components that need testing

These parts are best considered as:

- *Basic preparedness:* this focuses on individuals and communities, looking at personal equipment and knowledge readiness, as well as supplies and communications systems, and anything else that makes for better management practices and recovery. This can be supported by regular tabletop exercises and live drills where appropriate.
- *Hazards identification – natural and technological.* A hazards assessment should always be performed as part of preparedness and training, to identify potential disasters in a community (e.g. large mining town disaster, nuclear power station disaster etc.) and to assess the capacity and ability of the local services to cope with a potential incident.
- *Terrain considerations and political/social issues* – potential targets and areas where issues are likely to be 'aired' through terrorist activity or strike action.
- *Clinical activation* of an incident and the process that needs to be followed, including the acquisition and movement of logistics.
- *Recovering from disasters:* this should always focus on seeking help and assistance with coping, returning to normality, assisting others and health and safety issues.

2.12 Resources

Firefighting Resources of California Organized for Potential Emergencies (FIRESCOPE). Available at www.firescope.org. (Useful to understand the reasons and process that led to the development of the ICS.)

International Search and Rescue Advisory Group (INSARAG). *Guidelines and methodology manual.* Available at www.usar.nl.upload/docs/insarag_guidelines_july_2006.pdf. (A comprehensive guideline for international rescue and relief work.)

Major incident medical management and support. 2nd edition, BMJ Books, 2002.

Ciottone GR (ed.) *Disaster medicine*, 3rd edition, Philadelphia: Mosby Elsevier, 2006.

2.13 References

1. Advanced Life Support Group. *Major incident medical management and support.* London: BMJ Books; 2002.
2. Bigley GA, Roberts KH. The Incident Command System: high reliability organizing for complex and volatile task environments. *Academy of Management Journal* 2001;44:1281–1300.
3. Briggs SM. Regional interoperability: making systems connect in complex disasters. *Journal of Trauma* 2009;67:S88–S90.
4. Buck DA, Trainor JE, Aguirre BE. A critical evaluation of the Incident Command System and NIMS. *Journal of Homeland Security and Emergency Management* 2006;3(3).
5. Chan TC, Killeen J, Griswold W, Lenert L. Information technology and emergency medical care during disasters. *Academic Emergency Medicine* 2004;11(11):1229–36.
6. FIRESCOPE (Firefighting Resources of California Organized for Potential Emergencies). Available from: www.firescope.org.
7. Global Disaster Alert and Coordination System. Available from: ocha.unog.ch/virtualosocc.
8. Howitt AM, Leonard HB. A command system for all agencies? *Crisis/Response* 2005;1(2):40–3.
9. Lindell MK; Perry RW, Prater CS. Organizing response to disasters with the Incident Command System/Incident Management System (ICS/IMS). International Workshop on Emergency Response and Rescue 2005.
10. Moynihan DP. From intercrisis to intracrisis learning, *Journal of Contingencies and Crisis Management* 2009;17(3):189–98.
11. Stumpf J. Incident Command System: the history and need. *The Internet Journal of Rescue and Disaster Medicine* 2000;2(1).
12. United Nations. UN General Assembly Resolution 57/150, 16 December 2002. Strengthening the effectiveness and coordination of international urban search and rescue assistance. Available from: www.ifrc.org/Docs/idrl/I238EN.pdf.
13. Minnie J. Managing disasters with standard business tools and software. *ESSA/Occupational Risk* 2009;1(7):8–13
14. Fick P. Emergency contact centres: where inefficiency can cost lives. *ESSA/Occupational Risk* 2009;1(7):17–18
15. Communication control systems vs. PABX's/ACD's. *ESSA/Occupational Risk* 2009;1(8):12–14
16. Advanced Life Support Group. *Major incident medical management and support: the practical approach at the scene (MIMMS).* 2nd edition. London: BMJ Books; 2002.
17. Hodgetts TJ, Brett A. Chapter 47. Major incidents. In: Greaves I, Porter K. *Pre-hospital medicine.* London: Arnold; 1999. pp. 557–67
18. International rules for radio communications. Available from: www.howtodothings.com/electronics/how-to-use-radio-communication-procedures. Accessed 29 June 2010.
19. Republic of South Africa. Telecommunications Act 13 of 2000. Pretoria: Government Printer; 2000.

20. Public safety wireless network. Comparison of conventional and trunked systems. May 1999. US Dept of Homeland Security, Washington, DC.
21. Mustard T, Blakemore J. Site communications. Hand signals for emergency scenes. Available from: www.elcosh.org/en/document/422/d000413/site-communications.html. Accessed 30 June 2010. Stevens Publishing; 2000.
22. Emergency Medicine Society of South Africa. Practice guidelines, number 3/2008. Major Incident Management System. Priorities, communications and triage.
23. Hardcastle TC. Heat exhaustion and heat stroke: when Hot is NOT. Emergency Services SA/*Occupational Risk* 2010;1(9):6–7
24. Advanced Life Support Group. *Major incident medical management and support: the practical approach at the scene (MIMMS)*. 2nd edition. London: BMJ Books; 2002.
25. Stoy WA, Centre for Emergency Medicine. Chapter 32. Special response situations. *Mosby's EMT-Basic textbook*, Mosby Yearbook, St. Louis, MO; 1996.
26. FEMA. Emergency incident rehabilitation. FA114, July 1992. US Fire Administration 0-B-06-005, June 2006, Washington, DC.
27. US Enviromental Protection Agency. *Excessive heat events guidebook*. EPA 430-B-06-005, June 2006, Washington, DC.
28. Weekes R. Chapter 21: Scene approach, assessment and safety. In: Greaves I, Porter K. *Pre-hospital medicine*. London: Arnold; 1999.
29. Bates, D. Safety at major incidents, part 1. Available from: www.homeland1.com/homeland-security-products/bio-agent-identification-monitoring/articles/403921-safety-at-major-incidents-part-1/. Accessed 29 June 2010.
30. EPA. PPE Classification. Available from: www.ehso.com/OSHA_PPE_EPA_Levels.htm#. Accessed 29 June 2010.
31. Guidelines for rescue training. *Prehospital and Disaster Medicine* 1993; 8(2):151–6.
32. Wallis LA *et al*. The Cape triage score: a new triage system for South Africa. Proposal from the Cape Triage Group. *Emergency Medicine Journal* 2006; 23:149–153.
33. Kennedy K, Aghababian R, Gans L, *et al*. Triage: techniques and applications in decision making. *Annals of Emergency Medicine* 1996; 28:136–144.
34. Garner A, Lee A, Harrison K, *et al*. Comparative analysis of multiple-casualty incident triage algorithms. *Annals of Emergency Medicine* 2001; 38(5):541–8.
35. Hines S, Payne A, Edmondson J, Heightman AJ. Bombs under London. The EMS response plan that worked. *Journal of Emergency Medical Services* 2005; 30(8):58–60, 62, 64–7.
36. Wallis LA, Carley S. Validation of the paediatric triage tape. *Emergency Medicine Journal* 2006;23(1):47–50.
37. Hodgetts TJ, Hall J, Maconochie I, *et al*. Paediatric triage tape. *Pre-Hospital Immediate Care* 1998; 2:155–9.
38. Romig LE. Pediatric triage. A system to JumpSTART your triage of young patients at MCIs. *Journal of Emergency Medical Services* 2002; 27(7):52–8, 60–3.
39. Sacco WJ, Navin DM, Fiedler KE, *et al*. Precise formulation and evidence-based application of resource-constrained triage. *Academic Emergency Medicine* 2005; 12(8):759–70.

40. Gebhart ME, Pence R. START triage: does it work? *Disaster Management and Response* July–Sept 2007; 5(3):68–73.
41. Asaeda G. The day that the START triage system came to a STOP: observations from theWorld Trade Center disaster. *Academic Emergency Medicine* 2002; 9(3):255–6.
42. Cook L. The World Trade Center attack. The paramedicresponse: an insider's view. *Critical Care (London)*. 2001; 5(6):301–3.
43. Teague DC. Mass casualties in the Oklahoma City bombing. *Clinical Orthopedics and Related Research* 2004; (422):77–81.
44. Schultz CH, Koenig KL, Noji EK. A medical disaster response to reduce immediate mortality after an earthquake. *New England Journal of Medicine* 1996; 334(7):438–44.
45. Benson M, Koenig KL, Schultz CH. Disaster triage: START, then SAVE – a new method of dynamic triage for victims of a catastrophic earthquake. *Prehospital and Disaster Medicine* 1996; 11(2):117–24.
46. Hodgetts TJ. Triage: a position statement. Available from: ec.europa.eu/ environment/civil/prote/pdfdocs/disaster_med_final_2002/d6.pdf. Accessed 24 June 2010.
47. Nocera A, Garner A. An Australian mass casualty incident triage system for the future based upon triage mistakes of the past: the Homebush Triage Standard. *Australia New Zealand Journal of Surgery* 1999; 69(8):603–8.
48. Centers for Disease Control and Prevention. SALT Triage. For: Terrorism Injuries Information, Dissemination, and Exchange Project. Atlanta, GA; 22 September 2007.
49. Romig LE. Pediatric triage. A system to JumpSTART your triage of young patients at MCIs. *Journal of Emergency Medical Services* 2002; 27(7):52–8, 60–3.
50. Veatch RM. Disaster preparedness and triage: justice and the common good. *Mount Sinai Journal of Medicine* July 2005; 72(4):236–41
51. Bogucki S, Jubanyik K. Triage, rationing and palliative care in disaster planning. *Biosecurity and Bioterrorism* June 2009; 7(2):221–4

3

Major Incident Management in the Hospital Environment

*T Ligthelm, J Augustyn, P Brysiewicz, J Goosen, S Hattingh
and M Toubkin*

Objectives

By the end of this chapter, the reader will be able to:

- compile an executable major incident plan for a hospital;
- effectively command a hospital in a major incident;
- know how to maintain efficient communication during a major incident;
- know how to ensure safety within a hospital during a major incident;
- execute surgical triage to prioritise surgical intervention;
- understand optimal utilisation of scarce resources such as ventilators in a major incident;
- know how to provide best possible definitive care within a hospital in a major incident, including:
    - establishing an efficient management hierarchy;
    - utilising job cards to enhance operational activities;
    - allocating staff judiciously to execute activities;
- successfully identify, discharge and reunite victims with next-of-kin following a major incident;
- identify the essential hospital equipment required for a major incident;
- understand how to prepare and maintain operational-ready staff members to manage a major incident well through comprehensive training and exercises;
- evaluate hospital readiness for major incidents on a regular basis.

3.1 Introduction

Healthcare facilities are generally perceived to be safe areas where optimal care is provided and patients are accommodated in a supportive optimal care environment. However, this idealistic scenario can be easily disrupted by various situations, such as fire, extreme weather conditions or transport-related incidents such as a plane crash, necessitating emergency measures to receive large numbers of injured or sick patients requiring drastic measures to save lives.

It is essential that healthcare facilities plan to function optimally in extreme situations with large numbers of casualties, requiring extraordinary measures to save as many lives as possible. These plans must be developed and tested with the participation of as many staff members as possible to ensure that everyone is acquainted with the essential elements of the plan. These plans should also be an integral plan of the chief executive's management plans.

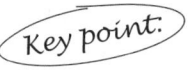 **Hospitals must plan and practise to manage major incidents effectively.**

3.2 Planning

Planning for major incidents includes coordinating which areas of the facility will be utilised, aligning all the appropriate resources to address the incident, and coordinating the functions through effective command to ensure that the hospital functions optimally. During major incidents, difficulties mostly arise from failure to coordinate resources, not a lack of resources.

A written, detailed Major Incident Plan is, however, not the same as being prepared – only practice makes perfect. Therefore the effectiveness of the planning needs to be assessed regularly to ensure readiness. Reviewing a bad weekend is perhaps worth as much as practising an artificial scenario.

Area allocation

No hospital is designed to manage major incidents. Internally, any or all of the human resources, equipment or infrastructure may be compromised during a major incident (e.g. strikes of healthcare personnel, power supply failure, fire etc.). Externally, extraordinary measures often need to be taken to deal with the numbers, complexity or type of patients presenting as a result of the incident. This all requires detailed and comprehensive planning to enable a healthcare facility to be ready to manage a major incident.

Globally, common problem areas identified in managing major incidents by hospitals include communication and power failures, water shortage and contamination, physical damage, hazardous material exposure, unorganised evacuations and resource allocation shortages. To deal with these situations, a hospital has to rapidly expand and reorganise its capabilities to meet the requirements of the situation. At present, there is little evidence on how to plan for these expansions – only frameworks and experience. Analysing local experience may be of value and more productive.

Area allocations are inseparably linked to staffing, equipment and infrastructure. The term 'surge' deals with the expansion measures to accommodate a sudden influx of patients.

- *Surge capacity* reflects the ability of a healthcare system's ability to rapidly expand normal services to meet the increased demand for qualified personnel, medical care and public health, in the event of a major incident.

- *Facility-based surge capacity* refers to the actions taken at the healthcare facility that allow for the augmentation of services within the structure of the facility.
- *Area allocation* refers to all the activities performed to rapidly provide added space, staffed and equipped to deal with patient requirements, to the best possible degree, and to receive and allocate those mobilised to deal with the threat, so that the transition from normal to extraordinary activities proceed to the best benefit of patients in hospital, and those presenting.

The hospital needs to plan where it proposes to receive patients and expand to (decanting, reserve space), with whom (personnel), how (operational plan), with what (resources) and when (time). Before mobilising reserve space, existing facilities need to be utilised optimally, since these are equipped, staffed and trained to deal with a rapid increase in workload.

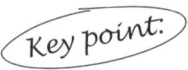 **To reach surge capacity, hospitals must identify which areas will be utilised to address which functions.**

Creating space: decanting

Decanting is the process whereby suitable patients are moved to lower levels of care appropriate to the situation to clear space for new casualties. In constrained health systems, slang terms such as 'finding beds', 'clearing casualty' or 'finding movers' describe the activities encompassed in the term 'surge'. These informal systems need to be recognised and refined, as they are usually successful in creating capacity.

The best area in which to manage major incidents is the existing emergency centre: it is familiar, equipped and purpose-designed. Clearing this area for new (decanting) and potentially unstable patients and utilising alternative space for minor patients is hugely valuable in managing space.

Typically, 10% to 20% of a hospital's operating bed capacity can be mobilised within a few hours using strategies including expedited disposition of patients, clearing the emergency centre of ambulatory patients, transferring patient to other facilities and other alternative measures. Up to an additional 10% of bed capacity can be mobilised by converting the hospital's existing 'flat space' (such as hallways, lobbies and conference rooms) into emergency bed space.

Principles of decanting

The aim of decanting is to provide space and infrastructure where nursing staff can care for patients. At worst, medical practitioners can assess patients with the minimum facilities, but the nursing staff require space and equipment to render long-term care.

Time to decant patients is essential to successfully managing major incidents. Expanded roles need to be practised regularly. Practising these roles during normal workloads expands skills and tests systems.

All activities of patient care need expanded space for major incidents. Each hospital area must be designated, and each must practise a routine role and an expanded role.

Unidirectional flow through the hospital speeds the care process. Every patient contact needs to be the final for that purpose (e.g. assessment, treatment, medication, pick-up and out).

Counselling and comforting uninjured survivors is much increased during major incidents, and large areas need to be allocated for this.

Obstructions to creating space

Typical obstructions to decanting patients include:

- Shortage of low-level resources, sucking in high-level resources to do the job: for example, lack of cleaners to turn around beds, lack of porters etc. All of these distract caregivers from their primary task.
- Conversion of treatment areas into storage or office space, making it impossible to revert to treatment space.
- Inefficient or unavailable inter-hospital transport during a major incident, leaving the identified patients stuck in the higher-level facilities
- Learned ignorance – an apparent inability to cope with new or expanded responsibility.

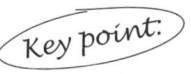 **To reach the surge capacity, decanting must be properly planned.**

Allocating space

Table 3.1 summarises the activities for which space must be allocated.

Table 3.1: Area requirements during a major incident

Action	Requirements	Possible area
Routing and Parking	Unidirectional flow One entrance, many points of dispersal Single point (control, direction)	
Traffic Control Point	Clear routing or route maps handed out Pre-prepared route markers are positioned	
Ambulance Route and Patient Route (including private vehicles carrying patients)	Clearly indicated Lead to drop-off point and triage area Additional planning may be required to address larger vehicles used in a major incidents, such as major incident buses	Existing patient routes to emergency areas

Action	Requirements	Possible area
Helicopter Route	Civil Aviation Authority requirements Additional planning may be required to accommodate large military helicopters (often mobilised in a major incident) Easy transport to triage area	Existing or an adequate size and approved space to accommodate large helicopters
Drop-off Zone Separate areas for: 1. Patients (casualties) arriving by various means of transport	Good lighting Crowd control Firm surface for austere weather conditions Access to Triage Area	Ambulance stop Parking area
2. Walking patients often arriving by mass transport such as buses	Easy walking via triage to Priority 3: Green treatment area	Entrance lobby Any area close to P3 area
3. Uninjured survivors (worried, well)	Easy walking distance Closest to reconciliation area	Administrative entrance Public visitors' entrance Visitors' area, recreation hall or large area for information
Media	Secure route to avoid media straying into sensitive areas Closest to press venue	Press liaison area, lecture room, chapel or other suitable area
Additional Staff – Hospital	Security-controlled entrance to confirm staff status	Own working area
Additional Staff – External Backup and Volunteers	Security-controlled entrance to additional staff registration venue Rapid integration Rapid orientation	Training centre, information desk, human resource management offices
Command	Space for coordination, conferences Existing and alternative communications Direct contact with emergency room, theatre, ICU, press Secure access	Existing management suites or boardroom
Tactical Command	Mobile Alternative communications	Centered in emergency centres ⮕

Action	Requirements	Possible area
Triage Area	Immediate proximity to drop-off points First patient contact with hospital Covered Space Adequate lighting and emergency lighting Same floor level as drop-off-point and Priority 1: Red treatment area Unidirectional flow	Ambulance drop-off point, entrance lobby
Priority 1 Treatment Area (Red Area)	Space Equipped to resuscitate (medical gas, suction, oxygen in all bays etc.) Advanced resuscitation equipment in all bays (airway, breathing, circulation) Pre-packed emergency trolleys to provide additional capability	Existing emergency centre (P1 and P2 areas)
Priority 2 Treatment Areas (Yellow Area)	Oxygen, suction, medical gas Equipped to assess Pre-packed mobile trolleys	Emergency centre Existing P3 areas
Priority 3 Treatment Areas (Green Area)	Oxygen Clinical assessment Minor treatment (dressings, suturing) Dressing and suture packs Emergency crash-cart for patients who may collapse (mis-triaged)	Outpatient department, physiotherapy department, patient ward if no other space available
Theatre	Existing theatres usually sufficient once elective lists cancelled	Existing theatre(s) If inadequate, consider labour wards
Radiology	Transferring patients on and off radiology tables is the single biggest delaying factor Requesting non-essential radiology shifts the major incident from the scene to the radiology department Unidirectional flow	Increase throughput by providing teams to transfer patients Essential radiology only

Action	Requirements	Possible area
Pharmacy for Priority 3 Discharged Patients	Close to Priority 3 treatment area Pre-stocked Expanded as required	Existing outpatient pharmacy or a temporary capability
Pickup Points for: Discharged Patients and Uninjured Survivors	Traffic control point Unidirectional flow Space (much expanded)	Public parking area
Reuniting, Grieving and Counselling Including Comforting and Counselling Uninjured Survivors	Vastly expanded space as holding area Privacy for counselling Basic hospitality Furnishing and comfort with adequate ablution facilities	Outpatients department, recreation hall or ancillary health departments (for example, occupational therapy)
Staff Rest and Recovery	Privacy and comfort Facility for counselling and debriefing Familiarity Basic hygiene (toilet, shower, sleep)	Staff restaurant Departmental offices/ sleepover Nurses home
Decanting	Traffic control Covered loading space Proximity to wards Away from emergency room and ambulance entrance	Service entrance/exit
Mortuary	Overflow can usually be accommo-dated for up to 24 hours in existing air-conditioning space Existing cold storage in vicinity May need to accommodate body identification capability and access to relatives	Existing Expand to use existing floor space Ensure capacity for ex-panded air-conditioning area or cooler areas such as cold storage space or cooler trucks
Major incident Storeroom	Pre-determined stock Specialist items such as triage tags and additional spine boards Provide stock to cover period from activation until standard stores can provide stock Stock rotated to prevent expiry	Emergency stock room
Priority 4 Patients	Privacy Access to family Access to counselling	Low care ward

Action	Requirements	Possible area
Pharmacy	Man and expand emergency centre dispensary Restock critical areas Re-order stock, ensure reserve maintained	Pharmacy
Communications Capability	Backup not dependent on existing land lines, mobile networks Preferably dedicated broadband	Existing switchboard Mobile radios to key personnel
Media Briefing Area (free flow of information minimises snooping) Opportunity to build positive image	Space Connectivity Lighting Audio-visual Hospitality	Lecture facility

3.3   Command

Command is a function vested in an individual, whereby that individual will plan, organise, lead and control the organisational activities through, and with, others so that the desired result is achieved.

Commanders can and must work through, and with, other people (major incident committee, command group etc.), and accountability for the outcome is never to be delegated.

Components of a hospital incident command structure include:

- *Strategic command:* managing relations with higher levels of management (e.g. provincial authorities), referred to as *gold command*;
- *Operational command:* managing the incident within the hospital, referred to as *silver command*;
- *Tactical command:* managing areas within the hospital, referred to as *bronze command*.

Planning

Planning is the work managers do to predetermine a course of action. It includes establishing guidelines for planning, risk analysis, analysis of strengths, weakness, opportunities and threats, identifying key goals, developing a plan to achieve those goals, auditing and refining the plan.

Planning is not the product of individual effort; it follows on the structured efforts of all involved, preferably a major incident committee.

Guidelines for planning

Guidelines for effective planning include the following areas:

- *Strategic needs:* the requirements of higher authority, stated in a mission statement and strategic plan for the province, region and hospital.
- *Inevitability:* major incidents are inevitable.
- *All hazards:* a stadium filled with spectators can deliver a mass of casualties due to a spectator rush, an explosion in a gas cooker, an epidemic of food poisoning or violence emanating from spectators in a tavern etc.
- *Imagine the unimaginable:* by employing an organised thinking process, the unimaginable can become the imagined, the predicted and part of the plan.
- *Bypass:* victims will bypass emergency medical services to the nearest and most familiar hospital. Plan to receive all priorities, with lowest priorities arriving first.
- *Communication:* channels of communication, if not damaged, become rapidly overloaded – and your hospital may be overlooked in the chain of communication.
- *Burnout:* staff burnout is common, particularly with constant exposure to violence in an emergency centre. Expect difficulties in finding staff during a high-risk event. At least the command group can ensure protective gear, emotional support, crèches, etc. beforehand – loyalty creates loyalty.
- *Redundancy:* expect the primary plan to fail, and build in alternatives to every component of the plan. There is no science to the predictive value of Murphy's law.
- *Standard procedures:* rely on standard procedures whenever possible. A major incident is not the time to introduce new systems of management or care. Those providing care are challenged enough doing their job, and should not have to supervise new, untrained and unskilled assistants during a major incident.
- *Records:* maintaining records is usually the first element of care to be lost during a major incident, and the last to be caught up with. Administrative systems should be simple enough to be operational at normally busy times, and in order to function during major incidents. Triage cards should be used daily.
- *Degraded services:* ensure that staff are legally protected to do the best for the most by means of protocols and guidelines providing legal cover for expanded scopes of practice and degraded standards of care. This is best achieved by establishing protocols for clinical care during major incidents, where lower levels of care are stated explicitly.

Organising

Organising is the work managers do to arrange and relate work to be done, so that it can be performed most effectively by people. Principles of organising include:

- *Structure:* strategies, plans and performance indicators do not just happen. They need to be planned and practised. A well-functioning major incident committee creates the framework.
- *Enthusiasm:* organisations harbour layers of resistance to change, whether due to fear of change, or fear of losing control. Resistance can be overcome by bypassing resistance, addressing fears and, as a last resort, by coercion. Presentations, lectures and positive feedback are powerful tools.

- *Common message:* a common message allows people to understand, adopt and practise the plan. Examples are a single system of triage, surge over weekends, measuring and improving time. Teaching and feedback create the common new language.
- *Success:* success breeds success. Analysis, feedback and correction allow opportunities to catch people doing things well, and to build confidence. Each hospital needs to develop a set of guidelines based on what worked in the past, and what should work in the future.

Leading

Leading is the work managers perform to influence people to take effective action. The terms 'command' and 'leadership' are often used interchangeably. Leadership refers to the style of command.

Requirements for leadership

The requirements for leadership include the following:

- *Credibility:* whoever is in command must have commanded successfully in the past, and have a sound technical knowledge.
- *Detachment:* the aim of leadership is to get the whole job done, not to be sucked into patient care, or a similar urgent activity.
- *Communication:* leaders must be able to convey their message clearly to minimise misunderstanding, and build in feedback. They need to seek information to maintain an overview.
- *Visibility:* the command group cannot be in the thick of things, but need to place themselves in a visible and accessible area. The fluidity of the situation calls for a style of managing by wandering around (rapid, on-the-spot analysis, goal-setting, decision-making, feedback and control), so that decision-making loops are shortened.
- *Networking:* commanders need to be able to expand services rapidly. This often involves calling up old favours, and obtaining cooperation from reluctant providers. Public figures are valuable allies during major incidents.
- *Coordination:* very often, the first casualty is the plan. Goals and requirements change, and all involved need to be apprised of their altered responsibilities. Frequent, quick and informal coordinating conferences are essential.
- *Structure:* a typical command group would consist of the strategic commander (political power, e.g. chief executive officer), operational commander, the person in charge of the discipline most affected, nursing decision-makers and a public liaison officer. Command groups must be small, and know each other well.
- *Reserve:* nobody is indestructible, and focusing command around individuals implies that the mass casualties can be managed only as long as the commander can stay on her/his feet. Deputies need to command beforehand.
- *Training:* commanders are not born – existing talents need to be developed. Technical excellence and seniority do not ensure sound command. Formal management training is essential for heads of units or departments.

Scope of command

The scope of command (things to plan beforehand, and to act on at the time) includes a simple mnemonic (CO-S-TR). The CO-S-TR model is a simple conceptual tool for hospital incident command personnel to prioritise initial incident actions in order to adequately address key components of surge capacity. 'CO' stands for command, control, communications and coordination, and ensures that an incident management structure is implemented. 'S' considers the logistical requirements for staff, stuff, space and special (event-specific) considerations. 'TR' comprises tracking, triage, treatment and transportation – basic patient care and patient movement functions. This comprehensive yet simple approach is designed to be implemented in the immediate aftermath of an incident, and complements the incident command system by aiding effective incident assessment and surge capacity responses at the healthcare-facility level.

Controlling

Controlling is the work managers perform to assess and regulate work in progress and to assess results achieved. Prior to the major incident, leadership will be challenged to maintain the necessary enthusiasm and initiative to ensure adequate standards of planning, training and re-evaluation – best achieved through a major incident committee. The major incident committee needs to represent all the major clinical and managerial disciplines of the hospital, and needs to be at an appropriate level to authorise actions within the hospital. The committee must have the support of top management to be effective.

A major function of the committee is to develop standards of performance. The Pareto principle states that 20% of effort produces 80% of reward. These 20% of results constitute the key performance indicators of any endeavour. Key performance indicators for hospital command include:

- Ability to predict overload and prepare accordingly (e.g. particularly busy weekends);
- Time to mobilise appropriate reserves of staff and consumables for major events;
- Time to decant patients who can be moved from critical areas (from ICU to ward, high care to ward, terminating theatre lists, moving patients to other facilities);
- Time and capability to expand the hierarchy to manage the event;
- Time for normal work to return to normal;
- Preventable mortality after a major incident.

Phases of command

Command consists of planning, preparation and training: this is largely the work of a major incident committee, backed up by higher levels of management.

Incident command is the work of the strategic, operational and tactical commanders.

Hospitals differ from scenes of major medical events, in that they are required to continue functioning at an altered level during the event, and normally immediately thereafter. Few can afford backlogs of elective admissions and elective lists.

As the major incident recedes, so the return to normal levels of activity must increase, along with audit, review and modification of major incident plans. Again, a well-functioning major incident committee is the strongest tool to identify lessons learnt, and to initiate corrective action.

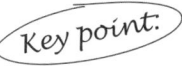 **For a hospital to function effectively in a major incident, effective command must be established and leadership demonstrated to coordinate activities optimally.**

Expanding hierarchies

A key concept in the command of a hospital's response to a major incident is the ability to function effectively with key roles filled even at minimal staffing levels (e.g. at 02h00). In order to ensure that such roles are identified and filled appropriately, an Incident Command System (ICS) is used. The key roles in the ICS, as adopted in South Africa, are shown in Figure 3.1.

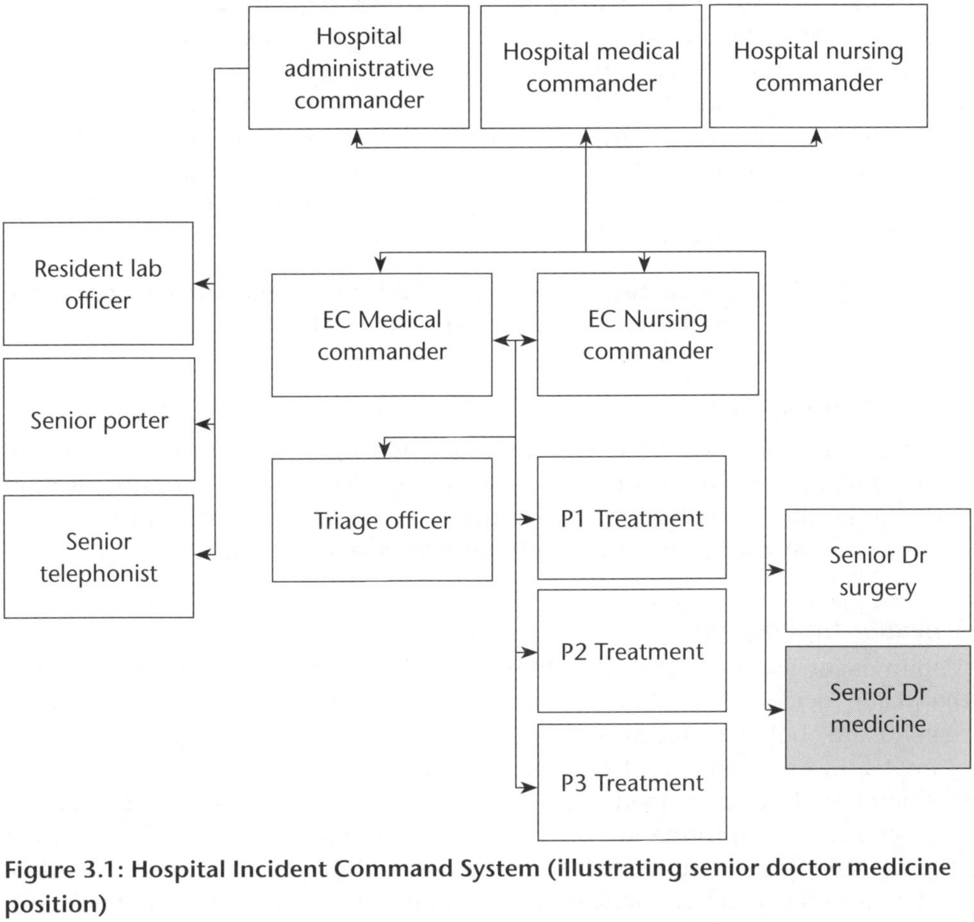

Figure 3.1: Hospital Incident Command System (illustrating senior doctor medicine position)

In most instances, when the hospital is faced with a major incident, the allocation of personnel to tasks becomes an area that creates logistical problems. This is partly due to the lack of coordinated major incident response experience among staff, and partly due to high rates of staff turnover.

Ensuring that action cards are developed early in the institution's planning phase will benefit the efficiency of the teams and assist in the coordinated command structure: an example of action cards is available for free download at www.emssa.org.za.

In many instances, hospitals make the mistake of allocating specific individuals to the roles, which results in mayhem if that individual is not on duty during the activation. All roles should be allocated to posts rather than individuals.

The key roles to be filled at the outset of response are the Hospital Coordination Team (HCT). This team comprises the Hospital Nursing Commander, the Hospital Medical Commander and the Hospital Administrative Commander (HAC). The HAC is typically in overall command, but this can be subject to local variation. This team should be kept small, with distinct areas of responsibility, to ensure efficiency in the management of all areas of the hospital.

In order for a hospital to function at its best in the event of a major incident, HCTs should exercise their management roles on a regular basis, ensuring that staff understand the top–down command structure for major incident response.

The HCT is responsible for ensuring that all actions are coordinated, structured and safe. Once command is established, roles can be allocated according to the hierarchy principle. Essentially, this is the allocation of major-incident tasks according to the needs of the institution, the nature of the major incident and available staff capabilities. As more staff arrive, more roles can be allocated; in the meantime, one person may be filling several key roles.

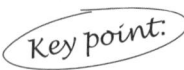 **A hierarchical structure should be established for command; critical first-line positions should be filled first.**

3.4 Communication

Facilitating efficient and effective communication is a cornerstone for successful management of a major incident or major incident. This includes communication with the hospital, communication by the hospital with its staff and resources, communication with relatives and communication with the media.

Activating the hospital

A point of entry must be identified to place the hospital on stand-by or to activate the Major Incident Plan. Most often, this point of first contact is the hospital switchboard, but it could also be any other prior identified department – for example, the emergency centre of the hospital. It is critical that the personnel at this point are briefed, trained and provided with a plan on how to respond to a message and what information to obtain. The identified point must be staffed at all times, and it is recommended that the standard METHANE set of information, used by the emergency services, is used to obtain information from a caller:

- *Major incident stand-by or declared.* Through proper pre-planning and liaison, the process of placing the hospital on stand-by, or to activate the Major Incident Plan by the emergency services, is determined. This activation will only be accepted from an official source such as the ambulance service.
- *Exact location of the event.* This gives the hospital an idea of distance and timelines before patients will reach the facility, and is important if a medical team is requested on site.
- *Type of incident.* Information on what exactly happened gives the hospital a indication of the nature of patients to expect, and gives an indication of possible requirements, such as mass burns management.
- *Hazards.* The hazards present on scene may influence the response of the hospital: for example, chemical hazards on site will result in decontamination on scene, and therefore patients will arrive wet and cold at the hospital.
- *Access.* Information on routes of access to the scene gives an indication on how quickly, and with what type of transport, patients may arrive.
- *Number of patients.* An estimate of the number of patients on scene guides the hospital in its response and influences the number of resources to be activated by the hospital.
- *Emergency services on scene or activated* to the scene gives an indication of whether fairly stabilised, or totally unstable, patients can be expected.

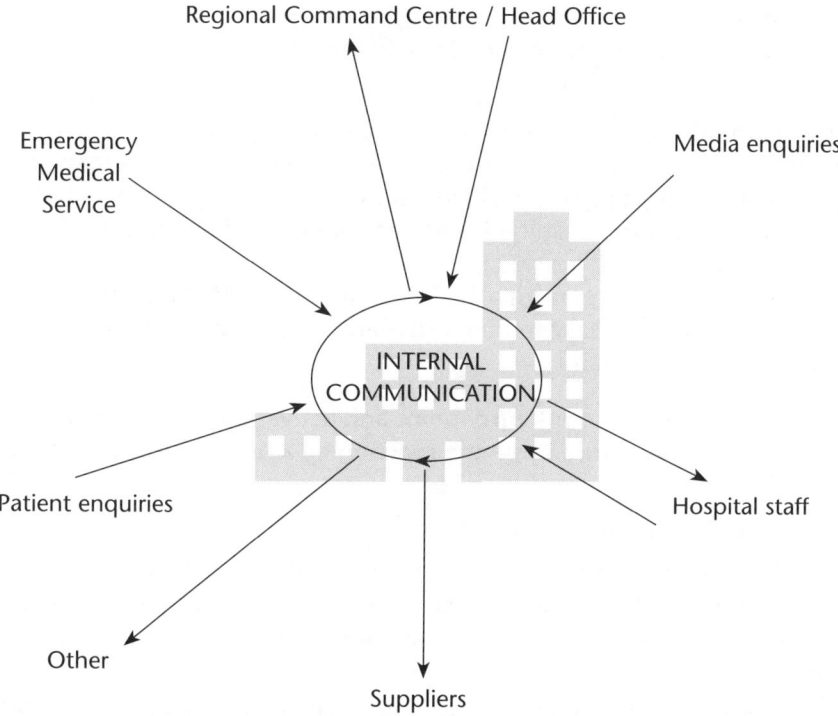

Figure 3.2: Hospital communication during a major incident

Additionally, the contact details of the caller need to be recorded so that the call can be verified and to obtain more information, if required. Hospitals often receive hoax calls to activate the Major Incident Plan. It is recommended that the switchboard/contact point immediately calls the caller back at the given phone number to verify the number and the information. Thereafter, the local ambulance service can be contacted to confirm the information.

It is recommended that a point such as the switchboard is used to receive and activate the hospital's plan, rather than a specific individual such as the CEO or the nursing service manager. Often, the planned individual is not readily available, and valuable time is wasted by trying to trace an individual.

The switchboard is authorised to activate the first phase of the plan, such as preparing the triage area and the emergency centre. Then a senior official can be contacted to authorise the activation of a second phase of actions, such as stopping theatre lists.

The switchboard, on receiving a major incident message, must react in a planned and structured way:

- Confirm the authenticity of the call, if the call source is not known to the receiver.
- Inform critical role-players within the hospital in order of their need to manage the situation, such as security to clear and control the entrance first, and then:
  - Triage officer;
  - Senior porter, to provide portering services;
  - Emergency centre to prepare for patients;
  - Nursing service manager.

The order, and the role-players, to be informed will depend on the hospital's own plan, and will include staff members on duty as well as staff that may be off duty. It is crucial that the complete and clear message is communicated to all the role-players, specifying if the hospital is only on stand-by for a major incident or if the plan is activated.

This communication is normally done using the telephone and/or cellphone networks, but it is necessary to plan alternative modes of communication should the telephone network fail.

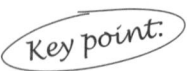 **An efficient entry point and activation process must be planned to ensure optimum reaction by a hospital to a major incident.**

Activation of personnel

A logical action following the activation of the plan is to call out resources to manage the situation. Management must determine in advance who should be called, and in which order, to implement the plan. Various systems can be used:

- Key role-players, such as members of management, and key functionaries should be called by a central caller(s), such as the switchboard, in order of priority. Reaching each of these critical staff should be recorded, so that management can be updated on who has been reached and is on their way, and who cannot be reached and therefore a replacement must be appointed.

- Additional personnel can be activated using a cascade system: for example, the member in charge of the section on duty calls the chief of the department at home; the chief calls two senior members; these two each call two more; and the system cascades until all required staff are activated. For such a system to be effective, accurate planning is required, together with frequent updating and distribution of contact details. As soon as such a cascade is activated, it cannot be stopped.
- Different technological devices are available to assist in the activation of large groups of staff, such as pre-grouped calling systems on the cellphone network, group pager activation and, even in smaller communities, an audible siren system. Whatever technology is planned, a back-up plan must be in place to address a failure of the system.

Using the mass media to activate hospital staff to report, such as a broadcast over the regional radio network, must be a last resort, as it causes mass panic reactions and results in the hospital been swamped by curious spectators, and enquiries from the public and the media.

Measures must be planned to limit use of telephone lines by staff to free capacity for vital communication. Placing pre-paid telephone cards in central places within the hospital will allow on-duty staff to use call boxes in the hospital to call off-duty staff and lighten the load on the switchboard.

It is important to plan specific reporting point(s) for staff members at the hospital, so that their presence can be recorded and efforts to reach them can be stopped.

Command communication

Establishing command is an integral priority action in managing any major incident. Command is optimally established in a specific location within the hospital from where all activities are coordinated and actions planned: for example, the boardroom at the management's offices. It is, however, essential that this command centre is in contact with all role-players to be able to respond on situation and address problems.

Communication is normally achieved using the hospital's internal telephone network and external telephone links. This is then backed up with radio communication with critical external, and often internal, role-players.

A telephone network has a limited capability, however, and can be easily overwhelmed. It is also possible that the total network, including the cellphone network, can fail. Planning a back-up system of messengers and other alternatives is necessary.

It is essential to plan the internal communication towards the command centre to prevent an overload and to streamline communication. A basic measure is to install a duplicate plug on each member of the command team's office telephone line in the boardroom or command centre. Each member of management can then unplug their office phone and plug it in again in the boardroom and function as normal in a centralised location.

A second plan is to install a number of additional telephones in the command centre, for incoming calls. The different departments of the hospital are then allocated to these numbers, and each department is informed of only the one number used for that department to communicate with the command centre.

Special emergency lines must be identified, with these numbers only made known to key managers.

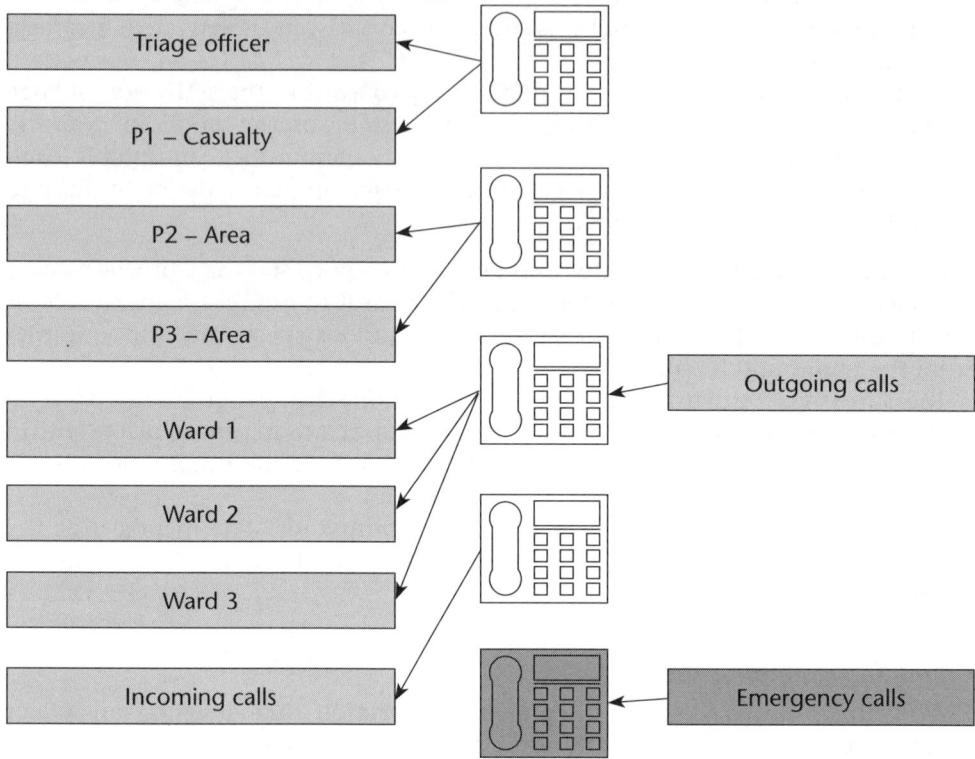

Figure 3.3: Example of a hospital command centre's communication plan

The command centre should also have access to electronic communication capabilities such as e-mail. This is essential to transmit information such as patient name lists or plans from the head office. A fax machine is also a basic necessity.

Internal communication by the command centre to the staff is critical to keep staff informed on what is expected and actions that are taken. This will counter rumours within the hospital and will assist in maintaining morale.

The command centre is the central point for channelling communication and for coordinating messages. A record of messages received, and actions taken, by the command centre is a useful tool to coordinate actions and to confirm decisions taken.

Public enquiries

It is vital to establish a patient information centre, to which all enquiries about patients can be channelled early in a major incident. Depending on the size of the hospital, this centre should have applicable communication capabilities. It is preferable that the patient information centre's telephone lines should function on a separate system to avoid overloading of the hospital system. These telephone numbers and physical location are then communicated over the mass media as early as possible.

Such a centre should also be equipped with e-mail capabilities, as relatives of international patients may only have access to an e-mail system to enquire about their relatives.

Media communication

Establishment of an effective method for communicating with the media is addressed in the section on challenges. It is worthwhile considering setting up special phone lines for the media to use.

Communication system failure

Effective communication is indispensable in the successful managing of a major incident. However, management must plan for a failure in the basic communication systems of the hospital. This may be caused by the major incident, such as an earthquake destroying the telephone network, or even by an overload of the number of people trying to reach the hospital.

Planning additional emergency communication is an integral part of major incident planning. Radio communication is often the alternative of choice. It is, however, important that equipment is properly maintained and checked regularly, and that staff are trained and experienced in using radio communication. Radio links also use infrastructure, such as repeaters and antennas, that may be damaged in the major incident. It will, however, only link the hospital with specific key institutions and not necessarily all the role-players required. A radio network may link the hospital with the emergency medical service but it is unlikely to extend to the supplier from which food must be ordered. Additional communication back-ups must therefore be planned.

A messenger system, both inside and outside the hospital, is a low-technology option. External messenger systems will depend for their execution on planning for adequate vehicles, fuel and manpower, and will depend on the accessibility of the roads to reach the destinations. Using a basic carbon-type book in which to write messages, and having the recipient signing for it and then tearing out a copy, will prevent much confusion and assist in keeping a record of instructions given.

Specific direct telephone lines between the hospital and critical institution (so-called major incident phones) often use alternative cables and may provide critical capabilities if other systems fail.

The use of alternative modes of external communication to support the hospital is possible. These include satellite phones or military capabilities to establish a communication centre within the hospital, linking it to external higher-level command centres. The use of radio amateur long-distance capabilities has proven vital in the past to link outlying hospitals with the rest of the country.

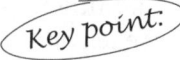 **Communication in a major incident includes planning for the activation of personnel, effective internal liaison and communication with the media and the next-of-kin of casualties. This may require innovative measures to address failures in the regular systems.**

3.5 Safety

Safety and security are interlinked processes in managing a major incident. Personal safety is paramount to managing the major incident, and not to become part of the problem! The basic concept is to take the necessary precautions to ensure optimal personal safety, safety of the environment and then safety of the survivors:

1. Self
2. Scene/environment
3. Survivors/patients

Security

Security is the responsibility of all staff members and not only that of security personnel.

Access control

To be able to maintain structure and order within the hospital, and to be able to treat patients effectively, it is essential to establish effective access control as soon as notification of a possible major incident is received. If not controlled, the entire hospital will be swamped by curious onlookers, hysterical relatives, the media and even criminal elements. All entrances to the facility must be closed and staffed. Only patients and staff members are allowed to enter the complex. Patients are channelled to the predetermined entrance leading to the receiving and triage capability, while staff members are channelled to the staff reporting point to record their presence.

Ambulance staff, volunteer first-aiders and members of the public accompanying patients are channelled towards the receiving capability; a second line of access control must prevent access into treatment facilities.

Staff members not identifiable through reliable identification cards must be channelled to a separate staff entrance, where allocated human resource managers can check their information against the staff database and issue temporary identification.

Relatives and members of the public are channelled to a separate information and reunion capability, to which information on all survivors reaching the hospital is channelled and identification processes of unknown/unconscious victims are initiated.

As soon as volunteers are required, a separate volunteer recruiting entrance is established and all volunteers are channelled to this entrance for documentation and the issuing of a daily identification card.

The media is immediately guided to a media information centre where media briefings are held.

Traffic control

Orderly, well-managed traffic flow is one of the pillars of major incident management at a hospital.

Management must identify the appropriate entrance preferred for all arriving patients. This may not necessarily be the normal ambulance entrance, as this often leads directly to flooding of the emergency centre. An appropriate entrance needs to be identified, where adequate space for reception, transfer to hospital gurneys and triage is available. It is recommended that large clear signs are prepared in advance, to be placed in position as soon as the major incident or Major Incident Plan is activated, to guide ambulances and other vehicles to this entrance.

Adequate parking must be available for vehicles to off-load patients and should preferably have a circular flow to leave the area. Pitfalls include allowing vehicles to drive right up to the door, park and then block all other movement, or drivers leaving their vehicles and getting involved in off-loading, and even treating, patients, leaving the vehicles blocking the parking space. A firm control over vehicles arriving and off-loading is essential, as is having adequate porter staff/ volunteers to manhandle the stretchers. Patients must be transferred to hospital gurneys as soon as possible in order to return ambulance stretchers to vehicles, allowing ambulances to return to the scene.

It is essential to plan for large vehicles such as major incident buses, trucks or passenger buses arriving at the hospital with patients. If the identified entrance has a height restriction, alternative plans must be made.

Planning must be done to receive large numbers of patients by helicopter. It is essential to plan landing space for helicopters, including large military helicopters that are often used in major incidents. Small heliports may not be suitable for large helicopters which require alternative arrangements. Often, various helicopters arrive at a major incident scene and start ferrying patients to the hospitals; this requires the hospital to plan a semi-permanent presence at the helicopter landing area to off-load and receive patients at a much higher tempo than usual, often requiring 'hot' off-loading (with the rotors running). This requires training and very strict security to prevent over-eager photographers or relatives reaching the helicopters. The purpose must be to off-load as quickly and effectively as possible to allow the helicopter to take off and free the landing zone for the next helicopter.

Patient luggage and valuables

A significant challenge in a major incident situation is the control and management of patients' luggage and valuables on arrival at the hospital. Particularly in large transport-related incidents, this may entail large volumes of luggage. In a military incident, this may also include weapons.

Pre-planning for numbering patients is a standard process in major incident management. It is recommended that large transparent pre-numbered plastic bags are added to the prepared major-incident files for clothing. Patients need to be undressed as soon as possible (especially Priority 1 and 2 patients); clothing must then be sealed in the bags and stored in a safe area under direct security supervision. This clothing is often used as evidence in post-major incident investigations. It is recommended that non-transparent bags are not used, as these are often confused with refuse and incinerated!

Preparing similar pre-numbered luggage tags that can be attached to all large pieces of arriving luggage assists in managing these. Luggage is then removed and stored under the direct supervision of security staff.

Patients' valuables and money offer a further security challenge in a major incident. It is recommended that a special sealable valuable-item bag is pre-numbered and placed in the prepared major-incident file. Valuables and money are then sealed in the bags as soon as possible. Locked large postbox-type bins must be prepositioned in strategic positions in the reception and initial treatment areas. These sealed bags are then posted in the bins; afterwards, under security-controlled circumstances, these bins are unlocked and the content of each bag registered. As this often also becomes part of evidence, and may be critical in identification processes, precautions such as gloves are recommended when handling personal items.

Unaccompanied children

A serious security risk is unaccompanied children arriving at the hospital after a major incident as they can very easily get lost in the chaos, and may even be taken by paedophiles. Adequate security control of all children leaving the hospital is critical. The use of trained security staff, supported by skilled social workers is essential; allowing children to leave the hospital with alleged relatives, is a security responsibility.

Safety

Safety of the staff and the environment is a challenging task in major incident management.

Staff safety

Ensuring that the staff are safe by providing adequate personal protective equipment (PPE) is an integral part of the plan. It is essential that management obtain as much information as possible on the major incident to identify any hazards that may be transferred to the hospital. This is of critical important in chemical, biological or radiation incidents. Adequate PPE to protect staff must be available.

This is of critical importance if a medical team from the hospital is sent to the scene. It is essential to plan to provide, or obtain, adequate identifiable full protection for such a team. This should provide protection, functionality and durability as well as comfort.

Normally, the emergency services implement decontamination processes on the scene, but it is possible that bystanders may rush contaminated patients directly to the hospital. Plans to decontaminate patients before entering the facility must be in place, and may often be as basic as washing them down with fire hoses in the parking area and removing all contaminated clothing. Whatever the plan, adequate PPE for staff must be available.

Environmental safety

The safety of the hospital needs to be assessed immediately after a major incident. This is specifically important in natural disasters, but may also be applicable in riot situations, faction fights and chemical incidents in the area.

A safety assessment often requires specialist advice. Hospitals or hospital groups must identify in advance adequately skilled engineers who can be contacted to evaluate the structural integrity of a hospital after a natural major incident. Using engineers who know the structure of the building will enhance the process.

Advice from specialists on gas clouds and their movement, radiation distribution or other environmental hazards must be part of the initial reaction of the hospital, to ensure that safety is not compromised. It is, however, emphasised that any major incident situation will have a risk factor, but this needs to be assessed to determine optimal action from the hospital.

If in danger, it may be necessary to evacuate the hospital and use temporary facilities until the building is secure to use.

Inadequate safety and security may be the cause for the failure of the major incident response plan within the hospital.

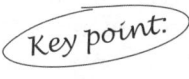 **Safety includes own, patient and environmental safety. It includes protection measures to protect staff and patients, and to ensure security of possessions, children and vulnerable groups.**

3.6 Triage

Triage is discussed in detail in Chapter 2. The focus of this section is on triage after the initial emergency care of patients.

In a major incident, a dedicated triage officer should be allocated to the reception area in front of the emergency centre. The Triage Sort is recommended as the best means of triage, although in the event of a sudden flood of patients arriving, the Triage Sieve may be used.

Surgical triage

Triage means sorting patients according to priority of treatment. Surgical triage aims to identify the priority of surgical intervention.

Aims

The aim of surgical triage is to identify those who need urgent surgical control of haemorrhage, contamination and/or evacuation of surface collections over the brain. The only ophthalmologic emergency requiring surgery within the hour is retrobulbar haematoma. Maxillofacial surgeons, reconstructive surgeons, ear nose and throat surgeons, urologists etc. are indispensable assistants during major incidents.

Failure to control contamination adequately and timeously leads to major incidents, particularly after earthquakes, military operations etc. Patients pay with their lives and limbs for the civilian luxury of delayed or inadequate control of contamination (soft tissue, compound fractures, hollow visceral perforations). Delaying drainage of intra-cranial haematomas will result in increased mortality, but, perhaps worse, will also create more vegetative patients to care for.

Time is the enemy of neurosurgical and orthopaedics patients as much as for those bleeding. For these, equipment needs must be downgraded significantly. The challenge for neuro- and orthopaedic surgeons is to debride early, debride extensively and to drain the clots. The rest can be done later.

Systems of triage

Because patients can and do bypass any and all of the triage points at the scene, and because disease is a dynamic process in which the patient's response may improve or deteriorate and rarely stay the same, the degree of threat to a patient will change over time. Triage is therefore never entirely accurate, and needs to be repeated at every stage of care.

Systems of surgical triage

The system of triage employed is dependent on the situation. Improvements in the accuracy of triage systems increase the time required to assess, the amount of technology and the complexity of decision-making. Patients accorded the lowest priority (Priority 4) (Priority 1 hold/moribund) for surgery require the most complex decision-making. In sequence of speed and in reverse order of complexity, these systems of triage are:

- *Triage Sieve:* performed on scene, as a minimum on arrival, and anytime thereafter when a large group of patients need to be triaged quickly.
- *Triage Sort:* performed on arrival after initial Triage Sieve.
- *Mechanism of injury* often combined with Triage Sort to increase accuracy of triage.
- *South African Triage Scale:* an accurate and simple system of triage that is ideal for day-to-day use in emergency centres and clinics to prioritise patient arrivals, but is perhaps too complex and slow for use in a major incident.

After initial triage to identify Priority 1 patients, surgeons need to decide on the priority of surgery, using the following criteria:

- Threats to life identified during the primary survey;
- Haemodynamic instability to determine the urgency of surgical control of haemorrhage;
- Possibility of non-operative intervention;
- Patients not for further intervention (P4).

In a private sector facility, it is essential that the major incident committee agrees in advance which surgeon(s) will be used to prioritise patients for surgery, and ensures that all surgeons utilising the facility agree with the arrangement.

Threats to life

These are identified during the primary survey. A few critical questions may determine the urgency of surgical intervention within minutes:

- Is the airway threatened?
- Are there any of five threats to life present in the chest?
- Is the patient shocked, and which class of shock is present?
- Is the Glasgow Coma Scale below 13, and are there localising signs (brain, spinal cord)?
- Is the patient hypothermic?
- Is there a threat to a limb (pulseless limb, compartment syndrome)?
- Is the patient haemodynamically stable or not?

Haemodynamic instability

The parameters to determine the need for urgent surgery show variable predictability, but are ignored at the peril of the patient. These are:

- Non-responders to resuscitation (Ringers lactate 200ml rapidly ivi), and no improvement in systolic blood pressure. Immediate surgical control is required.
- Transient responders to resuscitation (initial improvement in systolic blood pressure). In major incidents, treat as unstable.
- Systolic blood pressure < 90 mm Hg at any stage prior to resuscitation.
- Base deficit> –5 mmol/l, serum lactate > 2.5 mmol/l.
- The latter two parameters suggest a 40% to 45% risk of urgent, life-saving surgery.

Possibility of non-operative intervention

A mass casualty event is not the time for the extremes of non-operative management. Non-operative management requires intensive care, close observation, careful decision-making, and often angio-embolisation; all of these are resource-intensive. It is better to look and see than to wait and see.

Patients not for resuscitation

Experience assists in identifying those with a probability of survival of less than 10% on arrival, including: intubated without sedation, Glasgow Coma Scale < 5, fixed dilated pupils, trans-hemispheric gunshot, arrival with cardio-pulmonary resuscitation in progress, high quadriplegia, arterial base deficit > –15 mmol/L, etc. Resuscitating patients burnt beyond the criteria for acceptance to the local burns unit merely transfers the place of death. Patients in these categories should be accorded a full primary survey, have the decision verified by a senior second opinion, to allow proper counselling of the family.

Based on the above criteria, the patients are prioritised for surgical interventions in order of seriousness. The patients can be numbered T1 to T... to indicate order for surgery. It is, however, essential that continuous clinical assessment and monitoring is maintained, as a patient's condition may deteriorate, requiring an 'upgrade' in position on the surgical priority list. As most of the surgeons will be involved in the theatres, it is essential to identify clinicians in advance that would monitor the patients pre-op and post-op until the surgeons become available to resume this function. Use Triage Sort and assessment of the degree of haemodynamic instability for quick re-evaluation.

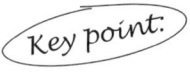 **Surgical triage ensures that the surgical capacity of the hospital is used to do the most for the most by prioritising surgical interventions using clinical parameters.**

Ventilator triage

Ventilator triage consists of all the activities to provide the best intensive care for the most present or presenting during a mass casualty event, including decanting, surge, limiting admissions to those with the best prognosis and excluding those with the worst prognosis. There are never enough ventilators in any facility. The aim is to select (triage) those with the best prognosis for ventilation.

Even recovery rooms and ventilated ward beds can be used to provide intensive care. Staffing can be expanded using clear ranges of upper and lower limits of parameters, so that inexperienced staff spend more time monitoring and providing basic care, and so that experienced staff can supervise several ventilated patients.

Ventilators are a scarce resource in a major incident. Healthcare facilities must plan how this resource may be substituted in a major incident by establishing a database of where ventilators can be obtained, keeping a record of all ventilators in the complex and possibly mothballing all phased-out ventilators to provide additional capabilities when required.

Decanting

The Sequential Organ Failure Assessment (SOFA) during the first few days of ICU admission is a good indicator of prognosis. Both the mean and highest SOFA scores are particularly useful predictors of outcome. The SOFA was adopted as the main standard of ventilator triage for the H1N1 influenza epidemic, but is accurate enough for all ICU patients. Table 3.2 shows how it is calculated.

Table 3.2: Sequential Organ Failure Assessment (SOFA)

Respiratory System	PaO2/FiO2 (mm Hg),	SOFA score
	< 400	1
	< 300	2
	< 200 and mechanically ventilated	3
	< 100 and mechanically ventilated	4
Glasgow Coma score	13–14	1
	10–12	2
	6–9	3
	< 6	4

Cardiovascular System	Mean Arterial Pressure OR administration of vasopressors required, SOFA score	
	MAP < 70mm/Hg	1
	dopamine <= 5 OR dobutamine (any dose)	2
	dopamine > 5 OR epinephrine <= 0.1 OR nor epinephrine <= 0.1	3
	dopamine > 15 OR epinephrine > 0.1 OR nor epinephrine > 0.1 (vasopressor drug doses in mcg/kg/min)	4
Bilirubin (mg/dl)	1.2–1.9	1
	2.0–5.9	2
	6.0–11.9	3
	> 12.0	4
Coagulation	Platelets×103/mcl	
	< 150	1
	< 100	2
	< 50	3
	< 20	4
Renal System	Creatinine (mg/dl) (or urine output)	
	1.2–1.9	1
	2.0–3.4	2
	3.5–4.9 (or < 500 ml/d)	3
	> 5.0 (or < 200 ml/d)	4

Table 3.3 shows how the SOFA is used.

Table 3.3: SOFA score

Blue: Exclusion criteria met or SOFA score > 11	Manage medically Provide palliative care as needed Discharge from critical care
Red: SOFA score 7 or single-organ failure	Highest priority
Orange: SOFA score 8–11	Intermediate priority
Green: No significant organ failure	Defer or discharge Reassess as needed

* If an exclusion criterion is met or the SOFA score is > 11 any time from the initial assessment to 48 hours afterward, change the triage code to Blue.

Limiting admissions

Detailed inclusion and exclusion criteria used in the triage protocol for critical care during an influenza pandemic (or major incident) are given below.

Inclusion criteria

The patient must have one of the following:

- Requirement for invasive ventilatory support: refractory hypoxemia (SpO2 < 90% on non-rebreather mask or FIO2 > 0.85.
- Respiratory acidosis (pH <7.2), clinical evidence of impending respiratory failure, inability to protect or maintain airway;
- Hypotension (systolic blood pressure < 90 mm Hg or relative hypotension) with clinical evidence of shock (altered level of consciousness, decreased urine output or other evidence of end-organ failure) refractory to volume resuscitation requiring vasopressor or inotrope support that cannot be managed in ward.

It is essential for healthcare facilities to determine surge capacity for ventilated patients in advance. This includes identifying additional space in the facility that is equipped with the resources to ventilate a patient. This will depend on the type of ventilators used – some ventilators require medical air to drive them. Identification of all medical air outlets in the complex is therefore required. The available ventilators are then allocated using the above criteria to ensure this scarce resource is allocated to the most appropriate patients with the optimum prognosis.

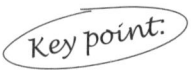 **Ventilator triage ensures that the scarce resource is used optimally for the most appropriate patients.**

3.7 Definitive care

Once triage has taken place at the front door of the hospital, definitive care begins. For the majority of patients, this is completed in the emergency centre. However, for a number of patients definitive care means admission to a hospital bed, with intensive care and/or operating theatre time. It is not the aim of this text to detail the correct clinical care to be performed. However, management principles will allow effective and efficient use of hospital resources to care for these patients, while minimising the impact on the day-to-day running of the hospital.

Patient tracking

One of the most urgent problems facing emergency personnel responding to a major incident is the overwhelming number of patients who need to be monitored and tracked from the scene of the major incident to the hospital. Patient tracking in this context refers to tracking which patient, with which condition, has been sent to which hospital, and then knowing where they currently are within the hospital. Whatever technology is used, it is essential that such systems can track patients accurately without getting in the way of the emergency treatment. There is currently a shortage of research-based literature on patient identification and tracking technologies used during major incidents.

There are two main types of patient tracking currently in use: the paper system (using paper tags, cards and charts) and electronic systems (bar codes, Wi-Fi networks, etc.). The paper system is cheap and easy to implement, and many emergency personnel are familiar with its use. In recent years, there have been numerous advances in bar coding, wireless networking, medical sensors etc., which have create many new possibilities for the ways in which patient tracking can take place at the scene of a major incident. Using a hand-held computer, emergency personnel can perform the identification process during triage, scan the bar code or electronic triage tag and attach it to the patient. These hand-held devices then transmit patient data (including photographs of the injury) directly to a database where it is then immediately accessible to multiple providers and healthcare facilities. As the patient moves through the system, emergency personnel scan the bar code and access up-to-the-minute information on the patient, as well as the patient's current location. The effectiveness of wireless electronic tracking devices to track victims in a large-scale major incident drill has been shown to be as effective as paper systems.

The minimum patient tracking information required is:

- Time patient arrived in hospital;
- Patient hospital number and time patient numbered;
- Time patient triaged;
- Triage code;
- Patient details (name, age etc.) or patient identifier (may use photographs);
- Identified injuries;
- Contamination/decontamination;
- Vital signs;
- Any treatment administered (including time it was administered);
- Time when the patient leaves the emergency centre and where they are transferred to – for example, theatre, X-ray – and if they return;
- Clinical team responsible;
- Were the next of kin informed?

This information must be recorded either on paper or electronically.

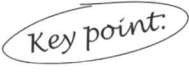 **Measures need to be implemented to track the movement of patients from the scene(s) of an incident to hospitals, and within the hospitals to ensure enquiries can be answered, next-of-kin guided and facilities optimally utilised.**

Psychological support

Major incidents are traumatic events which can result in many mental and physical health consequences. In recent years, there has been increased awareness of promoting the mental health of society. However, there are many victims of major incidents suffering from psychological and emotional injuries who receive little or no treatment. These people live injured, impaired lives, and their scars are often inherited by future generations. Psychological support for emergency personnel exposed to traumatic events is just as essential, although such personnel often disregard their own psychological needs. This may hamper team cohesiveness, and unit and individual functioning, as well as result in failure to assist the victims and survivors of a major incident. Post-traumatic stress disorder (PTSD) or other psychological reactions may not be visible at the onset, or even months or years after the major incident, but often comes in the form of distorted behaviour such as alcohol and drug abuse, sleeplessness and depression. Unfortunately, psychological support services for emergency personnel and the survivors/victims of a major incident are frequently neglected.

There is no universal recipe to deal with the psychological impact of major incidents as the psychological support for emergency personnel and survivors during and after major incidents is different.

The psychological support needed during a major incident will depend on:

- Major incident characteristics (intentional, unintentional or natural);
- Individual's characteristics (training, previous experience, proximity to the victims);
- Response characteristics (large-scale deployment, support, leadership, type of involvement).

Psychological support should start at the scene of the major incident and continue after the admission phase to hospital, and even after discharge from the hospital.

Debriefing and counselling

Debriefing is not counselling, psychotherapy or a substitute for counselling or therapy. While debriefing uses some of the basic communication skills or micro counselling skills which are used in counselling, such as empathy, active listening, nonverbal rapport, reflecting, open questioning, paraphrasing and summarising, debriefing is different from counselling both in content and style.

Only those who were involved in the major incident as a victim or as a worker are debriefed. Debriefing is always voluntary and is always presented in a group. Debriefing is formal and must be undertaken by a trained debriefer. A debriefer can be anyone who has been trained and tested to do so, and is usually an appointed person who works within the hospital and is seen as a respected, trained and experienced person who is trusted by staff and patients.

Debriefing is highly structured, and the debriefer is in control of the process. The debriefer judges the end of the sections of the process and moves onto the next stage. This is managed in such a way that factual information can be delivered in detail without the participant being overwhelmed by emotional and other post-traumatic responses. Debriefers do not change the underlying meanings of behaviours, thoughts or feelings. Instructive information and advice is provided during the debriefing session to help traumatised persons to understand their reactions and to reduce the chance of further problems. Debriefing stands alone as a single psychological crisis intervention and is not part of ongoing therapy. The debriefing process is not magical amnesia, and it is not possible to remove all the pain and trauma experienced during a critical incident from a person's mind.

In comparison, the trauma counselling process is not managed by a counsellor in the same way that a debriefer manages a debriefing session. Much of the emphasis in counselling is on the identification of the underlying feelings or thinking which may be causing the psychological harm. This is a longer type of intervention and can be done one-to-one. Risk cases are identified during the debriefing and are then referred to a psychologist or a psychiatrist.

Trauma counselling, which is undertaken with individuals, requires a number of sessions to complete. In trauma counselling, there is a much greater potential for iatrogenic distress caused by counselling interventions than is the case with debriefing. It is therefore important that trauma therapy and counselling be undertaken only by competent licensed practitioners using effective methods of treatment, and not by peers or debriefers.

Rules to be followed when debriefing during major incidents

- Debriefing is formal and is arranged in definite steps, which follow in sequence. It is done to enable the person to integrate, at a cognitive and emotional level, the profound personal experiences induced by trauma.
- The debriefing process involves one-on-one situations or groups of victims recounting their impressions and understanding of the event in a systematic and structured format.
- The debriefing process is facilitated by a debriefing team leader. This process is designed to enable the victim to re-experience the incident in a controlled and safe environment so that he or she can make sense of it and become reconciled to the traumatic incident.
- Debriefing is NOT conducted during the active phases of a major incident. It is never started before 48 hours after the event, as the people involved must have first overcome the shock phase of the event in their own minds, as well as any physical injuries.

Table 3.4: Debriefing process

Sequence of Phases	Contents	Level
Introduction	Introduce team members Rules and process explained	Cognitive
Facts	What happened (What did they see, hear, smell, touch?)	Cognitive
Thoughts and impressions	First thoughts and decisions made Own impressions of incident	Cognitive/ emotional ⤵

Sequence of Phases	Contents	Level
Emotional reactions	Questions about thoughts lead to answers about feelings What was the worst thing about the incident? Reactions at the scene and later physical and psychological symptoms Emotional, physical and cognitive reactions	Emotional
Normalisation	Assessment of incident, commenting on reactions/ stress symptoms, anticipating guidance, advice on helpful coping	Emotional/ Cognitive
Future planning and coping	Educational aspects, questions answered Mobilising support from family, friends, children	Cognitive
Disengagement	Summing up Follow-up resources Referral information De-roleing	Cognitive

Psychological support for emergency personnel

Major incidents have different phases, and every phase has different types of support that should be provided (see Table 3.5).

Table 3.5: Major incident phases and support interventions

Phases	Type of Support Provided	Supporter
Pre-major-incident phase	Select debriefers and mental health professionals. Introduce psychological support team to the emergency team, get to know their roles and the type of support provided. Provide training and information about stress reactions, establish leadership, policies	Full team of supporters including peers, debriefers and mental health professionals
Heroic phase	Provide physical support and observe needs, remove irritations, ensure safety and provide basic needs to alleviate stress, crisis intervention	Peers and support team
Honeymoon phase	Provide support in the form of defusing and physical support	Peers and support team

Phases	Type of Support Provided	Supporter
Disillusionment phase	Defusing, individual interviews, consider debriefing depending on situation in major incident area, type and duration of major incident. Being there	Mental health professionals
Reconstruction phase	Debriefing, follow-up debriefing, consider cases for referral counselling, psychotherapy	Mental health professionals and referral to advance practitioners

Psychological support for survivors

This starts at the scene of the major incident and continues during admission and after discharge from hospital. Psychological support should be provided to all who have been involved in the major incident – whether they are admitted to hospital or not.

The guidelines to follow when providing psychological support for survivors of a major incident are as follows:

- Remove them from the scene and transfer to hospital (if necessary);
- Provide physical needs (shelter, safety, food);
- Reassurance;
- Survivors need to tell their stories as they perceive them – listen;
- Children need special intervention and supportive actions;
- Provide the contact details of support centres for survivors (both for those survivors who are admitted to hospital as well as those who are not);
- Medical evaluation – this starts at the major incident scene and continues in hospital;
- Provide accurate information;
- Assign a buddy;
- Limit exposure to scenes that may re-traumatise;
- Do not give false hope;
- Short periods of crisis intervention.

Challenges in providing psychological support

There are many critics who question the usefulness of debriefing. However, people, including researchers, often misunderstand, or wrongly apply, debriefing during major incidents. For example:

- Well-meaning individuals, entrepreneurs, those driven by adrenaline or those who thrive on attention from the media are often selected as 'debriefers'. These people may be harmful in the provision of all crisis interventions, including debriefing. Debriefing should not be forced. It is voluntary, and only for those who were directly involved in the crisis situation, including staff.
- Debriefing is not suitable for children, as they require more specialised interventions.

- Debriefing is NOT a therapy or type of counselling.
- Debriefing is NOT required for every single event in the line of duty of emergency personnel.
- Debriefing is a formal process provided by skilful and trained experienced mental health professionals.
- Debriefing is not conducted before at least 48–72 hours after an event.

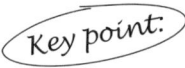 **Comprehensive counselling and debriefing is a structured and planned intervention to address the mental wellbeing of casualties and staff following a major incident. Specific rules need to be followed, utilising professionally trained staff and appropriate interventions.**

3.8 Discharge and reuniting

Patient discharge and reunification are vital aspects that require fine planning in major incident management. Proper patient discharge is an essential component of good patient care. In addition to this, efficient patient discharge practices ensure greater capacity for (potential) patient admissions, which is again essential in creating surge capacity.

Reception phase patient discharge

Frequently, the majority of survivors in (natural) incidents have fairly minor injuries. It follows then that these patients will be discharged home from the hospital on completion of their clinical care. In order to create efficient flow, ideally these patients should be discharged to a designated discharge area, so as to create greater capacity for further admissions to the emergency centre.

On discharge, patients should receive information as with any routine discharge. Pre-prepared printed information (such as wound care advice and plaster cast information) should be handed to patients and explained. Printed information should also be given regarding where trauma debriefing and counselling may be obtained. Debriefing and counselling should, however, not be enforced immediately. Patients should also receive information that provides the hospital's telephone contact number, as well as any other pertinent numbers (such as the local police or a centralised major incident enquiry point).

Discharge point

The discharge point (discharge lounge) should be located outside the emergency centre, away from the public eye and the press. If possible, the lounge could be situated adjacent to the hospital's enquiry area to facilitate reunification with next-of-kin.

The discharge point functions to:

- Remove patients from the busyness of the emergency centre on completion of their medical management;
- Allow patients to contemplate the events and what has happened to them;

- Allow patients to interact with other survivors (which assists with emotional recovery);
- Enjoy refreshments;
- Be reunited with next-of-kin;
- Be supported emotionally by nursing staff or counsellors within a secure area and removed from the press;
- Ensure that patients receive follow-up after discharge;
- Discharge in-hospital patients;
- Check that patients have transport or accommodation, and, if not, hand them over to major incident management staff to provide.

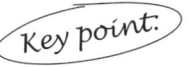 **Patients involved in a major incident who are admitted to the discharge point require psychological first aid.**

Enquiry management

A public enquiry point should be set up where the public and next-of-kin may direct enquiries regarding patients involved in the major incident. This area should be well away from patient receiving and treatment areas, but accessible to the public. A senior staff member should oversee the area and ensure that only *'bona fide* enquirers' are accompanied to the patient discharge point or clinical area. Staff manning this area should be kept up to date continuously by the command centre as to patients' locations. The enquiry point should be manned by staff capable of managing enquiries from members of the public who are distressed and often very aggressive.

Persons enquiring after patients who are not located at the hospital should be directed to a centralised major incident enquiry office or be provided with a telephone number where all major incident victims' movements should be tracked.

Bereavement area

Enquiries may be received where the person may (unknown to the next-of-kin) have died. The management of this situation should be well planned. Tips include:

- The news should not be given at the enquiries desk, nor in any other public place.
- Only staff trained in conveying such bad news should manage such situations.
- The next-of-kin should be taken to a private area away from public areas, to be given the news.
- A designated bereavement area may be created to allow next-of-kin to be allowed to come to terms with the news. Support personnel (such as nurses, social workers or clergy) should be on hand to provide emotional support.
- Persons leaving the bereavement area should ideally be allowed to leave the hospital avoiding the public and press.

Paediatric considerations

Children are particularly vulnerable during major incidents, and require special considerations to ensure they receive suitable care in major incidents. Besides specific considerations in managing primary injuries related to the incident, secondary injuries and medical conditions (including communicable diseases, gastroenteritis and dehydration) must be prevented at all cost. Intentional secondary injuries may be sustained through abuse or neglect.

In large-scale incidents, children may be separated from their primary guardians, and so they require special care. Unaccompanied paediatric patients should be kept together, and specific persons should be assigned to their care. Reuniting children with their parents quickly should be a priority as the mental health of the family is better preserved, the acute effects of community panic and upheaval are reduced and the effects of post-traumatic stress are minimised.

It may be necessary to plan specific areas to care for uninjured children until they can be reunited with their legal guardians. Aspects to address include proper security to ensure that children do not get lost; that they are kept entertained by using televisions or games; and that stressors should be addressed and identification be confirmed. It is often necessary to take pictures of uninjured and discharged children to enable identification by next-of-kin.

The identification of discharged children and the positive confirmation that the person collecting the child is the legal guardian require special planning. In the event of major incidents involving children, it is good practice to get a social worker and/or the police's child protection unit involved to oversee the identification of adults collecting the children, as the misuse of major incidents by paedophiles is a well-documented phenomenon.

Reverse triage – creating surge capacity

A brief explanation regarding in-patient discharge cannot be excluded. In order to create surge capacity, reverse triage may be undertaken. Reverse triage includes the earlier safe discharge of current inpatients so that greater capacity is created to manage those with greater needs. These patients may then be discharged to home or step-down facilities, or may even be transferred to other facilities. Patients who are able to be discharged home should be discharged via the discharge point so that beds can be vacated swiftly. Care should be taken to ensure that discharged patients are:

- Properly briefed on possible complications;
- Provided with the appropriate medicine or script for the medicine;
- Informed when to return for follow-up (should it be indicated);
- Supported by accurate record-keeping (this is critical to prevent medico-legal risks).

Patient identification and reunification

Efficient patient tracking throughout a major incident should be a priority so that reunification with next-of-kin may be expedited. In a large-scale major incident, where patients may be distributed among several hospitals, a system should be in place whereby all patients' names are submitted to a centralised major incident enquiry centre. A database should then be constructed, with all patients' conditions and the hospitals to which they have been admitted. In such an event, the public should be directed (by the media, for example) to contact or visit the centre so that a massive influx of enquiries at hospitals may be avoided. The next-of-kin would then be able to enquire as to their loved one's location and be directed to the relevant hospital.

Unidentified patients (unconscious or deceased) may present as a challenge during a chaotic major incident response. However, their identification may be expedited as follows:

- Digital photographs may be taken of victims and sent to the centralised database. All enquiries regarding missing persons may then be directed to the central database and identification facilitated at this point. In large-scale incidents, the photographs may even be placed on a restricted internet site so that controlled access may be available for persons located some distance from the incident.
- Where digital photographs may not be able to be taken, preprinted patient identity cards and patient enquiry cards may assist in reunification. Preprinted patient identity cards should be available at all emergency centres (ideally located within the hospitals' major incident pre-prepared supplies and folders). In case of unidentified unconscious or deceased persons, the identity card should be completed as soon as possible at the treating hospital, listing all identifying features, such as sex, height, weight, estimated age, dental features, birthmarks or tattoos, clothing details (type and colours) and any other identifying features. The information should then be forwarded to the centralised major incident centre so that the information may be entered into the database. Public enquirers, on the other hand, should then be asked to complete the patient enquiry cards on their arrival at the major incident centre. Information can then be compared and matched so that positive identification of individuals may be facilitated.

Key point: **Ensure that you are aware of the system your community utilises in identifying unidentified persons involved in a major incident. Enter this information into your Major Incident Plan.**

A large percentage of patients who have been involved in a major incident will be discharged from the emergency centre. Although the reception phase may appear to be chaotic at times, efficient patient discharge will assist in creating greater surge capacity as well as reducing the patients' trauma of the event.

Key point: **Discharge from a hospital in a major incident requires structured planning to ensure that administrative, clinical and emotional support processes are addressed. Survivors and discharged patients must be reunited with relatives and receive appropriate care.**

3.9   Equipment

Hospitals are complex facilities that may be the weak link in the major incident response system due to their failure to plan. Because equipment needed for major incidents is often redundant until needed, needs constant maintenance, is expensive and generates no revenue, it is difficult to get hospital administrators to understand the need for the expenditure.

Hospitals are among the first institutions to be affected by a major incident, either internal or external, and this places a very heavy workload on its services. Almost all hospitals are unable to acquire and deploy the resources that may be needed to respond appropriately to large-scale major incidents. Therefore it is imperative that, when planning for a major incident, particular attention is paid to critical elements in the hospital, such as emergency exits, fire detection and suppression systems, electricity and generator systems, the water supply system, the medical gas and vacuum systems and the communication systems. If these critical elements have not been maintained and incorporated into the hospital's planned response, the institution may not be able to provide care to existing patients or surge patients during major incidents.

Preparedness for a major incident involves purchasing essential equipment required to orchestrate an appropriate response. Equipment to enable staff to function in a major incident response is essential, and will denote the institution's commitment to preparedness. It is essential that the hospital staff also have an understanding of the scope and availability of essential equipment for a planned structured response.

Most major-incident planners are aware that, while it is impossible to keep all the equipment and supplies needed for every major incident a hospital has to deal with, there are some essential basics that need to be purchased, while the rest should be planned regionally or collectively so that capacity is available and can be accessed if needed. Some of the essential hospital equipment has been listed in the following sections. It is by no means a complete list, but offers practical advice to hospital planners and can be added to as needed.

General equipment

Most hospitals maintain a disaster or major incident storeroom, with equipment and stock for a major incident. Most often, the quantity of stock is determined by arbitrary guidelines. As a rule of thumb, major incident storerooms should provide the stock the emergency centre requires from the time of activation of the Major Incident Plan until the main supply line (pharmacy or medical store) can deliver the required stock to the department. Based on the number of bays that can be utilised (surge capacity), the quantities can be calculated and then stockpiled. Rotation of stock is critical to ensure that stock does not expire.

Additional job cards

All services or medical institutions should have at least four full duplicate job card systems available for additional staff usage or for use in areas that are not normally used as patient areas.

In the confusion of major incidents, staff often misplace their major incident job cards; these should be immediately replaced so that all staff are very clear with regard to their responsibilities. The additional sets of job cards should be stored in separate locations to address possible damage to hospital structures.

The use of the job card system also makes it easier for staff controlling areas to ensure that all required actions are being carried out.

Alternative communication devices

Communication during a major incident is one of the most important aspects of the plan, and alternative communication devices must be immediately available.

Very few institutions make plans for mass communication in their hospitals; they tend to rely on the traditional communication methods used on a day-to-day basis. It is well known that traditional methods of communication (telephones and cellphones) become unstable and unreliable during major incidents, as discussed in the section on communication.

The hospital coordination team must have alternative methods of immediately informing staff and occupants of the hospital important information, this may include megaphones (bullhorns), public address systems or even something as basic as a whistle.

Blankets

In all major incident responses, whether internal or external, additional blankets are required in the hospital. Blankets can also be used to prepare additional areas for patients to lie on in the event that the hospital runs out of physical bed space.

Because hospital blankets are often in normal use, with very few spare, it is recommended that a stock of lightweight but warm, brightly coloured blankets be purchased and stored in a major incident storage area.

The reason for the bright colour is to identify patients that have been evacuated from a hospital simply by giving them a blanket on evacuation.

Chalk

Chalk is not often remembered when planning for a major incident, but is a vital piece of equipment in instances where a hospital is being evacuated. Closing and marking the doors of areas fully evacuated will assist emergency workers who have to search the hospital. Chalk is also a valuable communication tool for other staff passing an evacuated area.

Triage tags

All hospital units should have sufficient triage tags for the patients in their unit, and all patients who are evacuated in a major incident should be triaged and counted at the door prior to evacuation. The number and colour of triage tags issued must be reported to the command centre when the unit has been evacuated. Priority 1: Red patients who cannot be evacuated are then identified again using chalk on the doors so that assistance from evacuation staff is planned and is as efficient as possible. A simple message on the door for rescue services, such as 'x 3 red x 1 staff', is vital information that can save lives. These same triage tags can be deployed to the emergency centre in the event of an external major incident.

Clipboards with pens attached

Documentation is essential in all major incident responses, but keeping a written record is not easy when staff are on the move. A simple solution such as an abundant supply of clipboards in strategic areas of the hospital allows for documentation by all staff. Although this is not life-saving equipment, the documentation of all procedures during a major incident response is vital. Boards can contain a specific colour of paper used only for major incident recording, and the boards can be hung in strategic places so that any staff member wishing to document needs only to find the next board. Important messages can also be placed on the boards if communication systems are not functional.

Regular collection of all completed records and the collation of the information at the command centre or even after the major incident will prove invaluable for the hospital coordination team.

Emergency lighting systems

Emergency lighting systems should be available in all hospital units, in the event of a total power failure. These units can be placed either on the walls, or floors of the institution. Portable lighting that can be worn on the head by staff should also be purchased, and is preferable to hand-held lighting systems. By wearing the light source on the head, staff are then able to function in the dark using both hands. Emergency lighting of all evacuation routes is also paramount for every healthcare institution.

Extension cords

One of the least-considered essential items for a hospital major incident equipment list are extension cords and multi plugs. These items are essential when supplying external power to essential units, such as theatre and intensive care.

Portable generators

Although all hospitals are required to have generator back-up in the event of a power failure, generators are only machines and can also break down. This may place critical areas in the hospital in very difficult situations. A portable generator that can be placed right outside a critical unit, such as ICU or theatre, may provide the emergency support needed until the restoration of emergency power to the hospital.

In the event of an evacuation, portable generators can also be used outside the hospital to supply power to vital equipment, such as incubators, or even lighting to the area of evacuation.

Mattresses

Lightweight foam mattresses are always needed for both internal and external major incident responses, and, like the blanket purchases, are essential for any major incident. If purchased with handles, as found on most camping mattresses, they can also be used to drag patients out of the hospital during an evacuation (or even to carry lightweight patients).

Hand-held radios

The provision of radios represents the most important budget spend for any institution that is serious about its preparation for major incidents. Without adequate communication, the command and control function of major incident response is impossible. This has been confirmed in many post-incident reports, which highlight the fact that an inability to communicate is one of the main causes of failure to execute an adequate response.

When purchasing radios, expert advice must be obtained to ensure that the units are adequate for the needs of the institution. Hospitals that purchase hand-held radios often forget to purchase a base station for the command centre; a base station improves the quality and area of communication and eliminates any dead spots. Headsets for operational staff are also essential, as they cut out unnecessary noise and allow staff to work and listen to instructions at the same time, also freeing up both hands for staff to continue working.

Bringing the radios out in the event of a major incident is also problematic, as staff are then unsure of how they operate, and their role in the communication cascade. It is thus recommended that the radios be permanently installed in all functional units. The hospital can then adopt the policy of a radio day once a week, allowing staff to become comfortable with the use of the radios when not under pressure. Equipment for use in major incidents should always be purchased with adequate maintenance cover, replacement contracts and training commitments.

Staff identification tabards

All major incident staff with command and control functions should be identified by wearing brightly coloured emergency vests. The role of each staff member must be clearly visible on the vest. This makes the command and control function of a major incident much easier, as there is no confusion regarding the command roles. Staff then know from whom to take instructions, and to whom to report matters.

Staff identification cards

All other staff working in the hospital should be issued with a major incident identification card. These cards can be colour-coded according to qualification and role. This system helps to ensure that staff are in the areas to which they are allocated, and that only authorised personnel are in the institution during a major incident response. It also makes the job of the security teams much easier when only authorised staff are in critical areas.

Stair chairs

In all hospitals or institutions from which people or patients have to be evacuated down stairs, there should be a sufficient numbers of stair chairs. This prevents staff from having to carry patients down stairs with the potential risk of falling and injury to both the patients and staff. During a major incident, stair chairs may also be used to move patients from lower floors to wards in the event of a power failure that renders lifts useless.

Surge capacity hospital inventory list

A simple but essential piece of equipment for a major incident response is an inventory list of all equipment in the hospital. This vital information can be used when trying to manage patients either being evacuated from the hospital or being admitted to the hospital.

Major incident command centre equipment

In order to run an efficient command and control system, the hospital coordination team should have a dedicated store of essential equipment; this can either be in a dedicated centre or in a portable system that can be moved where needed. Listed below are some of the essential pieces of equipment:

- Portable phones that can be plugged into any phone line in any command centre (If a dedicated command centre is being used, provision should be made for at least four dedicated major incident lines, four data lines and a fax line.);
- Portable computer;
- Printer;
- Data projector;
- Notice boards (white boards);
- Staff identification tags;
- Hospital plans.

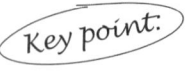 **To enable a hospital to address a major incident, sufficient equipment and stock is required. To ensure that equipment and stock is functional, rotation is essential.**

3.10 Training and exercises

All hospitals require a well-prepared major incident management plan, but, for it to be effective, the plan must be disseminated to the persons who will need to implement it when the incident strikes. Typically, though, few parties will voluntarily read a hefty written plan. Training, therefore, is probably the most critical aspect in preparation for major incident management in the hospital.

All hospital personnel require varied degrees of training in the major incident plan, so that they are absolutely clear as to their potential role when major incidents occur. Major incident management must be seen as a collaborative effort by all personnel, incorporating all hospital personnel, clinical and non-clinical. All staff should receive training, not as a once-off exercise, but continuously at predetermined intervals. All attendance of such training should be documented at all times.

Hospitals should have an active major incident management committee to take ownership of preparedness and management. The committee should include managers from all services, including administration, nursing, emergency medicine, pharmaceutical, infection control/risk management, human resources and public relations. It is this committee that should ensure that all personnel are kept abreast of the hospital's response plan, as well as lessons learned from previous hospital incident responses. For training to be successful, it is imperative that hospital management understands the importance, and buys into the concept, of continuous major incident management training.

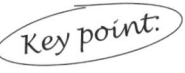 **Successful implementation of major incident management training requires a hospital management team's understanding of the following:**
- **The importance of major incident management;**
- **The pivotal role that senior management should fulfil;**
- **How an incident may affect the daily hospital operations.**

Effective training encompasses preparation, and should include:

- Analysing the environment and/or community in which the hospital is situated, so as to assist in developing appropriate training material. (This should, however, not deter the institution from taking the all-hazard approach.) Collaboration with community emergency and municipal services is extremely important in major incident preparedness, and will assist in managing incidents in a more coordinated fashion.
- Defining the target audience within the hospital, and the content that they should be taught. Hospital management may, for example, not be required to know how to use personal protective equipment (PPE) and perform decontamination, and may therefore only require knowledge thereof and to ensure that these facilities are available.
- Adapting training content to meet the training needs of the different job categories within the hospital.

Major incident management training within a hospital should focus on developing the following key competencies in healthcare workers (clinical and non-clinical):

- Recognising a major incident and implementing initial actions;
- Application of the principles of major incident management;
- Demonstration of major incident safety principles;
- Understanding of the hospital's major incident management plan, including the activation thereof, declaration as well as stand-down criteria;
- Demonstration of effective communications;
- Understanding of the major incident command and control system and the individual's role therein;
- Demonstration of the knowledge and skills required to fulfil each individual's role during an incident.

Competencies involve a combination of specific knowledge, attitudes and skills, and so major incident training does not simply imply knowledge transfer, but the development of skills to manage a major incident effectively.

Major incident training strategies

Orientation programmes

All orientation programmes for new employees should include an introduction to major incident management in the hospital. Clinical as well as non-clinical personnel should be oriented to managing internal incidents (such as fire or bomb threats), including reporting procedures and evacuation procedures and routes. External incidents that require an extraordinary response should be introduced, and personnel should be alerted to the fact that they become involved in one way or another. More in-depth orientation to new personnel's departmental responsibilities (during major incidents) may also be included during the orientation phase.

Formal major incident management courses

Formalised major incident management courses available include:

- *MIMMS:* Major Incident Medical Management and Support – the practical approach at the scene (focus is on the on-scene management);
- *HMIMMS:* Hospital Major Incident Medical Management and Support – the practical approach in the hospital (focus is on in-hospital personnel, both clinical and non-clinical).

Specialised training

A hospital-specific major incident management training course should be designed, and in-service training should be an ongoing process. The hospital's major incident management committee should review the incident plan at scheduled periods and accordingly ensure that all staff are up to date with appropriate training. It is essential that training content should be adapted as required after periodic major incident plan reviews and incident response/ exercise audits.

One extremely important principle of major incident management is that individuals' roles should closely reflect their normal roles and responsibilities. Having to perform new roles in times of crisis, especially when performed infrequently, creates much stress and will probably lead to failure.

Certain aspects in the major incident response are critical to its success, and so specialised training in the following aspects are recommended:

- Command and control;
- Triage;
- Press/media handling.

Mock drills

The benefits of performing exercises in major incident management are great. Organisations benefit by developing their emergency response and management capabilities, as well as being able to identify weaknesses and vulnerabilities. Individuals benefit by practising their individual roles within a safe environment, and teams are able to enhance teamwork and unification. While planning for a mock drill, key role-players should be informed of the intended exercise so as to prevent panic and chaos throughout the organisation.

Multi-agency exercises, where several emergency services are involved, are frequently seen at airports. Similar simulated exercises may be held in-hospital, where a large number of patients inundate the facility to practise and test its preparedness.

Drills should be conducted at least annually. They may be planned as well as unplanned, and need not always be protracted multi-agency exercises. Large-scale exercises may be conducted to practise community services' coordination, whereas smaller, department-specific exercises may be held to practise specific aspects of major incident management.

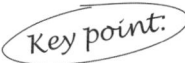 **When a disaster/major incident drill is planned:**
- **There should be clear objective(s);**
- **Management should define exactly what will be practised;**
- **A staff debriefing should be held.**

Communication problems are frequently encountered in large-scale major incidents. Research shows that hospital major-incident drills seldom include communication failure, and therefore drills should include practising using multiple modes of communication, such as cellular telephones, two-way radios, hospital public announcement systems and runners. Simple activation exercises may be held whereby the hospital switchboard is informed of an impending major incident and the communication telephone cascade tested through all departments and parties simply documenting the time of the message reaching them.

Simulated exercises allow practice in other aspects which may not be encountered all too frequently, such as:

- Management of a paediatric major incident;
- Wearing specialised personal protective clothing and learning the correct technique of donning such attire;
- Patient decontamination, as well as personnel decontamination procedures, in cases of personal protective clothing having been worn.

In order to evaluate training effectiveness, observers may be employed to study the simulation drill. However, they should be discreet, so as to decrease performance anxiety among participants. The drill may even be recorded on video for replay and evaluation and debriefing purposes. Observers should observe and document the following, which then serve as discussion points in the post-drill facilitated debriefing:

- Successes;
- Deficiencies requiring improvement;

- Further resources/equipment required;
- Alterations of the plan that are required.

Aspects requiring amendments in the major incident plan should be noted, and the plan adjusted accordingly as soon as possible.

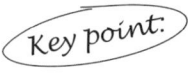 **Major incident plans should be tested and stressed so that weaknesses are identified that require revisions and improvements to the plan.**

Tabletop exercises

Exercises in major incident management need not always be simulated drills. Simulated exercises can be costly in terms of time, labour and infrastructure. For this reason, tabletop exercises have become extremely helpful in major incident training.

A tabletop exercise is simply a major incident drill on paper, whereby a scenario is given and a small group of people work around a table to discuss their management of the situation. The tabletop exercise may include a basic floor plan of the hospital or a fictitious hospital – such as that used in the HMIMMS course – as well as staff and patients (represented by cards or figures). The facilitator then takes the group through the phases of the response and the hospital floor plan is reconfigured for a major incident.

The group may consist of various staff from different departments or from a single department. Where the group consists of a multi-disciplinary team, all aspects of the response (clinical and non-clinical) may be discussed. Tabletops are powerful ways of illustrating and solving complex problems in major incident plans, and are particularly useful in demonstrating command, control and communication. Tabletop exercises are therefore crucial in training, in particular, the hospital command structure.

Computer-based simulations

A hospital's surge capacity and readiness for major incident management can be assessed through computer-based simulation exercises. Simulations such as these assist in identifying bottlenecks that may limit surge capacity.

'False' or 'stand-down' calls

Situations in which hospitals may be placed on stand-by for potentially receiving major incident survivors should be used as opportunities to practise the implementation of the major incident plan.

Hospitals, too, may become victims of major incidents and may someday require complete evacuation. Training for major incident management therefore should not only be limited to managing incoming incidents.

Training is an ongoing process. Employees should be kept updated on their roles and responsibilities through electronic mail, web page information, newsletters, posters and exercises. Complacency may lead to deleterious effects, and should therefore be avoided at all costs.

Rural communities are advised to focus training efforts on facets that may improve the hospital's response to any major incident. These aspects include command and control, communication and inter-agency cooperation. All forms of training, including tabletops, simulations or drills, should include as many local emergency services within the community, as smaller hospitals may require a community-wide response to a surge in major incidents.

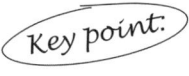 **A well-prepared plan will only succeed if staff are made aware of it through training.**

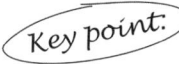 **Through formal and informal training and orientation, the readiness of an institution and its staff is ensured.**

Summary

Hospital response to a major incident or major incident is dependent upon adequate planning, preparation and training. Staff awareness of their role in the response plan is essential; ideally, they should do their normal daily functions in the event of a major incident.

3.11 Resources

Ciotone GR (ed.). *Major incident medicine*. 3rd edition. Philadelphia: Mosby Elsevier; 2006.

Powers R, Daily E. *Major incident nursing international*. Melbourne: Cambridge University Press; 2010.

International Critical Incident Stress Foundation Inc – www.icisf.org

3.12 References

1. Milsten A. Hospital response to acute-onset major incidents: A review. *Prehospital and Disaster Medicine* Jan–Mar 2000;15(1).
2. Nager AL, Khanna JD. Emergency department surge: models and practical implications. *Journal of Trauma: Injury, Infection and Critical Care* Aug 2009;67(2):S96–S99.
3. Hick J, Hanfling D, Burstein J, *et al*. Health care facility and community strategies for patient care surge capacity. *Annals of Emergency Medicine*. 2004;44:253–61.
4. Agency for Healthcare Research and Quality. Addressing surge capacity in a mass casualty event: surge capacity and health systems preparedness. Transcription of Web Conference; 2004.
5. Louis B. Allen Associates. Allen Seminar for Management. 1992.
6. Carley S, Mackway-Jones K. *Major incident medical management and support: the practical approach in the hospital*. Oxford: Blackwell Publishing Ltd; 2005.
7. Chaffee MW, Oster NS. The role of hospitals in major incident. In: Ciotone GR (ed.). *Major incident medicine*. Philadelphia: Mosby Elsevier; 2006.
8. Hick JL, Koenig KL, Barbish D, Bey TA. Surge capacity concepts for health care facilities: the CO-S-TR model for initial incident assessment. *Disaster Medicine and Public Health Preparedness* Sept 2008;2(Suppl 1):S 51–7.

9. Ennis-Holcombe K. Major incident communications. In: Ciotone G. (ed). *Major incident medicine*. Philadelphia: Mosby Elsevier; 2006. pp. 229–232.

10. Advanced Life Support Group. *Major incident medical management and support: the practical approach on scene*. 2nd ed. London: BMJ Books; 2002.

11. Budd C. Informatics and telecommunications in major incidents. In: Ciotone G. (ed.). *Major incident medicine*. Philadelphia: Mosby Elsevier; 2006. pp. 130–38.

12. Giannou C, Baldam M. *War surgery*. Geneva: International Committee of the Red Cross; 2009.

13. Advanced trauma life support for physicians. American College of Surgeons. 2008.

14. Bruijns SR, Wallis LA, Burch VC. A prospective evaluation of the Cape triage score in the emergency department of an urban public hospital in South Africa. *Emergency Medicine Journal*. July 2008;25(7):398–402.

15. Boffard KD (ed.) *Manual of definitive surgical trauma care*. London: Hodder Arnold/ International Association for Surgical Trauma and Intensive Care; 2003.

16. Convertino VA, Ryan KL, Rickards CA, Salinas J, McManus JG, Cooke WH, *et al*. Physiological and medical monitoring for en-route care of combat casualties. *Journal of Trauma*. April 2008;64(4 Suppl):S342–53.

17. Ferreira FL, Bota DP, Bross A, Melot C, Vincent JL. Serial evaluation of the SOFA score to predict outcome in critically ill patients. *Journal of the American Medical Association*. 2001;286:1754–58.

18. Christian MD, Hawryluck L, Wax RS, Cook T, Lazar NM, Herridge MS, *et al*. Development of a triage protocol for critical care during an influenza pandemic. *Canadian Medical Association Journal*. 2006;175(11):1377–81.

19. Vincent JL, Moreno R, Takala J, Willatts S, De Mendonca A, Bruining H, *et al*. The SOFA (Sepsis-related Organ Failure Assessment) score to describe organ dysfunction/failure. *Intensive Care Medicine*. July 1996;22(7):707–10.

20. Alm AM, Gao T, White D. Pervasive patient tracking for mass casualty incident response. *Journal of the American Medical Informatics Association* 2006:842.

21. Gao T, Hauenstein LK, Alm A, Crawford D, Sims CK, Husain A, *et al*. Vital signs monitoring and patient tracking over a wireless network. *Johns Hopkins APL Technical Digest* 2006;27(1):66–74.

22. McBride M. Wireless patient tracking in major incident management. *Health Management Technology*. July 2006; 9–12.

23. Buono CJ, Chan TC, Killeen J, Huang R, Brown S, Liu F, *et al*. Comparison of the effectiveness of wireless electronic tracking devices versus traditional paper systems to track victims in a large scale major incident. In AMIA Symposium Proceedings; 2007. p. 886.

24. Pate BL. Identifying and tracking major incident victims. State-of-the-art review. *Family and Community Health* 2008;31(1):23–4.

25. Hattingh SP. A model for training of peer debriefers in the emergency serices. Dissertation. Pretoria: University of South Africa; 2003.

26. Marcus EH. Major incident mental health services. 2000. Available from: www.ispub.com/journal/the_internet_journal_of_rescue_and_major_

incident_medicine/volume_1_number_2_58/article/major incident_mental_ health_services.html. Accessed 10 January 2010.

27. Mitchell JT. Critical incident stress debriefing (CISD). Available from: www. info-trauma.org/flash/media-e/mitchellCriticalIncidentStressDebriefing.pdf. [Online]. [cited 2010 Jan 10. Accessed 10 January 2010.

28. Mitchell JT. Maintaining the balance: a strategic support system for operations personnel and survivors. 2009. Available from: mediccom.org/public/tadmat/ training/NDMS/CISM.pdf. Accessed 10 December 2009.

29. Middaugh DJ. Maintaining management during major incident. *Medical and Surgical Nursing*. 2003;12(2):125–7.

30. Noji EK, Kelen GD. Major incident medicine services. Available from: www. accessmedicine.com/content.aspx?aID=585376. Accessed 11 December 2009.

31. Brandenburg MA, Watkins SM, Brandenburg KL, Schieche C. Operating Child-ID: Reunifying children with their legal guardians after Hurricane Katrina. *Major Incident Management and Response* 2007;31(3):277–87.

32. Weeks SM. Mobilisation of a nursing community after a major incident. *Perspectives in Psychiatric Care* 2007;43(1):22–9.

33. Kelen GD, Kraus CK, McCarthy ML, Hsu EB, Li G, Scheulen JJ, *et al*. Inpatient disposition classification for creation of hospital surge capacity: a multiphase study. *The Lancet* 2006;368:1984–90.

34. Pan American Health Organization, World Health Organization, ICRC. Management of dead bodies after major incidents. Washington, DC: Pan American Health Organization; 2006.

35. Hsu EB, Thomas TL, Bass EB, Whyne D, Kelen GD, Green GG. Healthcare worker competencies for major incident training. 2006. Available from: doi:10.1186/1472-6920-6-19. Accessed 29 November 2009.

36. Rogers B, Lawhorn E. Major incident preparedness: occupational and enviromental health professionals' response to Hurricanes Katrina and Rita. *American Association of Occupational Health Nurses Journal* 2007;55(5):197–207.

37. Wise GI. Preparing for major incident: a way of developing community relationships. *Major incident Management and Response* 2007;5:14–17.

38. Danna D, Bernard M, Jones J, Mathews P. Improvement in major incident planning and direction for nursing management. *The Journal of Nursing Administration* 2009; 39(10):423–31.

39. Fahlgren TL, Drenkard KN. Healthcare system major incident preparedness. Part 2. *The Journal of Nursing Administration* 2002;32(1):531–7.

40 Yale New Haven Health Center for Emergency Preparedness and Major Incident Response. Drills and Exercises. Available from: www.yalenewhavenhealth.org/ emergency/drills/index.html. Accessed 27 December 2009.

41. Fendya ML. When major incident strikes – care considerations for pediatric patients. *Journal of Trauma Nursing* 2006;13(4):161–5.

42. Douglas V. Developing major incident management modules: a collaborative approuch. *British Journal of Nursing* 2007;16(9):526–9.

43. Patillo MM. Mass casualty nursing course. *Nurse Educator* 2003;28(6):271–5.

44. Manley WG, Furbee PM, Coben JH, Smyth SK, Summers DE, Althouse RC, *et al*. Realities of major incident preparedness in rural hospitals. *Major Incident Management and Response* 2006;4(3):80–7.
45. Bernard M, Mathews PR. Evacuation of a maternal-newborn area during Hurricane Katrina. *American Journal of Maternal and Child Nursing* 2008;33(4):213–23.

4

Internal Major Incidents in the Hospital Environment

T Ligthelm, T Hardcastle and W Lubinga

Objectives

By the end of this chapter, the reader will be able to:

- optimise functioning of a healthcare facility during a disruption of essential supplies and services;
- maintain optimal functioning of a healthcare facility during an interruption of human resources;
- calculate the surge capacity of a healthcare facility;
- know how to react judiciously to a bomb threat;
- ensure optimum patient and staff safety during a bomb threat;
- optimise reaction to a fire in a hospital through effective command, basic fire fighting and coordinated evacuation;
- understand why hospital evacuation planning is necessary;
- know the indications for, and types of, hospital evacuation;
- understand the challenges and risks of working in the operation suite environment during an internal major incident;
- understand how major incidents can affect the function of the operation suite;
- understand the challenges and risks of working in the ICU environment during a major incident;
- understand the challenges of dealing with major incidents on specific hospital units;
- understand the challenges of dealing with special patient groups;
- understand the basics of isolation units and the complexities of moving patients with communicable disease during hospital evacuation.

4.1 Internal major incidents

Various internal incidents can disrupt the functioning of a healthcare facility and threaten the safety of patients and staff.

Planned versus unplanned disruption of functioning

Often, the factor disrupting the functioning of the facility is part of a planned action, allowing sufficient time to plan for the situation. Examples of this type of incident are major maintenance work to the oxygen supply to the hospital, requiring the discontinuation of piped oxygen supply throughout the total complex. When this is known in advance, the facility can activate its action plans well in advance and mitigate the effect of the cut-off on patient care by providing alternative sources of oxygen, such as cylinders in critical areas, and limiting the number of patients in the facility by stopping elective interventions. This will normally be addressed without any major discomfort to patients or loss of life.

However, when a disruption in oxygen is due to a burst main supply line from the oxygen bank to the hospital, the same actions need to be taken, but with no lead time or preparation, and will most probably cause loss of life.

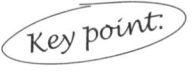 **Disruption in essential services is often planned or predictable due to maintenance or other reasons. This requires pre-planning to be able to keep a healthcare facility functioning optimally.**

Preparing for a planned disruption in essential services

As soon as the hospital is informed, or becomes aware, of an incident that may disrupt essential services, pre-planning must start. It is essential that planning is done as comprehensively as possible to allow for various complications that may develop within the system, and to compile additional action plans if indicated timelines are exceeded.

Limiting the dependency load within the facility

As soon as information is received on a planned disruption in services, an evaluation must be done to determine the impact on the functioning. If the impact of the planned action is significant, the most effective mitigating factor to consider is reducing the dependency load within the facility by reducing the number of patients within the facility. This is normally done by postponing elective surgery and placing limitations on admissions well in advance. To ensure cooperation from all clinical role-players, it is essential to communicate effectively, highlighting the reasons for the limitations and indicating the planned duration. A second option would be to transfer high-dependence patients, as a precaution, to other facilities.

Assessing the remaining dependence load

After implementing measures to limit new admissions and transferring high-dependency cases, it is necessary to assess and classify the remaining dependency load within the facility. This is done by classifying all the remaining patients into a simple classification system, providing management with clear options to implement should complications develop with the planned action.

Classifying dependence load

The first step would be to classify patients, indicating the impact of the disruption. For example, in case of a discontinuation of piped oxygen supply, classify patients indicating dependency on oxygen (see Table 4.1).

Table 4.1: Example of a dependency classification system for oxygen

Red: Totally depending, will not survive without continuous supply.

Orange: Partially dependent and can be supported with an oxygen generator or cylinder.

Yellow: Those that may require oxygen only occasionally, such as asthma patients, and for which a few cylinders may be placed centrally as an emergency resource.

Green: No dependency on oxygen.

With this information available, and updated continuously until the time the oxygen is turned off, management can now determine in advance, for example, to transfer all the Red patients to another hospital, or plan that those patients can be supplied for four hours with cylinders; but if the repair is not completed within the timeline an action plan will be activated to transfer these patients to predetermined and ready facilities in another hospital.

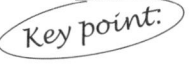 **Through a proper planning process, the dependency on a service can be classified and mitigating measures taken to address the requirements.**

4.2   Essential supplies disruption

A healthcare facility relies on numerous supplies to keep it functioning effectively. Although a disruption in the supply of some utilities may be uncomfortable, the disruption in certain essential supplies or utilities will totally disrupt the effective functioning of the facility and may threaten the safety of patients. This section will highlight some action plans to address these internal disasters, when the disruption is unplanned and uncompensated without the resources readily available to the facility. The term 'utility outages' are often used to describe these situations.

It is not possible to describe all possible essential supply disruptions that can occur within a healthcare facility. A proper risk assessment is recommended to identify the risks for the facility and then to compile flexible action plans that are able to accommodate various emergencies. Some of these essential supplies are electrical power, oxygen and medical gas, steam, suction, telephones, water and sewage. These are discussed in detail in the sections that follow.

Electrical power

Most modern hospitals are completely dependent on electrical power for effective and safe functioning. Although most hospitals are by law forced to have a back-up power system, these systems often supply only specific high-dependency areas or/and can also fail at a critical stage. It is therefore essential to compile action plans to address a complete power failure, especially over a prolonged period of time.

It is essential to identify – in advance, in a similar grading system – the dependency on electricity of all units within the facility. This must be done in collaboration with the clinical staff of the various units and can be graded using a colour-coded dependence grid or any other easily understandable system. An example is shown in Table 4.2:

Table 4.2: Example of dependency classification for electricity

Red: Completely dependency on electrical power, and loss of life will occur if not provided. An example is an intensive care unit with electrically driven ventilators.

Orange: Dependency on electricity, and loss of life will occur if not provided within 10 minutes after disruption. An example is an orthopaedic theatre complex in which non-major orthopaedic procedures are done with gas-driven anaesthetic machines.

Yellow: Dependency on electricity for effective functioning, but loss of life will not occur if not restored. An example is a general nursing unit with post-operative patients.

Green: No dependence on electricity at all: for example, an outpatient department that only operates during office hours and has adequate natural light.

If the emergency power supply of the facility does not supply the total complex, it is essential to identify and mark all power outlets supplied by the emergency supply. The areas covered by the emergency back-up must be compared with the colour-coded assessment of the needs, and, if required, adjustments to the distribution must be made. Emergency generators each have a specific capacity, and it is important for management to determine the capacity of the back-up generators and the current utilisation, in order to determine surge capacity in the system.

Some hospitals have a double back-up system, where the emergency power generating system is backed up by a battery supply, lasting a specific time. These facilities can differ from a small uninterrupted power supply (UPS) unit for a specific piece of equipment to large battery banks that provide full electrical power to sections of the facility. This type of supply normally supplies only very high-risk areas such as cardio-thoracic theatres. Management must have a clear picture of which areas are supplied with emergency power, and which areas do have an additional back-up system.

Normally, all areas classified as red in the above classification (see Table 4.2) will have at least emergency power supply. If some of these areas are not supplied, action plans must be made, to be activated immediately if a power failure occurs. For example, if an intensive care unit cannot be supplied with emergency power, bag-valve-mask units must be mounted with a battery torch at each bed. If a power failure occurs, the standard drill must be for additional nursing staff working in a low-risk area to run to the unit to assist with the manual ventilation of patients.

Action plans must also be compiled to optimally support the functioning of all the other orange and yellow areas. The nursery may be classified orange, as it is not possible to feed the babies in the dark. An action plan of mounting battery lights that provide adequate light for one hour in the nursery will change its classification to yellow. A second action plan to move the babies in the nursery within that one hour to the neonatal intensive care unit, which does have emergency power for temporary care, will change the nursery's classification to green.

Critical areas that must be assessed for the impact of a power failure include the following:

- Central vacuum pumps supplying piped vacuum systems, including the electrical control valves of these systems.
- Oxygen banks, oxygen generator plants, valves and alarm systems.
- Telephone switchboards normally have a limited-time battery supply/UPS system. (A back-up plan is essential to maintain communication within the facility.)
- Electrical doors, especially at the emergency department ambulance entrance. Knowledge of a manual override capability needs to be part of the action plans.
- Elevators/lifts: often, when the power fails, the hospital elevators are lowered automatically to ground level and open, or function at half-speed on the emergency power supply. A system must be in place to limit elevators functioning on emergency power for emergency use only, such as theatre cases, and to prevent visitors and staff from using them.
- Blood, frozen food or specimen storage: if not supplied by emergency power, isolation measures must be implemented to retain temperature for as long as possible. Some large hospitals' frozen food storage facilities are equipped with nitrogen tanks that can be activated manually to maintain temperature in case of a total power failure.
- Autoclaves: often, steam-driven autoclaves can be manually operated in the event of a power failure.
- Intercom and alarm systems, including patient bedside alarms, fire alarms, intercom systems for emergency warnings and evacuation alarms. All of these utilities must be covered in action plans to substitute the service with a manual-operated system or battery-driven system in case of a complete power failure.
- Computer-driven admission systems.

The total electrical consumption of the facility under normal working conditions must be determined. This will give management an indication of the emergency generator capacity to run the facility optimally if a network failure occurs. It is then possible to enter into an agreement with private generator-supply companies or government institutions to provide a mobile generator plant to the facility within an agreed period of time – for example, within six hours – to supply electricity to the facility during a long-term network failure. It is necessary to determine the technical detail of connecting such a generator plant to the existing cable network, and to isolate the generated supply from the network supply. If an additional mobile generator unit is planned, it is essential to be able to isolate the areas supplied by these units, and to prevent staff from switching on circuits which cannot be supplied by the additional facilities. This requires detailed pre-planning, including safety measures to protect staff, patients and equipment from power surges.

The positioning of the switch network and transformers in a facility needs careful consideration. In many situations, these critical pieces of electrical equipment are positioned in the basement of the building, which is normally the first area to be flooded. If housed at ground or below-ground level, the risk for flooding needs to be assessed with technical expert advice. If the risk exists, plans must be formulated to, for example, encase this equipment in a watertight compartment, or move it to higher ground (which is normally a very expensive challenge).

The availability of adequate emergency lighting, down to as basic as a flashlight with spare batteries per unit, is the absolute foundation of action plans for internal disasters. This must include battery-operated exit signs, stair lights and basic roof lighting throughout the facility.

Various other options are available to mitigate an electrical outage:

- Alternative heat sources for incubators, such as chemical heat-generating mattresses;
- Gas-driven emergency ventilators, as a short-term solution, to ventilate patients during a power failure.

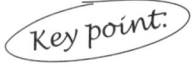 **Key point:** Evaluating the needs for electricity in advance helps management to keep the facility functioning at the best possible level if the supply is disrupted. Back-up systems need to be tested and evaluated on a regular basis, and emergency interventions planned for situations where back-ups fail.

Oxygen and medical gas supplies

Most modern healthcare facilities are totally dependent on the supply of oxygen and medical gases to render advanced care. A total failure in these supplies to an acute care facility will cause a serious internal disaster situation. Most modern facilities are neither equipped nor knowledgeable enough anymore to operate with cylinders or mobile tanks and regulators. A grading system similar to that in Table 4.2, to determine dependency on oxygen and other gases dependency, is suggested.

Depending on legislation in the country, various prescripts indicate what back-up gas supplies must normally be available on anaesthesia machines for use in operating theatres. These prescripts must be adhered to, regularly tested and all tests recorded for possible enquiries. As a basic requirement, an emergency oxygen cylinder, providing at least one hour's oxygen supply, must be immediately available on every anaesthesia machine.

In areas where patients are ventilated, alternative sources for oxygen and, if required, other medical gases must be planned. Manual ventilation capability with a bag-valve-mask will be the first line of defence. Depending on the type of ventilator used, additional oxygen must be planned. This can be cylinder-based, liquid oxygen tanks, oxygen concentrators using room air, or oxygen generators using chemical processes to generate oxygen. It is seldom possible to have this supply directly next to every bed in the ICU facility, due to size, space and maintenance requirements. Many ICU facilities are equipped with an emergency gas bank and an automatic switch-over system for when the main supply fails. These are very useful systems, but often the switch-over mechanism is electrically driven, which may require a manual override ability or a back-up power supply. However, the availability of an appropriate-size bag-valve-mask at the bed of each ventilated patient is non-negotiable.

It is necessary for management to do the following:

- Have clear data on the average need for gases, to be able to request emergency supplies in an external disaster situation.
- Be able to calculate the time the facility can function on its emergency oxygen supply before restocking will be required.
- Plan action drills for additional staff to assist in critical areas to ventilate patients manually.
- Other high-dependency areas, such as pulmonology, geriatric and internal medicine departments, must be identified and action plans formulated to supply these facilities as soon as possible with cylinder or tank supplies. It is often possible to isolate these high-dependency sections within the facility from the larger network of pipes, using cut-off valves, and then supply that isolated high-need area from a mobile tank. In chronic facilities, the use of chemical oxygen generator units may be a solution.
- The use of tanks with a multi-regulator, often used by the emergency services at a disaster scene, is also a possibility, on condition that all the patients can be brought into one venue. This is often the solution for neonatal and premature baby care units.
- The need to have a central supply of cylinders with regulators (or tanks) for an emergency during the oxygen outage must be planned. This can be part of the emergency trolley or crash-cart per floor of the building.
- Identify suppliers of small-volume oxygen equipment in the area and enter into emergency supply agreements to obtain additional equipment at short notice during a failure of the main supply. This often requires pre-planning for manpower to move and connect heavy cylinders within the facility and continuously replace empty cylinders. The need to ensure the safety of mobile cylinders, and to ensure that cylinders are stored in an upright position, is emphasised.

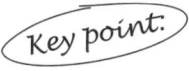 **Appreciating the need for gas supplies is a critical process to be able to introduce emergency interventions in a disruption. A basic triage and prioritisation system is used to distribute emergency supplies optimally.**

Steam supplies

Most hospitals are dependent on steam supplies for sterilisation, kitchen equipment and sometimes for cooling or heating systems. In particular, older facilities in less developed areas of the world are completely dependent on steam supplies for sterilisation and for cooking. Planning for a failure in steam kettle operations must be part of the internal disaster action plans.

Due to the high technical requirements involved in safely relaying pressurised steam through a pipe system, it has not been possible in the past to provide temporary emergency steam supplies within facilities.

It is therefore necessary to plan alternatives:

- Steam-operated autoclave sterilisation units cannot be operated at all without an external steam supply; therefore alternative methods for sterilising or disinfecting equipment need to be planned. (More modern units generate their own steam internally.) The use of mobile pressure cooker-type sterilisation pots on a gas stove, to sterilise theatre instrumentation, is a low-technology solution for the less developed parts of the world. The use of boiling is an acceptable alternative for instrumentation. However, dressing material, gowns and drapes cannot be sterilised in this way, and in a disaster situation disinfection by ironing is often the only possibility.

- Chemical sterilising solutions are commercially available, and, if not activated, often have a very long shelf life. Containers to submerge instrumentation, preferably on a removable grid, must be planned. This type of equipment can be centrally stockpiled for the total complex, but needs to be checked and, if possible, rotated regularly to ensure functionality when needed.

- Electrically driven mobile sterilisation units, often generating their own steam, are commercially available in the more developed parts of the world. The instructions from the suppliers must be kept with the unit to ensure the equipment is operated according to the manufacturer's instructions.

- The use of pre-sterilised disposable equipment is the easy-out solution for a lack of sterilisation capacity. This is, however, a very expensive solution, and seldom possible in the developing world. If used, plans must be in place to obtain these packs at short notice from suppliers.

- Cooking without steam can be impossible in certain facilities' kitchens if these are designed for steam supplies. (The same applies if the facilities are totally planned for natural gas supplies or electricity supplies.) To prepare meals, alternative solutions need to be planned. This will mainly depend on the size of the facility and the environment in which it is located. In a small facility, the use of mobile liquid gas cookers and stoves may be a solution, while in larger facilities the use of external options, such as a community centre's kitchen, may be a solution. In the developing world, the use of open fires may be the only available solution. Safety must be considered, especially with staff not used to operating alternative energy sources, such as gas.

- Cooling and/or heating systems in healthcare facilities often use steam or hot water for heating, and often use steam to operate air-conditioning chiller facilities. Depending on the climate of the area and the time of year, alternative plans need to be formulated. This risk may increase because of extreme weather conditions.

- Heating through alternative heat sources is possible, but needs pre-planned resources such as electrical heaters or gas heating systems.

- Cooling down air-conditioned buildings in a hot climate is an enormous challenge. Often, these buildings are designed with very little natural ventilation, and often without windows that can open. If it is not structurally possible to open windows, evacuation may be the only alternative.

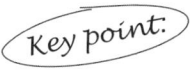 **Steam is used to drive various critical functions within a healthcare facility, and pre-planning is required to provide alternatives for those functions.**

Suction facilities

Piped, centrally operated suction systems are essential, especially for acute care and intensive care. These systems often depend on electricity to drive the central vacuum pump(s), and may fail due to mechanical defects in the system. In the event of structural damage to the facility, the piping may be damaged. Often, suction pumps are housed in the basement, and are therefore prone to flooding.

A colour grading system, similar to that used in Table 4.2, is recommended to determine the dependency of the total facility on a central suction supply.

Management must make staff aware of the position of cut-off valves that isolate a damaged area of the system, to enable the rest of the system to function.

Planning for alternative suction equipment is necessary. The most reliable alternative suction equipment remains manual-operated hand- or foot-suction devices. Although battery-driven apparatuses are available commercially, these machines have a limited battery time and then require electrical power to recharge the batteries. An extended power failure will make these machines useless.

Mobile electrically driven suction machines, with back-up power, are essential for operating theatre complexes. These machines can be stored centrally in the theatre complex and then distributed to the theatres in the event of a suction failure.

All emergency suction devices must be serviced and checked regularly.

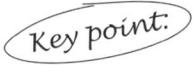 **Emergency suction capabilities include manual and electrically driven devices. Distributing the resources requires triage and prioritisation of the needs.**

Telephone outage

It is possible that a complete telephone outage can occur, affecting the healthcare facility or the surrounding area. This may be linked to an external situation, such as an earthquake, or to an internal situation caused by an external hazard such as flooding of the telephone control mechanisms. Often, a telephone outage is followed by cellphone outages due to overloading. This may leave the healthcare facility isolated, without the ability to contact outside resources.

The foundation of internal disaster planning is an effective, assessable, continuously updated database of all role-players, support agencies and staff, with their complete contact particulars, including mobile telephone numbers. To substitute for telephone outages, all physical addresses must be available so that contact can be established using messenger systems.

An effective messenger system, both internal and external (if needed), remains a foolproof solution for a communication failure. The need for additional human resources to be used as messengers needs to be appreciated and planned. Most institutions plan to use non-acute ancillary health and administrative staff as messengers – for example, occupational therapists. These can then be substituted by planned volunteers in a longer-duration situation. When an external messenger system is needed, the availability of vehicles, fuel and effective maps of the area are components that must be factored into planning.

The use of radio communication is a very effective alternative during a failure of the telephone and mobile phone network. This may include external long-distance links to community control-centre facilities, such as the fire brigade, and internal links, such as short-range mobile radios carried by all departmental heads. As a training drill to ensure skills in operating radios, some facilities in high-risk environments go so far as to actively disable their internal telephone network periodically to force staff to use radios. The use of amateur radio operators can provide the facility with a long-distance communication capability.

The use of the mass media, such as local or regional radio stations, to activate off-duty staff to report for duty is an option. This type of message, however, often causes panic and leads to a mass of volunteers also arriving at the facility, requiring pre-planning for access control before such a request is broadcast.

The availability of unlisted additional telephone lines, linked to alternative cables to the main telephone lines, has in the past often saved a facility. This can be substituted with direct magneto-type lines to the emergency services, such as the fire brigade. Particularly in developing countries with an unreliable telephone system, this type of link can be life-saving.

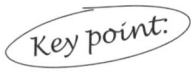 **Key point:** **Planning alternatives for telephone communication includes radio communication, intercoms and messengers. The use of alternative telephone communication, such as call boxes, must be analysed.**

Water supply failure

The water supply to the healthcare facility can be disrupted for various reasons. Depending on local legislation, most hospitals are obliged to carry an on-site emergency water reserve. It is essential that management determines the volume of the water reserve and how long it will supply normal needs. It has happened, however, that the main supply to a facility was disrupted and, by the time it was discovered, the emergency reserve was already depleted. Such a situation leaves the facility in a predicament to maintain hygiene and functional sanitation without water. A water reservoir containing enough water for 24 hours is recommended, with an alarm system to indicate any disruption in the main supply.

An action plan to substitute water supply at short notice is essential. Water can be brought in at various levels of purification, depending on suppliers and sources. In developed countries, the use of bottled water is an immediate option, while in a developing country water from a borehole may be the only source available.

Action plans must be in place for how to get water supplies to the facility. If a borehole is available on site, then the functionality of the pump, fuel for the pump and the piping are all aspects to consider.

Often, a facility's water supply functions from a reservoir on the top of the building, providing adequate pressure for systems in the building. These reservoirs are then supplied from the main water source on a continuous basis. Filling this reservoir from a borehole or water tanker is often very difficult, as it may be too high for normal pumps to pump the water into the reservoir. This often requires the use of relay-pumping by experts, often from the fire brigade, to get the water into the reservoir. This must be planned and practised to ensure that water can be pumped into the reservoir. The use of fire brigade riser installations are often of value to get water into the reservoir.

The emphasis in supplying water to a facility must be on volume rather than on purity. Basic chlorination of the borehole water in the reservoir may be sufficient to prevent transmission of any waterborne diseases. An alternative may be to pump unpurified water into the reservoir to keep the sanitation and hygiene system functioning, while providing separate purified drinking water or water purification tablets to all staff and patients. Warning notices not to drink tap water need to be pre-prepared and placed at all taps in the facility. Children, geriatric and psychiatric patients may require special measures to prevent them accidentally drinking 'polluted' water.

Emergency short-term solutions to provide water in the facility may include the use of water bunker trucks delivering water to central points around the facility and then moving containers of water to the various sections of the buildings. This may include buckets of water to flush toilets. This is an enormous, labour-intensive operation requiring pre-planning.

Although it was stated that emphasis should be placed on volume, rather than purity of water, the risk of polluting the brought-in water with dangerously contaminated containers needs to be emphasised. Often water bunker trucks are obtained from a reserve, such as used by the military. These trucks are often stored for extensive periods of time, emphasising the need to wash them out prior to use.

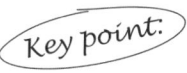 **The healthcare facility's daily water needs must be analysed in advance. The quantity of the reserve on site must be analysed and preferably coupled to an alarm system. Sources for emergency water need to be planned in advance, and the connecting of emergency supply trucks to the system should be investigated.**

Sewage system failure

Keeping a modern healthcare facility functioning with a failure in the sewage system is nearly impossible. Ground movement during earthquakes often cause underground sewage lines to be kinked and blocked. This may result in a total blockage in sewage drainage. If the blockage cannot be corrected, and alternative drainage for sewage cannot be established, evacuation of the facility must be considered. The challenge is that a situation such as an earthquake may result in the community relying on the healthcare facility to care for the victims, making evacuation nearly impossible.

The establishment of outside ground-draining toilet facilities or mobile toilet units at healthcare facilities has been done successfully in the past. However, it drastically influences the functionality of the facility. Mobile chemical tank toilets in the hospital facility have also been used in extreme situations in the past.

Alternative solutions for disposal of items such as placentas must be planned, as normal shredding systems will not be functional.

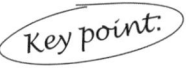 **Keeping a hospital functioning without a functioning sewage system is nearly impossible. Emergency measures are seldom able to meet requirements.**

4.3 Interruption in human resources

Healthcare facilities are fully dependent on available human resources to provide optimum care. Although the participation by healthcare professionals in labour action that disrupts patient care raises serious ethical questions, this has occurred in the past and will occur again in the future. In many countries, total walkouts by healthcare workers, sometimes associated with aggressive violent intimidation, have completely paralysed healthcare facilities, including acute care and critical care units. In these events, patients were left unattended in hospitals. These walkouts or strike actions do not only disrupt clinical care, but also interrupt housekeeping, cleaning, laundry and food services.

It is extremely challenging to keep a hospital functioning when violent intimidation is disrupting the facility. In some countries, including South Africa, total nursing and housekeeping strikes have occurred, with massive intimidation and, in some cases, violent removal of staff who preferred to work during the strike.

This section will deal only with action to address the need for the continuous care of patients during strike action, and not the labour relations actions associated with the situation. It must, however, be emphasised that the two aspects are always interlinked, and action to address patient suffering almost always has a counter action from the striking workforce. Actions can therefore never be taken in isolation.

It is essential for hospitals, in an environment where such action is possible, to plan to address this type of disruption. As this type of major labour action seldom occurs at a moment's notice, it is possible to implement actions in advance to address the massive disruption that will occur.

Limiting the dependency load

The first action to address a disruption in the availability of human resources is to limit the dependency load within the facility. This involves a coordinated effort to discharge as many patients as can safely and ethically be sent home. The impact of the mass discharges must be assessed, however. Record-keeping must be updated prior to discharge for medico-legal reasons. Discharged patients often need transport to get home, which may also be jeopardised due to wider strike actions. Next-of-kin should collect discharged patients from hospital as far as possible and, if needed, receive a written guideline on how to care for the patient at home. This should include warning signs that will necessitate re-admission to a hospital. Making discharge decisions when clinical staff are on strike is enormously challenging. One solution may be to use a special team to go from hospital to hospital to evaluate and triage patients.

Transfer of dependent patients to other healthcare facilities

When strike action is limited to a specific healthcare facility (or a group of healthcare facilities) closing the affected facility and transferring all in patients to another facility may be an option. However, the risk of a sympathetic strike by the receiving hospital's staff needs to be appreciated. Such mass transfers of patients requires extremely good coordination. Often, the situation in a striking hospital is chaotic, even unsafe and violent, making it very difficult to evacuate patients in an orderly manner.

It is suggested that triage be done on all patients to determine suitable modes of transport, and then the patients be removed to an interim hospital for re-triage and evaluation. Ambulance services are then activated from all surrounding towns to take patients from this facility to their specific hospitals.

It is suggested that patients be moved to further facilities in order to retain the capacity of the closest hospitals to take care of all new incoming emergency cases that would have been managed by the striking hospital.

There have been cases where strikers actively tried to disrupt care by destroying patient records or mixing records; therefore, patients need to be fully re-assessed on arrival at the receiving hospital before treatment is continued.

In the past, the temporary closure of the striking hospital, and the transfer of patients to other facilities, has proven to be the most sustainable solution. This immediately removes the patients as a bargaining chip for the strikers. However, in the event of a national or regional strike, this may not be achievable.

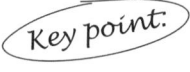 **Managing a healthcare facility without adequate human resources requires drastic measures to limit the dependency load as quickly as possible by limiting admissions, discharging patients where possible and transferring high-workload patients to alternative facilities.**

Protecting staff not participating in labour action

Effort must be made to protect staff not participating in the strike action. This may require a court interdict to prevent strikers from entering the grounds of the healthcare facility, but this is very difficult to enforce as it may not be possible to distinguish between striking intimidators and legitimate staff who want to work. Assembling staff who want to work at an alternative assembly point and then bussing them into the affected facility under armed escort has been necessary in the past, but holds the risk of intimidators using the approach to enter the facility and identify working staff members.

Active policing within the facility, and security at all entrances, must be planned to prevent unauthorised entry. This may require limiting the number of entrances into the facility to a minimum.

A special foolproof *ad hoc* identification system must be planned to identify non-striking workers and allow them into the facility for their next shift.

Countering false intimidator information

An active communication strategy must be planned to counter all information that may be used to intimidate workers. Intimidation is often focused on the healthcare professional's family or home. The moment information is picked up that, for example, 'Nurse X's house was burned down last night', the information must be actively followed up by management; if untrue, formal communication must be issued as soon as possible featuring Nurse X denying that her house was raised and even including pictures of her house. A single false message like this may result in a hospital's total staff staying away from work out of fear that their families will be targeted next by intimidators.

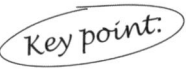 **Measures to assist staff who are willing to work includes protection and countering false information as quickly as possible.**

Establishing a volunteer support system

If there is a risk that a facility's human resource supply may be disrupted, active effort must be made to establish a volunteer support system to provide at least basic levels of care, such as feeding and housekeeping, during a disruption. This is critically important, especially for geriatric or psychiatric facilities and facilities for the disabled. Such a system needs time to build up and cannot be started during an incident. Useful approaches are to use existing community groups, such as women's organisations from churches and service clubs, and to link each group to a specific unit or ward of the facility. These groups can be invited over in advance to become involved in the ward, regularly visit the facility and assist with such tasks as reading to patients or doing shopping for basic necessities. During a disruption in the regular human resources, such a group could then fulfil essential support functions.

In case of intimidation, volunteers must be very carefully screened and protected on arrival at the facility. Safe parking for private vehicles must be planned, as staff vehicles are an easy target for aggression and attempts to intimidate workers.

A special volunteer recruitment point must be established, with secure parking facilities. The administrative information required from volunteers must be planned in advance, including legal advice on the use of indemnity documents to be signed by all volunteers. Volunteers must also be provided with temporary identification, which is renewed on a daily basis.

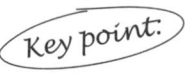 **Use of volunteers/temporary staff during an interruption in human resources requires proper planning and control to prevent intimidation.**

4.4 Surge capacity

Surge capacity is defined as the additional capacity, both physical and human, that is available within a facility to address an influx of additional patients. This capacity is often used as the buffer between a compensated major incident and an uncompensated disaster.

The surge capacity forms an integral part of the disaster planning of the facility, both for internal and external disasters. Surge capacity will always depend on time available to activate and prepare such additional facilities. For planning purposes, surge capacity is grouped into facilities that can be made available immediately, within six hours of notification, within twelve hours of notification and within 24 hours of notification.

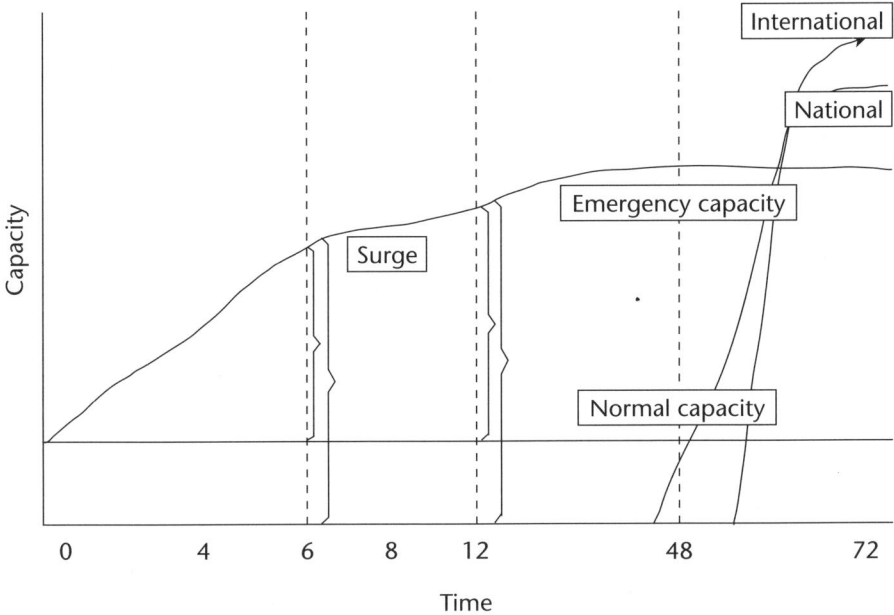

Figure 4.1: Surge capacity

The additional facilities that can be activated within a healthcare facility need to be determined in advance. It is necessary to accurately calculate the capability of a facility to accept additional patients, over and above the normal capability of the facility. To ensure that the information from different facilities can be compared in a central database per region, and even per country, a simple classification system is used, giving criteria for comparison. All facilities are classified into immediately available, can be made available within six hours, available within twelve hours and available after 24 hours.

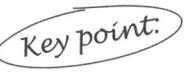 **Surge capacity refers to the additional space that can be made available within a facility to provide space for increased needs and numbers.**

Components of surge capacity

- *Space:* it is important to keep in mind that space is only one element of a surge capacity in a healthcare facility.
- *Staff:* the provision of staff to take care of the additional patients must be appreciated in detail. This may include volunteers that are available to the facility.

119

- *Equipment:* this is the third facet of surge capacity, and requires a detailed appreciation to ensure that acceptable levels of care can be provided for the additional patients. This includes catering capability and ablution facilities.

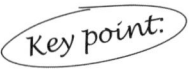 **Surge capacity consists of space, staff to provide care and equipment required.**

Limiting factors in surge capacity

Providing optimum care is not only dependent on space and resources, but also on making the resources available timeously for care. Therefore there are certain limitations to providing optimum levels of care.

Trauma patients

For a trauma patient, the optimum care is in making competent surgical capabilities available. Therefore the surge capacity of a healthcare facility for trauma patients *is limited by the capacity of the surgical facilities.* The space and equipment available must therefore be balanced with the availability of surgical capacity.

Calculating available theatre capacity

Surgery needs to be done within optimum cut-off times for optimal prognosis. It must be emphasised that this is a planning concept to determine optimum care, and not an absolute. This concept is used extensively in military planning processes to determine requirements on the battlefield. The concept can, however, be used as a guideline for disaster surge capacity calculation. In uncompensated disaster situations – for example the 2004 tsunami situation in the Indian Ocean – these norms will be ideal but unlikely to be achieved.

The available number of theatres, or areas that can be used as theatres within a facility needs to be determined. Determine for what triage category the theatre is suitable – for example, certain theatres will be suitable for Priority 1 critical patient-type surgery, whereas other theatres are only suitable for minor Priority 3 patients.

The equipment and staffing for the number of theatres must be confirmed. This would include the availability of anaesthesia machines and gases for anaesthesia. The requisite number of staff must be determined to staff all the planned theatres, with sufficient replacement staff to allow for rest periods if at all possible.

Sterilisation turn-around times need to be confirmed. It is essential to ensure that basic instrumentation can be returned sterilised to the theatre within the time planned for surgery (see planning norm below). If instrumentation can't be returned within the planned time, an additional set of instruments must be available.

Operating time required per triage category for the facility must be estimated by the surgical team. This will differ from facility to facility depending on the skills of the team and the support systems available. As a guideline, military planning norms for trauma patients are as follows:

- *Priority 1:* 3 hours/patient;
- *Priority 2:* 2 hours/patient;
- *Priority 3:* 30 min/patient (if surgery is required).

Optimum cut-off times need to be determined. Again, this will differ from country to country. Surgery within 24 hours may be an acceptable situation for a very poor underdeveloped country, but will be totally unacceptable for a developed country. As a guideline, a military planning norm is:

- *Priority 1:* surgery must be completed within 6 hours from time of injury;
- *Priority 2:* 12 hours;
- *Priority 3:* 24 hours.

> *Note on theatre capacity*
> Theatre capacity: (Ideal cut-off time – time elapsed since injury by time the patient reaches theatre) ÷ (Time needed for surgery per triage category) x (*N* of theatres earmarked for the triage category) = Capacity per triage priority.

The facility should be able to calculate the theatre capacity for Priority 1, for Priority 2 and for Priority 3 patients. This is the optimal surge capacity for trauma patients.

Medical patients

For medical patients, the *limiting factors will be space, equipment and staff.*

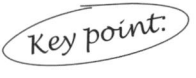 **Surge capacity for trauma patients is limited by the surgical capability available, and for medical patients by space, staff and equipment.**

Calculating surge capacity

To be able to compare the surge capacity of facilities to admit patients, a simple classification system is used. The space available is graded according to utilisation for the triage priorities.

   Space is needed for the full pathway of patient care within the facility, starting with the following:

- reception and triage space;
- resuscitation and treatment space;
- bed/accommodation space for hospitalisation.

Reception and triage space

Planning norm: 5 min/patient;
Space required: 6 m²/patient.

Additional requirements:

- emergency lighting.

Adequate infrastructure to receive patients:

- trolleys/gurneys;
- wheelchairs;
- floors at same level.

> *Note on reception capacity*
> Reception capacity: space available/m^2 ÷ 6 x (60min ÷ 5) = capacity/hour

Surge capacity resuscitation and treatment

Priority 1 – Space to resuscitate one Priority 1 patient prior to admission

Space required: 7 m^2/patient.

Additional requirements:

- emergency lighting;
- oxygen outlet (x 2);
- suction (x 1);
- power outlet (x 4);
- overhead IV hook (x 4).

> *Note on resuscitation capacity*
> Resuscitation capacity: (60 ÷ facility's throughput time) x *N* bays = capacity/hour Priority 1 patients
> (Planning norm throughput time: 28 min/patient)

Priority 2 – Space to stabilise/treat one Priority 2 patient prior to admission

Space required: 5 m^2/patient.

Additional requirements:

- emergency lighting.

Direct access to:

- oxygen;
- suction;
- overhead IV hooks (x 2).

> *Note on emergency care capacity*
> Emergency care capacity: (60 ÷ facility's throughput time) x *N* spaces = capacity/hour Priority 2 patients
> (Planning norm throughput time: 17 min/patient)

Priority 3 – Space to stabilise/treat one Priority 3 patient prior to admission or discharge

Space required: 5 m^2/patient.

Additional requirements:

- lighting;
- access to resuscitation equipment;
- consider utilising surge capacity space.

Note on treatment capacity
Treatment capacity: (60 ÷ facility's throughput time) x N areas = capacity/hour
Priority 3 patients
(Planning norm throughput time: 10 min/patient)

Surge capacity space for hospitalisation (admission of patients)

Priority 1 – Space suitable to nurse a Priority 1 patient requiring ICU care

Space: 8 m²;
Spacing: 2.5 m nose-to-nose (prefer 4 m).

Additional requirements:

- infusion hooks (x 4);
- oxygen outlet (x 2);
- medical air outlet (x 1);
- suction outlet (x 2);
- power supply (x 6) with 2 on back-up supply;
- emergency lighting.

Minimum equipment guidelines:

- ventilator (x 1);
- monitoring system (x 1).

Priority 2 – Space suitable to nurse a Priority 2 patient

Space: 6 m²;
Spacing: 1.5 m nose-to-nose (prefer 2 m).

Additional requirements:

- infusion hooks (x 2);
- access to oxygen and suction;
- ablution facilities;
- emergency lighting.

Priority 3 – Space suitable to nurse a Priority 3 patient

Space: 6 m²;
Spacing: 1.5 m nose-to-nose;
Ablution facilities.

Additional requirements:

- basic emergency lighting.

Ablution facilities:

Showers/baths: 1/12 patients;
Urinals: 1/20 patients;
Toilet: 1/12 patients (maximum 1/20 patients);
Basins: 1/12 patients.

Linen:

1 rotation set/day/patient;
2 sets/bed.

Utilising this classification system, it is possible to calculate the surge capacity of a particular facility. Within each of the categories, the number of beds or treatment areas that can be made available immediately, after six hours, after twelve hours and after 24 hours (and even later) must be calculated. It is re-emphasised that the available space and minimum requirements must not be used in isolation to determine surge capacity. It must be linked to the availability of staff and equipment within fixed timelines to ensure optimum care. For trauma patients, the determining factor remains the availability of theatre/additional theatre facilities.

Calculating surge capacity provides management with a predetermined additional capacity to be able to address requirements in an external disaster, or in an internal disaster where certain facilities must be evacuated.

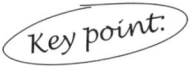 **Using predetermined criteria, the surge capacity of the healthcare facility can be calculated at various points in the treatment process. A mismatch between components needs special planning to optimise the surge capacity.**

4.5 Bomb threats

Bomb threats, or threats of any other disrupting action, may sometimes be sent to a healthcare facility. This can be as part of an intimidation agenda, often by disgruntled employees; as a propaganda action from a group or organisation; as an effort to disrupt functioning and cause chaos; and even as a dysfunctional form of humour. A bomb threat is, however, extremely disrupting, and should not be ignored.

In other public buildings, a bomb threat is normally managed through an evacuation of the entire building, followed by systematic surging. However, this is not possible for a healthcare facility, as evacuation can often cause loss of life, even without an explosion. It is essential that healthcare facilities use safe and accountable methods to manage a bomb threat, without causing more harm to patients.

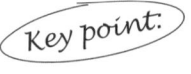 **Hospitals should plan an accountable and safe method to respond to a bomb threat, as evacuation may cause more harm to patients.**

Receiving a bomb threat

Bomb threats may be received in any department of the facility and by any member of staff. Most often, these threats are received telephonically, but can also be received by electronic mail or even by post.

It is therefore essential that all staff members are trained in the basic steps of how to react to a bomb threat.

It is essential for the receiver to obtain maximum information from the informer to enable optimum judgment of the risk. An effective way of addressing this requirement is to provide *pro forma* questionnaires with the information that must ideally be obtained from the caller at all telephones. Often these callers do not hold on that long out of fear that the call can be traced; it is therefore necessary to obtain essential information as quickly as possible. There is a myth that such a call can be traced while somebody keeps the caller talking; this is unfortunately no longer possible with modern communication equipment.

The information that should be obtained is as follows:

- Write down the exact words.
- Obtain maximum information:
  - Why is the explosive device placed?
  - Where is it?
  - What time will it explode?
  - What type of explosive was used/what kind of bomb is it?
  - What does it look like?
  - Can it be disarmed, and how?
- Maximum information on the caller:
  - Name (seldom given, and if given often false)
  - Language proficiency and accent
  - Speech deficiencies
  - Emotional condition of the caller
  - Age of caller
  - Gender
  - Intoxicated?

The purpose of obtaining the information is focused on determining the seriousness of the threat and the possible legal action that follow from identifying the caller. In most countries, it is a criminal offence to make a bomb threat, and it often results in a court case.

The reaction to a bomb threat will differ based on circumstances. A bomb threat in a country that is undergoing a terrorist or guerrilla war will be considered a far more serious threat than a similar call in a stable country town. However, the threat cannot be ignored, and the protection and safety services need to advise the hospital management on actions to be taken.

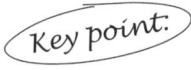 **When receiving a bomb threat, maximum information must be obtained to assist management, law enforcement agencies and emergency services in making informed decisions on how to react.**

Reporting a bomb threat (or suspicious object)

Any bomb threat, or suspicious object, needs to be reported immediately within the facility and then to the appropriate authority.

Each facility should identify a central point to which all emergencies within the institution are reported. It is essential that such a point is staffed 24 hours a day by competent staff who are clearly briefed on actions that need to be taken.

Examples are the telephone switchboard of the institution, or the control room of the security department. It is an option to write out the actions to be taken in the event of a bomb threat or a fire on large notices that are mounted on the wall in the control point. This will ensure that personnel are always aware of the actions that should be taken, and removes the need to search for the procedure in case of an emergency.

As soon as the internal reporting is done, the emergency needs to be reported to the appropriate external authorities. In most countries, bomb threats and suspicious objects are handled by the police. The central reporting point within the institution must inform the authorities and then activate the internal plan.

Every effort must be made to prevent panic and chaos within the institution. When the threat arises from an individual's dysfunctional sense of humour, the caller often waits for the chaos that follows his or her threat.

The internal plan normally includes the activation of the manager on duty at that time and the informing of all appropriate units or sections to search their respective areas with their own staff resources. Depending on the situation and the nature of the threat, the order of activation may differ, but is normally from the highest-risk areas to the lowest-risk areas.

All other emergency services, such as the fire brigade and emergency medical service, must be informed and placed on stand-by during the search procedure. Local procedures will dictate whether such services are called out to the healthcare facility or remain on stand-by while the facility's staff search the premises.

Searching healthcare facilities

It is physically impossible for the protection services/police to search the entire facility effectively within a realistic timeframe. Members of the external services do not know the layout, or the various activities within the facility. It is therefore essential for staff, especially nursing staff, within the boundaries of safety, to search the specific unit in which they are working for any unusual package. For example, a suitcase in the duty office may be known to belong to a discharged patient, while a similar suitcase in an empty room is obviously out of place and therefore highly suspicious.

Security authorities/police can report to the central control point during this internal search and wait for feedback from the various areas. In the meantime, police can assist with the searching of the public areas, such as waiting rooms, cafeteria facilities and admission offices of the facility.

It must be emphasised that an explosive device can be camouflaged in any format, from a device camouflaged as a loaf of bread and booby traps within incubators to commercial explosives and even military limpet mines attached to oxygen piping.

Under no circumstances must any suspicious objects be touched or moved by non-qualified members of the staff or the public! Any suspicious object must be reported immediately to the central control point who should then summon the experts to investigate it.

Special attention must be given to high-risk areas where an explosion will create the maximum disruptive effect. Examples include electrical distribution boxes, medical gas control valves and emergency stand-by services such as back-up generators. Risk areas also include service and pipe shafts, where an explosion will disrupt the services and reticulation to various floors of the building and where the airflow from the explosion wave can damage various levels.

The highest risk is with vehicles parked close to the structure of the building and in basement parking areas. A car or truck bomb can do massive damage to any healthcare facility. If at all possible, owners of vehicles in high-risk areas must be identified to try and confirm that the vehicle is not a risk. However, this is nearly impossible, and the only solution is prevention through effective daily access control to parking areas.

The entire nursing unit needs to be systematically searched by on-duty nursing staff, taking their own safety into account.

The facility management must plan to search non-nursing sections: for example, waiting rooms, admission offices and radiography departments – especially after hours, when these facilities may be closed. Such areas can be searched by internal security staff or other hospital employees.

As soon as any suspicious object is identified, it must be reported immediately to the central control point for inspection by the security authorities, such as the police.

If nothing suspicious is found, this fact must also be reported, so that an overall checklist for 'all clear' is completed by the security authority for the entire complex.

The emphasis is placed on a sensible search of the total facility without unnecessary risk for personnel.

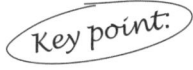 **It is impossible for external agencies to search an entire hospital effectively in a reasonable time. Staff must assist and search their area of responsibility within the margins of safety and to report back to the command point. Police and dogs can be used to search public areas and to investigate any suspicious objects found in the building.**

Explosive devices within the healthcare facilities

As soon as any suspicious object is identified, or a specific high-risk area is identified from the information received from the caller or informant, security authorities/police should be summoned to the area:

- Patients and staff must be evacuated immediately from the direct surroundings of the object, without causing panic. Discretion should be used, and expert advice from police should be followed. Hospital staff must refrain from any unilateral decisions in this crisis situation, and must adhere to the recommendation from the police. As a rule of thumb, patients and staff are evacuated so that there are at least two solid walls between the object and patients. Patients on the floor area directly above and below the object must also be evacuated. The guidance of the police should be followed strictly. In the case of a suspicious vehicle, the entire building may need to be evacuated.
- It must be taken into account that the evacuation of an entire facility may take several hours. Therefore, the command to evacuate an entire facility must be based on accurate reliable technical advice, and must be given by an authorised

person. Depending on a country's legislation, this command will be given by a police officer or an explosives expert from the armed forces.

Under no circumstances should the suspicious object or vehicle be disturbed or an effort made to disarm it by a non-expert.

To assist security authorities in their search, all lights must be left on in all areas that have been evacuated.

To enhance the spread of the airwave in the case of an explosion, all windows and doors are left open. If practical, curtains can be left closed to limit flying glass in the event of an explosion. It must be emphasised that this protection effect is very limited and is of value only with small explosive devices.

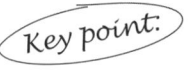 **If a suspicious object is found, patients and staff should be evacuated to areas of safety. Basic measures such as leaving lights on and windows open will assist in managing the situation. In multi-storey buildings the areas directly above and below the suspicious object should be evacuated as well.**

Activation of emergency services

As soon as any suspicious object is identified, and the police have confirmed the risk, all emergency services must be activated to respond to the facility. Police and fire frigade need to advise facility management on the need to evacuate the entire building based on specialist knowledge.

In the event of an explosion, the entire complex needs to be evaluated by a structural engineer and the fire brigade, to determine structural damage. The fire brigade must also advise the management on the safest route of evacuation, as areas for planned assembly may not be structurally safe to use.

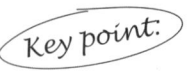 **If the risk is confirmed, all emergency services must be activated and all resources mobilised to address the situation.**

All clear

After a comprehensive search, a decision must be made in collaboration with the experts, normally the police. If nothing is found, and the police agree, an 'all clear' message must be distributed to the entire facility. If this is done in coded form, it is essential that all staff members understand the message as a stand-down, all-clear instruction and not an evacuation order.

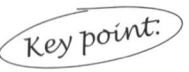 **Only after confirmation that the building is safe by the police must an all-clear message be communicated.**

Summary

When a bomb threat is received, a hospital needs to be able to react judiciously and obtain the maximum information. The hospital must plan to support the law enforcement agencies and emergency services effectively to ensure patient and staff safety and to react timeously to prevent a catastrophe.

4.6   Fire in a healthcare facility

A fire in a healthcare facility is an enormously destructive situation, and must be prevented at all costs.

Basic fire prevention

The increase in the use of technology within healthcare facilities, especially operating theatres – for example, high-technology diagnostic equipment, surgical lasers, fibre-optic light sources and alcohol-based disinfectants – dramatically increases the risk for fire.

A healthcare facility must be inspected regularly, as determined by local legislation, to ensure fire prevention measures are in place. Due to the risk in a healthcare facility, inspections by qualified fire prevention and safety personnel must be done more regularly than is required for industry. A suggestion would be every six months, but not less than annually. Fire alarm systems should be tested monthly and results of all tests formally recorded.

Inspection should include all firefighting equipment, fire alarm systems and all escape routes in the facility. All signs to indicate escape routes, emergency lighting of escape routes, escape devices and protective devices, such as smoke masks should also be checked.

High-risk incidents that have caused catastrophes in the past include the blockage of fire escape routes by stored surplus equipment and fire escapes being locked for security reasons.

Clear policies for the maintenance of equipment and infrastructure must be in place to prevent fire. This includes, for example, employing only qualified electricians to maintain all electrical appliances.

Good housekeeping and storage practices need to be adhered to throughout the total complex to prevent fire risks.

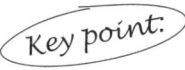 **Good housekeeping and regular inspection is the basis for fire prevention in a hospital.**

Fire alarms within healthcare facilities

Most modern healthcare facilities are equipped with automatic smoke-detecting and fire alarm systems. Although these systems are an enormous benefit, facilities must not rely on these systems only. A manual back-up is essential. In less developed countries, facilities are not necessarily equipped with such facilities, and rely totally on a person, staff or patient, to raise the alarm in case of a fire.

Immediately a fire (or a fire risk) is discovered, the alarm must be raised. It is essential that each staff member in the facility knows the procedure to report a fire. It is also essential that, if automatic alarm systems are installed, it is still confirmed that the alarm has been raised and emergency services activated. An example of such a manual method is a fire alarm notice with a reporting emergency number that is mounted next to every telephone in the total facility.

Many healthcare facilities may be equipped with manually activated fire alarm systems. These systems differ technically, but most systems include a glass panel that must be broken, resulting in the activation of an alarm at a central point within the facility or at the fire brigade. In certain older systems, the alarms are mounted outside the buildings in alarm boxes that need to be activated. Again, it is emphasised that staff members be trained in how to use the system, and never to rely only on a single alarm system. Always confirm that the automatic or manual alarm system message was received by the fire brigade.

Some healthcare facilities are also equipped with smoke-detectors that activate an alarm system as soon as the sensor detects smoke. Although these systems are very useful for the early detection of fire, they are not fail-proof. It is therefore essential that such systems are backed up with a fire reporting telephone number posted throughout the complex.

Immediately a fire alarm is received, the local fire brigade must be activated. Never waste time trying to extinguish the fire before activating the fire brigade. It is safer to activate the fire brigade, and then try to extinguish the fire. If successful, the fire brigade still needs to inspect the area to determine if it is safe.

Fire brigades normally have a standard predetermined turn-out for alarms from a healthcare facility, based on the risk of the building. This would normally include a command element to establish incident command, major fire pumps and hydraulic/ladder equipment based on the height of the building.

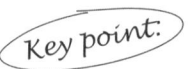 **The fire alarm must be raised as soon as possible and the fire brigade activated irrespective of the size of the fire.**

Command

A fire in a healthcare facility is usually classified as a major incident, and various emergency services are activated. This includes the fire brigade as the main responder; ambulance services to assist with casualties and to transport evacuated patients; police for crowd control; and maintenance staff to assist with the unique risks in a hospital fire, such as the oxygen supply.

Incident command

The various role-players responding to a healthcare facility fire need to establish a joint incident command immediately. This is done according to the standard Incident Command System applicable in the country.

It is useful to identify in advance a specific point, outside the building, where incident command will be situated in collaboration with the major role-players. This position is then communicated to all role-players in advance, forms part of the formal fire alarm message from the facility and is included in training. Particularly in large hospital complexes, this position can be predetermined close to approach routes and far enough away from the building for safety.

An alternative position, or positions, must also be identified for the unforeseen situation in which the primary position cannot be used.

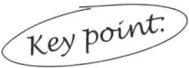 **A specific point for incident command must be pre-planned and an effective incident command established.**

Communication

Effective communication with rescue personnel is essential, but this must be supplemented with effective communication with personnel still in the building, patients evacuating the building, and management of the institution.

Various forms of communication are available, but a basic form of public address system audible inside the building has proven to be essential.

Liaison with the fire brigade

Depending on applicable legislation, in most countries the fire brigade is in charge of any fire situation, including those in a healthcare facility. This necessitates close cooperation between management and the fire brigade during planning, training and in case of a fire.

The fire brigade representative should be a member of the emergency planning committee of the institution and should guide the management in all decisions on evacuation routes, alarms, training and drills.

It is essential that management make the hospital facilities available to the fire brigade for training exercises, as this will enhance cooperation and will be extremely valuable in a fire.

Basic firefighting for healthcare professionals

The safety of patients, visitors and fellow staff is a key responsibility of healthcare facilities. This includes comprehensive measures to ensure fire prevention, but also includes basic measures such as good housekeeping, safe storage of combustible material and proper maintenance of equipment and installations. Although firefighting is an advanced science which requires specialised knowledge and skills, basic fire fighting measures by a healthcare professional may prevent a small incident from developing into a catastrophic inferno threatening the lives of patients, staff and visitors. If a small incident is discovered early and managed correctly, it can be extinguished with a low-risk intervention. It is, however, reiterated that raising the alarm is the first and most important function of the healthcare professional, thereafter ensuring that patients are removed from immediate danger, before attempting to extinguish the fire. This sequence of events often occurs simultaneously, with various members of the staff executing the different functions.

Combustion theory

In order to understand how a fire extinguisher works, it is important that the healthcare professional has a basic knowledge of combustion.

Four elements are needed for combustion, namely:

- *Fuel or combustible material:* this is any combustible material from linen, curtains and flammable liquids such as alcohol-based hand-cleaning solution to storerooms of dressings and protective clothing;
- *Heat:* adequate heat to raise the fuel or combustible material to ignition temperature. Multiple sources of heat are present in the healthcare facility, including cigarette butts, heaters, electrical motors to drive various pieces of equipment, sparks from an electrical short circuit, maintenance equipment such as welding torches, and chemical reactions in oily rags.
- *Oxygen:* required to sustain combustion. Not only is this element present in the atmosphere, but is often in a higher concentration in the healthcare facility.
- *Exothermic chemical reaction:* This chemical chain reaction occurs when the other three elements combine.

These four components form the fire tetrahedron of combustion (see Figure 4.2).

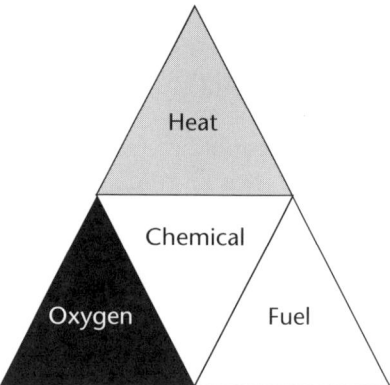

Figure 4.2: Fire tetrahedron

Basic fire prevention involves keeping these four components separate from one another. As oxygen and fuel are continuously in contact with one another in the environment, the basic measure for healthcare professionals is to isolate heat from the fuel and oxygen to prevent a chemical chain reaction from taking place.

Fire extinguishers used in healthcare facilities

Theoretically, fire extinguishers put out fire by removing one or more components of the fire tetrahedron. For example, applying water to the fire will remove the heat component of the tetrahedron, by cooling the material down to below the ignition temperature. Spraying the fire with a carbon dioxide (CO_2) extinguisher will remove the oxygen component of the tetrahedron.

Combustion or fire is defined as a process involving rapid oxidation at elevated temperatures accompanied by the evolution of heated gaseous products of combustion, and the emission of visible and invisible radiation.

The combustion process occurs in two modes:

- Flaming;
- Non-flaming, smouldering or glowing embers.

In the flaming mode, heat transferred from the flame to the fuel surface continues to drive off more volatile gases and perpetuates the combustion process. Continued burning in the flaming mode requires a high burning rate, and the heat loss associated with the transfer of heat from the flame area by conduction, convection and radiation must be less than the energy output of the fire. If the heat loss is greater than the energy output of the fire, the fire will extinguish.

This leads to the three stages of fire:

- *The incipient stage:* in this stage, preheating, distillation and pyrolysis are in process. If preheating is discontinued, the development of fire is stopped.
- *Smouldering stage:* fully developed pyrolysis that begins with ignition and includes the initial stages of combustion. Invisible aerosol and visible smoke particles are generated and transported away from the source by moderate convection patterns and background air movement. This process, if stopped, will prevent the development of fire.
- *Flame stage:* the flaming stage is a rapid reaction to a fully developed fire. Heat transfer occurs predominantly from radiation and convection from the flame.

Fire has been categorised into five classes, based on the material involved:

- *Class A:* involving organic solids such as paper, linen and wood;
- *Class B:* involving flammable liquids;
- *Class C:* involving flammable gases;
- *Class D:* involving metals;
- *Class F:* involving cooking oil.

The class, or type, of fire will determine the type of extinguisher that can be used to extinguish the fire. Within a healthcare facility, the identification of the risks and the placement of the appropriate type of extinguisher is the responsibility of the safety coordinator. This should be done and reviewed on a continuous structured basis by an expert(s), possibly from the local fire brigade. It is essential that the appropriate type of extinguisher is mounted in the appropriate areas of the facility based on the assessment of the risks that are present.

Extinguishing is done using basic techniques to remove the most appropriate component, or components, of the fire tetrahedron.

The three basic techniques applicable to a healthcare professional are:

- *Smothering:* this extinguishing technique removes the oxygen component from the tetrahedron. By putting a lid on a pot of burning oil in the hospital kitchen, the oxygen supply to the fire is cut off and the fire is extinguished. Using a blanket to cover a patient who is on fire limits the oxygen supply to the fire so drastically that the rapid reaction cannot continue and the fire is extinguished.
- *Starving:* this extinguishing technique removes the combustible material or fuel from the fire. Moving other combustible material away from a burning wastepaper basket, for example, will prevent the fire from spreading, and it will be extinguished as soon as all the material in the basket has been combusted.
- *Cooling:* in this technique, the combustible material is cooled to below the ignition temperature and the fire is extinguished. For example, in spraying a

linen room on fire with water from a fire hose, the linen in the room will be cooled to below the ignition temperature and the fire will be extinguished.

Extinguishing systems

As indicated, the type of extinguisher used is dependent on the classes of fire, and therefore the type of material or fuel involved. The appropriate type of extinguisher should be selected by a firefighting expert and mounted in the area concerned.

Three basic types of extinguishing systems are normally used within a healthcare facility – excluding laboratories, where more specialised equipment is often needed. These systems are decribed below. It is essential that staff are aware of where extinguishers are mounted in the facility and how to access these in an emergency. It is preferable that extinguishers be mounted at eye level and their positions marked with approved signs.

Water

Water is still the most available extinguisher in a healthcare facility. In the event of a fire, water can be delivered through various systems, such as a mounted automatic overhead sprayer system, an installed fire hose on a spool reel in a ward or by using a patient's jug of drinking water to extinguish a burning cigarette butt in a wastepaper basket. Water can safely be used on most fires in a healthcare facility. Automatic sprinkler systems are activated automatically when a fire is detected by the various types of sensors. Most healthcare facilities also have fire hoses on a spool reel available for use by non-firefighting experts, such as nursing staff.

These hoses are actually nothing more than high-volume and -pressure garden hoses. Various models are installed in facilities based on systems and legislation applicable in the country concerned. However, there are certain basic similarities: the hose is wound on a spool, with the end of the hose threaded through. The operator aims at the base of the fire, and uses S-movements to spray the water over all the burning material. This will cool the material down and extinguish the fire.

A fire hose reel must not be confused with high-pressure canvas-type fire hoses sometimes available within healthcare facilities. The use of these fire hoses requires proper training, and should preferably be used by professional firefighters only.

Water must never be used on live electrical currents as it conducts electricity and will cause the operator to be electrocuted. Water is also not suitable for use on burning liquids as it will often spread the liquid over a large area.

Dry powder

The type of extinguisher most frequently used in a healthcare facility is the dry powder chemical extinguisher. These extinguishers differ from country to country, but basically consist of a container filled with a dry chemical powder, forced out by a compressed air cylinder inside the container. These extinguishers can be used effectively to extinguish fires in a healthcare facility. However, the chemical powder will damage electronic equipment, and if alternatives are available it is not recommended that this type of extinguisher be used on electronic equipment.

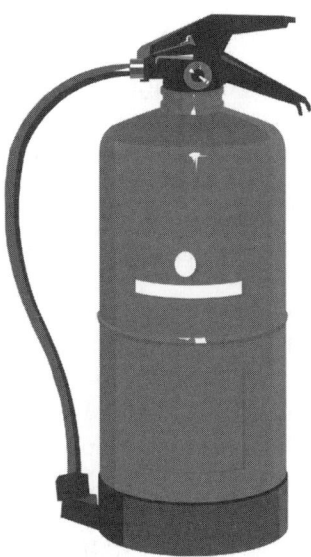

Figure 4.3: Dry powder extinguisher

Carbon dioxide

A carbon dioxide extinguisher is basically a cylinder of compressed carbon dioxide gas with a control and spray mechanism. These extinguishers are easy identified by the funnel-like hose with which the CO_2 is aimed at the fire. These extinguishers are not effective outdoors in windy conditions.

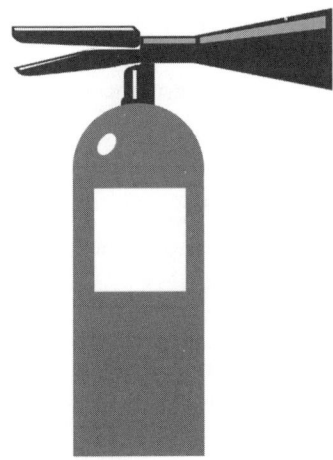

Figure 4.4: Carbon dioxide extinguisher

For extinguishers, including water hose reels, to be effective, they must be checked and serviced regularly, as determined by legislation. These service records must be retained for inspection and investigations if required. Staff must be trained in the prescribed signage used in the facility to mark the position of extinguishers and emergency exits. The orientation of all new staff should include orientation to the position of extinguishers and emergency exits from units.

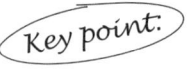 **Basic and appropriate firefighting equipment must be positioned according to governance, and hospital staff must be trained and exercised to use the equipment.**

Staff training

It is essential that all staff members are trained and certified competent to use the appropriate equipment in the facility. This section is not intended as a training course, but merely to provide introductory information. It is recommended that all healthcare workers attend formal training in the use of the specific type of extinguishers used in their facility. This training needs to be presented regularly, and staff refreshed in a controlled process. Depending on local legislation, a refresher training session is recommended at least every two years.

This section focuses on the use of standard fire extinguishers in a limited fire, to prevent spreading. It is not aimed at hospital staff using professional firefighting equipment. Firefighting is the role of professional firefighters; the role of healthcare staff should focus on raising the alarm, extinguishing a minor fire and thereafter, if not successful, evacuating patients to safety.

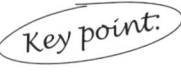 **Staff must be trained and exercised to prevent and fight a fire effectively and to raise the alarm immediately in case of a fire.**

Evacuation

Patients need to be evacuated to safety as orderly and efficiently as possible. Depending on the risk and the situation, this may necessitate evacuation of a specific ward, a specific floor or the entire complex. Healthcare professionals should be guided in this regard by the fire brigade.

Re-entry and recovery

After a fire, the area or entire facility should be inspected by the fire brigade and declared safe before re-entry.

Summary

Due to the nature of their operations and activities, hospitals do have a substantial fire risk. This requires continuous fire prevention monitoring and measures. As soon as a fire does occur, an early alarm will save many lives. Using basic firefighting techniques safely and efficiently can prevent a catastrophe. Staff must be trained and exercised to use equipment and evacuate patients efficiently.

4.7 Evacuation of a healthcare facility

Several recent disasters, notably the South Asian tsunami of 2004 and Hurricane Katrina in New Orleans, USA, have focused the attention of public health officials and policy-makers on hospital disaster planning. The World Health Organization (WHO) dedicated its 2009 World Health Day to the theme, 'Save lives. Make hospitals safe in emergencies', which includes both safe construction and disaster planning.

   The first consideration in hospital evacuations should always be the safety and wellbeing of patients and staff. In New Orleans, 127 people died in hospitals (over 10% of storm casualties) during or shortly after Katrina, with delayed evacuation playing a significant role. Furthermore, lack of an evacuation plan may put hospitals at odds with regulatory bodies and the courts: the Joint Commission in the USA requires hospitals to have an evacuation plan for accreditation. In Hurricane Katrina's aftermath, families have sued, claiming that the absence of evacuation plans led to their relatives' deaths.

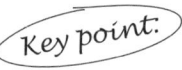 **Failure to include evacuation in a hospital disaster plan poses an unacceptable risk to patients and staff, and a legal risk for hospitals themselves.**

The state of hospital preparedness

Despite the global push for hospital disaster preparedness, hospitals continue to overlook planning for internal disasters and hospital evacuation. A review of published international literature on hospital evacuations identified 69 case studies, in which only four hospitals had a specific evacuation plan. A 2008 survey of 27 public hospitals in the Western Cape province in South Africa found that 93% of respondents had a general disaster plan, but that only 40% had a hospital evacuation plan. In the developing world, additional factors may hinder the development of effective hospital evacuation planning: for one, hospital officials may lack the time, resources and expertise to develop and drill hospital evacuation plans. Secondly, because many hospitals in the developing world consist of only one floor, the notion may arise that an evacuation plan is not necessary. Nevertheless regardless of hospital design, it has been noted that a significant bottleneck in hospital evacuation occurs in transporting patients to alternate care locations after extracting them from the hospital. Even when an evacuation plan exists, it may not be consulted during a disaster, because of a lack of familiarity or a lack of involvement in the process. Many authors, in developed and developing countries alike, comment on the apathy or indifference of hospital staff when it comes to a perceived rare event such as the evacuation of the hospital.

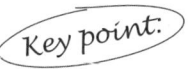 **The majority of hospitals around the world are unprepared to evacuate.**

Indications for evacuation

The motivation to evacuate a hospital may be internal or external. Impending external threats, such as hurricanes, wildfires, toxic spills or military attacks may prompt evacuation before systems critical to the hospital's function are affected. Internal threats, such as a fire or an armed intruder, may disable all or part of a hospital's ability to care for patients safely, while the community at large is unaffected. In the worst-case scenario of a combined internal-external disaster, a hospital faces the prospect of evacuating a surged volume of patients. A review of 275 hospital evacuation events in the USA revealed that over 50% stemmed from internal causes rather than external disasters. Internal fire ranked first among all causes, followed by internal hazardous materials spills, hurricanes, internal human threats and earthquakes. Other indications included floods, external fires and failures of the power or water supply. As evacuation carries its own inherent risks to patients, the grounds for evacuation must be sound and considered by the most experienced people at hand. Analysis of the response to the 1989 Loma Prieta earthquake in the USA revealed that some assessments for structural damage were conducted by security and nursing personnel, not hospital engineers. Repeatedly, case studies have identified a pattern of uncertain roles and responsibilities regarding the final decision to evacuate.

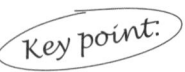 **Internal disasters (e.g. hospital fires) are a more common cause of hospital evacuations than external disasters (e.g. earthquakes).**

Types of evacuation

Evacuation may be categorised as horizontal or vertical, and as complete or partial. Horizontal evacuation signifies that patients are moved away from a hazard, such as a fire or hazardous fumes, on the same hospital floor. Vertical evacuation entails moving patients from one floor to another. In a partial evacuation, only some of the patients are moved, typically within the hospital. However, some hospitals in the USA conduct partial evacuations in response to the impending threat of a hurricane, during which they will transfer their non-critical patients to facilities outside the projected path of the storm. A complete evacuation may be horizontal or vertical depending on the physical layout of the hospital. Evacuations usually follow the regular triage order of prioritising the sickest patients. In some instances of perceived imminent structural collapse or other imminent danger, hospitals have successfully evacuated in reverse triage order: ambulatory patients first, followed by non-critical patients with limited mobility, and finally by those few needing the most resources.

An evacuation can be further categorised in terms of the destination of patients and staff. It may be to an internal location, to an external staging area (usually temporary), to other local hospitals or to non-health facilities that may function as field hospitals. In the case of an imminent structural threat, patients should be evacuated to a designated safe staging area, which may be either outdoors or in an adjacent building. From the staging area, patients may either be discharged or transferred to other facilities depending on their condition. In the case where all regional facilities are damaged or overwhelmed (e.g. massive earthquake, flood, etc.), patients may be transferred to a designated makeshift field hospital in a school, stadium or other safe public space. The final appearance of the evacuation will depend on the required speed and on the number of functional hospital systems. In the case of a pre-disaster evacuation (e.g. approaching storm or wildfire), lifts will continue to function and will greatly ease the vertical evacuation of patients. When electrical power fails, staff will need to carry patient downstairs and manually bag ventilated patients during evacuation.

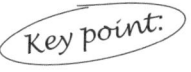 **Complete evacuations may be the most challenging in high-rise hospitals, but all facilities face the challenge of finding safe havens for their patients.**

Evacuation planning

All hospitals should have an evacuation plan as part of their broader disaster plan. Evacuation plans should provide criteria for the different types of evacuation, and specify where specialist input is desired, e.g. that of a structural engineer. The evacuation plan requires that maps of evacuation routes must be available to all patient-care areas. The plan should designate the order of the evacuation, the staging areas and the various destinations for transferred patients. Some hospitals stock specialised equipment for evacuation, such as rescue sleds or patient drag sheets. Other hospitals report performing well in evacuations by using backboards, mattresses and other routinely available supplies. Before the need arises, hospitals should negotiate mutual agreements with other facilities for accepting patients transferred during an evacuation. The remainder of the evacuation plan relies on the key components of the overall disaster plan: establishment of a command centre, establishment of clear lines of command and control, establishment of backup communications systems, etc. As for disaster planning as a whole, the evacuation plan should take a community-wide approach and involve local authorities (fire, police, etc.), patient transport services and other hospitals in the region. Perhaps above all, the plan should take into account various contingencies but remain flexible. It is better to have a good plan A, and a decent plan B, than a single perfect plan.

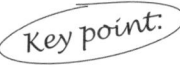 **Hospital evacuation planning requires a multi-disciplinary team, with the direct involvement of local and regional authorities.**

Evacuation plan evaluation

The consensus among experts is that disaster drills remain the best and only truly effective way to prepare hospitals for disasters and evacuations. However, little direct evidence provides a basis for this conclusion. Many note that, time and again, the same mistakes are made, and the same lessons learned, in disasters and evacuations. As a way forward, Schultz and colleagues propose a basic questionnaire and data collection tool to evaluate hospital evacuation plans and actual performance during an evacuation. This standardised data set provides a stronger basis for evaluating evacuation plans and their execution during a disaster.

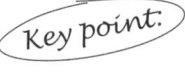 **Alhough no gold standard exists, frequent drilling gives the hospital its best chance at preparedness and at safe evacuation when necessary.**

4.8 Areas of special concern

Several parts of the hospital present particular concerns with respect to major incident response. These may be external major incidents in which the hospital is responding, or internal incidents whereby part of the hospital is directly affected. Such internal major incidents can be divided into three main groups, namely, functional incidents, external incidents requiring activation of the major incident plan and evacuation due to hazards.

Functional major incidents may not be a major incident for the general wards of a hospital, but may have a major impact on key areas. Much of the detail of these incidents has been dealt with at the start of this chapter.

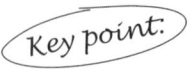 **Functional issues are the most common cause of internal incidents and may complicate external incidents and thus the ability of the hospital to manage those incidents.**

Operating theatre

The operation theatre is a unique challenge when there is either an external or internal major incident. Challenges in the operation theatre include the following:

- Patients with airway compromise (due to general anaesthesia) on ventilation systems;
- Circulatory instability;
- Large open wounds that restrict movement;
- Numerous flammable products in the theatre;
- Machinery which can fail to function, or ignites flammable materials;
- The need to move patients carefully and safely from the hospital beds.

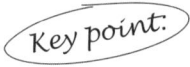 **The operating theatre environment has some of the most challenging components when dealing with major incidents.**

Functional major incidents

- *Power failure:* most power failures will be temporary as this area of the hospital is usually connected to the uninterruptible power supply (UPS) system, such that power will be restored within less than one minute. This type of incident becomes an issue only in a protracted power failure, where the battery back-up runs out, or the supply of diesel to the back-up generators runs short. Failure of back-up generators to 'kick in' during a power outage, especially during external major incidents that affect the entire community, such as floods, tornados and similar events, means that the limited UPS system will be overwhelmed after the usual 30-minute 'cover' period.
- *Water cut-off:* water is required for many activities in the operation theatre. When the water supply fails, the surgical teams are prevented from continuing normal work as this compromises sterility, with a risk of increased post-operative infection, and as sluice services and washing of reusable equipment are not possible.
- *Failure of oxygen, other gases or the vacuum-suction system:* most hospitals today have oxygen, medical air, compressed air and vacuum suction systems piped

to the operation theatre from a central point, often in the basement of the hospital near the engineering section. Any failure of the piping system, the pressurisation system or compromise of the integrity of the supply (internal quality or external resupply) will lead to decreases in pressure and will place patient safety at risk. Mobile back-up equipment must be readily available.

- *Failure of the heating or air conditioning system:* the operation theatre is a controlled environment: if it is too hot the staff suffer from dehydration and exhaustion; if it is too cold the patient can develop hypothermia and deranged physiology. Thus, when the heating or air conditioning systems fail, the only option may be to terminate all current surgery and transfer patients to other areas or other facilities.
- *Logistical failure from the consumable stores or equipment stores:* most hospitals rely on a regular supply of consumables from a central stores area or through regular external delivery. Failure of this delivery system, due to destruction or incapacity, can become a major internal incident due to an inability to undertake procedures or provide the necessary sundries to perform quality of care.
- *Staff incapacitation:* whether due to injury or inability to reach the hospital, staff incapacitation leads to inability to provide routine services and may also hamper the response to a major incident, whether internal or external.

External major incidents causing internal incidents in the operation suite

External major incidents occur on a regular basis, and these may require the institution of in-house hospital major incident plans, such as curtailing elective surgical procedures, clearing post-anaesthetic care areas to increase intensive/ critical care capacity and opening additional operating rooms to handle the expected surge of major emergency cases.

The operation suite is the service delivery hub of the surgical team. Many external major incidents are traumatic in nature and will therefore test the abilities of the operation suite team to adapt to the required mentality of 'damage control' surgery and to triage and treatment principles not usually seen in the day-to-day care of the surgical patient. This is made worse during protracted incidents, such as natural 'disasters' that tax the in-hospital teams' abilities to adapt, as the hospital itself is stressed to capacity, due to the patient surge combined with the challenges already highlighted under the preceding section.

The team therefore need to be prepared for the effects of external major incidents by means of the following:

- The hospital should have a simple pre-set major incident plan, for both internal and external incidents, with a hospital coordinator and a leadership team of senior people who will direct the hospital response to the incident. Communication is the key to success.
- The scrub teams in the operation suite will fall under the nursing hierarchy in the scheme of command. They most often will be involved with the subsequent treatment phase when the type of incident involves injured patients.

- Adequate hazard information should be communicated to the staff regarding potential for injury if there is any chemical, nuclear or biological contamination.
- Action cards should be provided for the members of the operation suite to detail the extent of their actions during a major incident.
- Operative teams to undertake the surgical procedures deemed necessary by the senior surgeon, in communication with the senior operation suite nursing staff, should be formed.
- Surgery is usually restricted to 'life or limb' salvage initially and comprehensive reconstructive procedures as time progresses.
- The ability to face internal major incidents may also prolong the ability of the hospital to recover from an external incident, if it leads to deficiencies of infrastructure and shortages of consumable supply.
- Regular drills and tabletop practices are essential for adequate preparation.

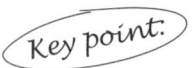 **It is essential that the operation suite and the operation room staff are part of a practised major incident plan.**

Evacuation due to hazards

Evacuation of a hospital is a stressful event, but even more so when the patient involved in the evacuation is under general anaesthesia with open wounds and a team of people responsible for that patient's life. An ethical issue is whether the safety of the team is paramount to that of the individual patient or whether the team is obligated to risk their lives for the patient, while still trying to mitigate the incident. Evacuation is made more challenging by the type of operative procedure being undertaken, the patient's clinical picture (e.g. elective versus emergency surgery, or open versus laparoscopic surgery) and finally the location of the operation suite in the hospital (floor level/lift access/stairwell size etc.).

Some operating tables are fixed and therefore require the movement of the patient to a gurney. Monitoring devices should be mobile and able to be rapidly displaced to the patient, to enable extrication. Connections to monitors and building services (medical gases, suction, electrical) should be disconnected. Chest drainage systems can be suspended from the bed frame (below heart level). Disconnect the suction line from the wall outlet if it is being used. Critical medications delivered through IV pumps attached to movable poles are usually supplied with battery backup, so a simple disconnection from the electrical outlet prepares them for transport without altering administration of the medication. Other IV bags can be removed from the pole, separated from the pump and then placed on the bed for evacuation. Disconnect ventilators from the ET tube and ventilate the patient manually with a bag-valve-mask and 100% mobile oxygen. All the infusion pumps, monitoring devices and ventilation devices should be mobile and able to be rapidly displaced to the patient, to enable extrication.

Situations where evacuation is considered are as follows:

- *Fire in the hospital:* Knowledge of fire suppression technique and activation of the warning system is essential.
- *Flood in the hospital:* this may be from internal pipe bursts or due to external community flooding.

- *Terrorist activity, bomb or hostage situation:* a bomb/physical threat plan is essential to handle these events, as evacuation is a last resort if the situation can be contained outside the operation suite.
- *Significant power failure* with failure of back-up generators necessitating evacuation to other facilities to enable ongoing patient care.

Evacuation plans should be area-specific, and should be tested with simulated patients to ensure that the plan is implementable when the need arises.

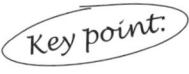 **Evacuation is a specific challenge for the operation suite and requires a regularly practised plan, including an all-hazards approach.**

Summary

Internal and external major incidents can affect the function of the operation suite and may necessitate evacuation or alternative management strategies. Planning for an 'all hazards' approach will prevent an incident from becoming a disaster.

4.9 Intensive care

Challenges in the ICU include the following:

- Patients with airway compromise on ventilation systems;
- Circulatory instability;
- Wounds that are at risk for infection, and wounds infected by rare or unusual organisms;
- The need to move patients carefully and safely on the hospital beds with numerous monitors and other ICU devices;
- Complex structures for communication, drug ordering, drug therapy and optimal maintenance of patient homeostasis and temperature regulation.

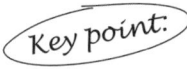 **ICUs offer both challenges and opportunities during major incidents.**

Functional major incidents

Functional major incidents include disruption of the infrastructural facilities required for daily optimal patient care and loss of the logistical resources to continue functioning during prolonged incidents:

- *Power failure:* most power failures should be temporary in the ICU, as this area of the hospital is usually connected to the UPS.
- *Water cut-off:* water is required for cleanliness in the ICU and to run devices such as dialysis machines.
- *Failure of oxygen, other gases or the vacuum-suction system:* most hospitals today have oxygen, medical air and vacuum suction systems piped to the ICU suite from a central point, as is the case in the operation suite.
- *Failure of the heating/cooling or air conditioning system:* the ICU suite is a controlled environment, and the same problems apply as in the operation suite. Hypothermia is of particular importance in trauma patients.

- *Logistical failure from the consumable stores or equipment stores:* most hospitals rely on regular supply of consumables from a central stores area or from regular external delivery, keeping only adequate stock for about 24–48 hours. Failure of this delivery system, due to destruction or incapacity, especially during protracted external incidents, can become a major internal incident due to an inability to provide the necessary sundries to perform quality of care.
- *Staff incapacitation:* a shortage of staff (due to an outbreak of food poisoning, for example, or due to gas leaks or explosions), leading to inability to provide routine services, may also hamper the response to a major incident, whether internally or externally. This will compound the existing worldwide shortage of trained staff in ICU areas.
- *Failure of communication and IT systems:* during most external acute incidents, and certainly during protracted external incidents, failure of telecommunications and computer services may result in the need for the use of radios or runners to provide feedback to other parts of the hospital. It is essential that all staff be familiar with correct radio procedure.
- *Lack of bed availability and lack of surge capacity:* ICUs are a scarce resource; in the USA the ratio of ICU beds and ventilators to patients is around 25 per 100 000 of the population. In South Africa and other developing countries, these figures are much lower. The ability to arrange for extra facilities, through expansion to other high-care and ICU areas, is limited but should be planned for in the major incident planning phase: prevention is better than cure.

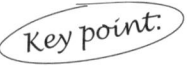 **Functional incidents, together with hazards such as fires, are by far the most common incidents affecting ICUs.**

External major incidents and the ICU

External major incidents occur on a regular basis, and these may require the institution of in-house hospital major incident plans, such as stopping elective surgical procedures, clearing post-anaesthetic care areas to increase intensive/critical care capacity and opening additional operation rooms to handle the expected surge of major emergency cases.

External major incidents may be traumatic in nature, although many will involve critically ill medical and paediatric patients. This is made worse during protracted incidents, such as natural disasters, which tax the in-hospital teams' abilities to adapt, as the hospital itself is stressed to capacity, due to the patient surge combined with the challenges already highlighted in the preceding section.

The team therefore needs to be prepared for the effects of external major incidents by means of the following:

- Knowledge of the local major incident plan, with a hospital coordination team who will direct the hospital response to this incident. Communication is the key to success.
- The ICU staff will fall under the nursing hierarchy in the scheme of command. They most often will be involved with the subsequent treatment phase when the type of incident involves many injured patients. This will involve application of strict triage criteria by the medical staff to decide when a critically ill patient

is offered an ICU bed. Often the standard of care normally provided will be reduced and the patients admitted will be those who are salvable, but with critically impaired organ systems.

- Action cards should be provided for the shift leaders of the ICU nursing staff to detail the extent of their actions during a major incident. Someone must coordinate the overall ICU nursing response with the reporting authority to the nursing service manager.
- ICU teams may be formed to undertake the inter-hospital transfers.
- Regular drills and table-top practices are essential for adequate preparation. The longest phase of the major incident is most likely to be the definitive care phase in the ICU, and this will delay the hospital recovery phase.
- Unlike the USA and Canada, developing countries do not have stockpiles of additional ventilators and other ICU equipment readily available. Knowledge of access to military resources and national resources may assist in alleviating the challenges of equipment shortage, such as the military deployable field hospital or the mobile hospital based in a train.

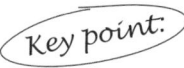 **External major incidents may overwhelm the normal ICU capacity. Team-based care is essential.**

Evacuation due to hazards

Evacuation of the ICU follows very similar principles to the evacuation of the operating suite, with similar command structures and triage decision processes to be followed.

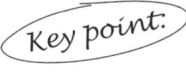 **Evacuation of an ICU will be most commonly due to fire, and next most likely due to an external threat. Planning for evacuation is essential.**

Conclusion

Internal and external major incidents can affect the function of the ICU and may necessitate evacuation or alternative management strategies. Planning for an 'all hazards' approach will prevent an incident from becoming a disaster.

Other areas of special concern

Hospitals faced with internal and external major incidents are often found to have planned mainly for adult patients in the wards, thus leading to challenges when patients of other age groups are also involved. The need to move patients carefully and safely from the hospital beds or transportation gurneys to assembly areas, or for ward consolidation, is only one aspect in which an 'all hazards' approach is essential.

It is essential that hospitals build into the in-house plans special considerations for the very young, the very old and the patient who presents a community health risk or a psychiatric challenge. A plan with a good command and control, addressing safety issues and with adequate paths for communication, will ensure appropriate situational assessment and will lead to correct triage, treatment and transport options for these high-risk patient groups.

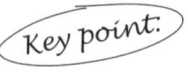 An all-hazards approach to hospital major incident planning must include specific plans for nurseries, paediatric wards, older persons, the mentally infirm and isolation wards.

Functional major incidents

Functional major incidents impact not only the daily functioning of the ward of a hospital, but may have a huge impact on overall infection control and patient comfort. These incidents affect all types of facility equally and are as discussed above:

- Power failure;
- Water cut-off;
- Failure of oxygen, other gases or the vacuum-suction system;
- Staff incapacitation;
- Failure of consumable and medication supply.

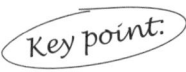 Nurseries and isolation areas are at particular risk of functional failure, while geriatric, psychiatric and paediatric wards may be less directly affected.

External major incidents causing internal incidents

In addition to the discussion above, such incidents may lead to the need for hospital evacuation and dealing with the challenges of the sub-groups of patients such as children, the aged and the psychiatrically infirm. The hospital should have a simple major incident plan, for both internal and external incidents, including an evacuation plan.

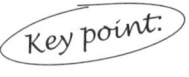 External major incidents may involve children and the aged. Adequate planning for these and other risk groups must be part of the all-hazards approach.

Specific issues relating to the nursery or children's wards

The issues for the nursery include the following:

- Babies have poor temperature regulation and the environment is often kept warmer than in general wards. Additionally, the need for a power supply for incubators and infusion pumps necessitates that battery back-up is provided during evacuation.
- Evacuation may preclude the administration of ultraviolet therapy to babies, leading to higher complication rates.
- Children's wards often have a mix of very frail children and reasonably well children, thus making evacuation a challenge.
- Children respond to fear by withdrawing, and may not follow instructions well during an evacuation, leading to confusion and further injury.

● For those in the 'well-baby' nursery, there is the potential advantage that the bassinets used to house the babies are a useful option for transporting two or three babies together during an evacuation.

Specific issues pertaining to the aged and geriatric wards

The aged suffer from physical challenges, such as poor vision, poor hearing and limited mobility. These issues may lead to difficulty in communicating the urgency of a situation to the aged or to mobilise them to evacuation status. Limited mobility makes the frail aged patient more prone to falls and further harm. The frail will require movement on gurneys or wheelchairs, thus leading to increased traffic and a decrease in corridor space for movement and evacuation. The diseases of maturity lead to polypharmacy and numerous chronic medications; abrupt withdrawal of these medications, due to unavailability during incidents, may result in rebound effects and increased morbidity.

Specific aspects of dealing with major incidents affecting the psychiatric wards

Psychiatric patients may be confined to wards within a general hospital or may be in specific psychiatric facilities. The challenge may be that the internal incident is itself the result of psychiatric disease (such as a hostage situation, fire-setting or suicide attempt) or that the incident is one that requires the movement of many sedated, medicated patients, who may be unresponsive due to the medication, who may misinterpret the situation and which may lead to outbursts of violence or panic episodes. The need for restraints and the risk of mixing psychiatric patients with other patients in assembly areas and temporary holding areas should be considered when planning for hospital incidents. Evacuation during major external incidents, such as a flood, is a challenge.

Specific challenges for patients with communicable diseases

Communicable disease emergencies are dealt with comprehensively in another section of this book. The unique environment of isolation wards and the specific equipment used to prevent cross-contamination of such diseases may present several challenges during a major incident. These wards generally have negative pressure ventilation to prevent external spread of contagion, separate changing facilities to prevent staff infection and the need for special protective garments and sometimes breathing apparatus to prevent staff contamination with droplet-spread agents. The patients may be severely ill and require ventilation or invasive therapeutic supportive agents that are difficult to transport readily.

The emergency services will often not have sufficient specially designed vehicles to transport these types of patients in the event of an evacuation. Movement of these patients places the staff and other patients at risk in assembly areas and potentially puts the entire community at risk when the agent involved is easily spread. The wearing of personal protective equipment may hamper movement and endanger staff further during evacuation. Finally, many isolation facilities are not designed for rapid access or egress, and this adds a further burden to the staff during a crisis.

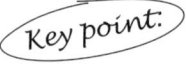 **Each of the numerous special-group wards in the hospital that are ordinarily considered 'general wards' may pose specific challenges and threats during major incidents.**

Evacuation due to hazards

The challenges as discussed with relation to the operating suite and ICU are relevant here; due consideration must be given in major incident plans for special risk groups such as children, the elderly and psychiatric patients.

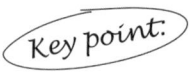 **Evacuation plans should be area-specific and should be tested with simulated patients to ensure that plans are implementable when the need arises.**

Summary

Internal and external major incidents may affect the function of hospital general wards as much as speciality care areas and may necessitate evacuation or alternative management strategies. Planning for an 'all hazards' approach will prevent an incident from becoming a disaster.

4.10 Resources

CBPP: Evacuation Planning for Hospitals, Draft Document, May 2006 (see full reference at no. 13) available from http://www.nyc.gov/html/doh/downloads/pdf/bhpp/bhpp-hospital-evac-plan.pdf (Useful checklist for hospital evacuation planning, and toolkit of forms necessary for planning and evacuation.)

Schultz CH *et al*: Benchmarking for hospital evacuation: A critical data collection tool (see full reference at no. 3) available at the journal website pdm.medicine.wisc.edu/ (The appendix contains the questionnaire and data collection tool.)

United Nations Development Program and Government of India, Guidelines for hospital emergency preparedness, available under resources and publications from safehospitals.info (See Annexures for Hospital evacuation plans and guidelines according to international best practices.)

World Health Organization Western Pacific Region Field manual for capacity assessment of health facilities in responding to emergencies, available under resources and publications from www.safehospitals.info (Tool contains several questions relevant to evacuation planning and preparedness.)

4.11 References

1. Ligthelm TJ. Hospital impact: internal disasters. In: Powers R, Daily E (editors). *Disaster nursing international*. Melbourne: Cambridge University Press; 2010. pp. 139–64.

2. Sternberg E, Lee GC, Huard D. US hospital evacuations 1971–1999. *Prehospital and Disaster Medicine* 2004;(2).
3. Restuccia MC. Hospital power putage. In: Ciottone MD (editor). *Disaster Medicine*. Philadelphia: Mosby Elsevier; 2006. pp. 897–900.
4. Lessons learned from a hospital evacuation during Tropical Storm Allison. Available from: www.semp.us/publications/biot_printview.php?BiotID=216. Accessed 17 May 2008.
5. Hospital emergency management plan. Available from: www.downstate.edu/emergency_medicine/pdf/KCHCSection01.pdf. Accessed 8 December 2008.
6. Malhortra SK, Nakra D. Smoke in the operating room complex: a rare incident of internal disaster. *Anesthesia & Analgesia*. 2006;(102).
7. Nates JL. Combined external and internal hospital disaster: impact and response in a Houston trauma center intensive care unit. *Critical Care Medicine*. 2004;3:686–690.
8. Reitherman R. Application of earthquake engineering information in hospital emergency response and recovery. Available from: host.uniroma3.it/dipartimenti/dis/ricerca/Hospitals/Articoli_pdf/r.0 1.eng.pdf. Accessed 8 December 2008.
9. US Dept of Defence. *Emergency war surgery*. 3rd edition. Washington, DC: Dept of Defence; 2004.
10. Dufour D, Kromen Jensen S, Owen-Smith M. *Surgery for victims of war*. Geneva: ICRC; 1998.
11. International Committtee of the Red Cross. *Hospitals for the war-wounded*. Geneva: ICRC; 1998.
12. International Committtee of the Red Cross. *War and public health*. Geneva: ICRC; n.d.
13. The Sphere Project. *The Sphere Project: humanitarian charter and minimum standards in disaster response*. Oxford: Oxfam Publishing; 2000.
14. USAID. Field operation guide for disaster assessment and response. 3rd edition. Washington, DC: USAID; 1998.
15. Ligthelm TJ. Hospital impact: internal disasters. In: Powers R, Daily E (eds). *Disaster nursing international*. Melbourne: Cambridge University Press; 2010. pp. 139–64.
16. Sternberg E, Lee GC, Huard D. US hospital evacuations 1971–1999. *Prehospital and Disaster Medicine*. 2004;(2).
17. The Cascade Hospital: Hospital Emergencies. Available from: http://www.geocities.com/Hollywood/Academy/8097/cascadehospital/hosp-codes.html. Accessed 31 December 2008.
18. Pan American Health Organization. Should hospitals be evacuated? Working group recommendations, San Salvador, 8–10 July 2003. Available from: www.disaster-info.net/hospital_disaster/assets/HospEvacuationRecommemdation.doc . Accessed 18 April 2008.
19. Wisconsin Department of Health & Family Services. Hospital disaster plan. Available from: dhs.wisconsin.gov/rl_dsl/Hospital/HospitalDisastrPlngGds.htm. Accessed 18 April 2008.
20. Ligthelm T. Hospital impact: internal disasters. In: Powers R, Daily E (eds). *Disaster nursing international*. Melbourne: Cambridge University Press; 2010.

21. The Fire Safety Advice Centre. Information about the fire triangle/tetrahedron and combustion. Available from: www.firesafe.org.uk/html/miscellaneous/firetria.htm. Accessed 8 December 2008.

22. The Fire Safety Advice Centre. Information about the fire triangle/tetrahedron and combustion. Available from: www.firesafe.org.uk/html/miscellaneous/firetria.htm. Accessed 8 December 2008.

23. World Health Organization. World Health Day. Available from: www.who.int/world-health-day/2009/en/index.html. Accessed 21 December 2009.

24. Brunkard J, Namulanda G, Ratard R. Katrina Deaths, Louisiana, 2005. *Disaster Medicine and Public Health Preparedness* 2008;2(4):215–23.

25. Schultz CH, Koenig KL, Auf der Heide E, Olson R. Benchmarking for hospital evacuation: a critical data collection tool. *Prehospital and Disaster Medicine* 2005;20(5):331–42.

26. McConnaughey J. Is lack of hospital evacuation plan medical malpractice? Available from: www.lsuhospitals.org/Media-Relations/InTheNews/04.13.07.pdf. Accessed 21 December 2009.

27. Bagaria J, Heggie C, Abrahams J, Murray V. Evacuation and sheltering of hospitals in emergencies: a review of international experience. *Prehospital and Disaster Medicine* 2009;24(5):461–7.

28. Stander M. Hospital disaster planning in the Western Cape: are we ready for 2010? MMED dissertation, University of Cape Town, 2008.

29. Gansterer A. Disaster management and its economic implications. Master's thesis, University of Vienna, 2008.

30. Milsten A. Hospital response to acute onset disaster: a review. *Prehospital and Disaster Medicine* 2004;15(1):32–45.

31. Sahdeo J. Surgical registrars' knowledge, attitude and practices regarding hospital disaster preparedeness across three tertiary hospitals in Gauteng. Master of Public Health research, University of Witwatersrand, 2008.

32. Sternberg E, Lee GC, Huard D. Counting crises: US hospital evacuations, 1971–1999. *Prehospital and Disaster Medicine* 2004;19(2):150–7.

33. Sexton KH, Alperin LM, Stobo JD: Lessons from Hurricane Rita: the University of Texas Medical Branch Hospital's evacuation. *Academic Emergency Medicine* 2007;82:792–6.

34. Schultz CH, Koenig KL, Lewis RJ. Implications of hospital evacuation after the Northridge, California, earthquake. *New England Journal of Medicine* 2003;348:1349–55.

35. Center for Bioterrorism Preparedness and Planning (CBPP) and Continuum Partners. Evacuation planning for hospitals. Draft document, May 2006. Available from: www.nyc.gov/html/doh/downloads/pdf/bhpp/bhpp-hospital-evac-plan.pdf. Accessed 21 December 2009.

36. Williams J, Nocera M, Casteel C. The effectiveness of disaster training for healthcare workers: a systematic review. *Annals of Emergency Medicine* 2008;52:211–22.

37. Roccaforte JD, Cushman JG. Disaster preparedness, triage and surge capacity for hospital definitive care areas: optimizing outcomes when demands exceed resources. *Journal of Anesthesiology Clinical Pharmacology* 2007;25:161–177.

38. Eiland JE, Pritchard DA, Stevens DA. Emergency preparedness – is your OR ready? *Association of Perioperative Registered Nurses Journal* 2004;79:1276–83.
39. Sternberg E. Planning for resilience in hospital internal disaster. *Prehospital and Disaster Medicine* 2003;18:291–300.
40. Hardcastle T. Operation room methodology for the trauma team in the modern era of damage control surgery. *South African Theatre Nurse Journal* 2009;34:8–12.
41. Hardcastle T. Major incidents and the operative team: how to be prepared. Ibid. 2009;34:28–31.
42. Republic of South Africa. Department of Health. Guidelines for the development of a disaster plan. 2nd Draft, 23 March 2001. Pretoria: Government Printer.
43. Carley S, Mackway-Jones K. *Major incident medical management and support. The practical approach in the hospital.* London: BMJ Books; 2005.
44. Salmon L. Fire in the OR – prevention and preparedness. *Association of Perioperative Registered Nurses Journal* 2004;80:42–54.
45. Mahoney EJ, Biffl WL, Cioffi WG. Mass-casualty incidents: how does an ICU prepare? *Journal of Intensive Care Medicine* 2008;23:219–235.
46. Bhagwangee S, Scribante J and the Council of the Critical Care Society of Southern Africa. National audit of critical care resources: how long before we act? *South African Journal of Critical Care* 2008;24:4–6.
47. Roccaforte JD, Cushman JG. Disaster preparedness, triage and surge capacity for hospital definitive care areas: optimizing outcomes when demands exceed resources. *Journal of Anesthesiology Clinical Pharmacology* 2007;25:161–77.
48. Sternberg E. Planning for resilience in hospital internal disaster. *Prehospital and Disaster Medicine* 2003;18:291–300.
49. Carley S, Mackway-Jones K. *Major incident medical management and support. The practical approach in the hospital.* London: BMJ Books; 2005.
50. Christian MD, Devereaux AV, Dichter JR, Geiling JA, Rubinson L. Definitive care for the critically ill during a disaster: current capabilities and limitations. *Chest* 2008;133:8S–17S.
51. Philips R, Butts F. Code red! Some tips on fighting fire in the ICU. *Health Facilities Management* 1996;9:40.
52. Manion P, Golden IJ. Vertical evacuation drill of an intensive care unit: design, implementation and evaluation. *Disaster Management and Response* 2004;2:14–19.
53. Roccaforte JD, Cushman JG. Disaster preparedness, triage and surge capacity for hospital definitive care areas: optimizing outcomes when demands exceed resources. *Journal of Anesthesiology Clinical Pharmacology* 2007;25:161–77.
54. Republic of South Africa. Department of Health. Guidelines for the development of a disaster plan. 2nd Draft, 23 March 2001. Pretoria: Government Printer.
55. Carley S, Mackway-Jones K. *Major incident medical management and support. The practical approach in the hospital.* London: BMJ Books; 2005.
56. Frank L, Epstein B, Adams S. Disaster preparedness for the ICN: evolution and testing of one unit's plan. *Pediatric Nursing* March–April 1993;19:122–7.
57. US Dept of Health and Human Services, Administration on Aging. Just in case. Emergency readiness for older adults and caregivers. Washington, DC: US Dept of Health and Human Services; n.d.

58. Thomas J, Lackey N. How to evacuate a psychiatric hospital: a Hurrican Katrina success story. *Journal of Psychosocial Nursing* 2008;46:35–40.
59. Schultz CH, Koenig KL, Auf der Heide E: Benchmarking for hospital evacuation: a critical data collection tool. *Prehospital and Disaster Medicine* 2005;20(5):331–42.
60. Cocanour CS, Allen SJ, Mazabob J, Sparks JW, Fischer CP, Romans J, Lally KP. Lessons learned from the evacuation of an urban teaching hospital. *Archives of Surgery* 2002;137:1141–5.

5

Mass Gatherings

W Smith

Objectives

By the end of this section, the reader will:

- understand that there is increased rate of medical presentations at mass gathering events;
- understand the necessity and the components of a thorough risk analysis;
- appreciate that medical planning for mass gatherings requires an integrated effort from all relevant role-players.

5.1   Introduction

There is no universally accepted definition of a mass gathering. Most definitions are based on number of people attending, but this can vary between 1 000 and an excess of 25 000, depending on the author. Regardless of exactly how they are defined, mass gatherings have been shown to have a higher presentation of patients compared to the general population, and have at times results in mass casualty situations. Wherever a large number of people gather in one defined area, there is an increased risk of a major incident.

5.2   Planning for a mass gathering

Medical planning for a mass gathering needs an integrated approach, involving all role-players in order for the medical response to occur smoothly. Below are some aspects to be considered in planning.

Event safety

The organising body needs to prepare for the event in accordance with national and local legislation and guidelines. This includes ensuring high standards in public health areas such as sanitation and food hygiene.

A risk assessment should be undertaken for each proposed mass gathering. This is essential as it informs planning for aspects such as the number and category of medical personnel that should be available. Important factors in risk assessment and planning are covered in the section on risk assessment and medical resource deployment.

Consulting valuable resources, such as parties with experience in previous or similar events, local services such as emergency services, who have knowledge of the local environment or data collected at similar events in the past, will provide useful information for planning.

5.3 Medical resources

Medical resources at a mass gathering fulfil two roles. The first is that of providing care for individual patients presenting during the event, whether due to injury sustained at the event, illness developing during the event or exacerbation of an existing disease. Immediate essential care should be available at the event, as well as the capacity to transfer patients to definitive care centres.

Depending on the event, it will likely be covered by a multi-disciplinary medical team comprising volunteer first-aiders, paramedics and doctors. Planning and training should involve the whole team to ensure a standardised response. It is also suggested that standardised protocols for common presentations be put in place and emergency drills practised regularly.

The second role is to form the initial response to a major incident. There should be prearranged, structured roles and actions for medical personnel in the event of a major incident. These roles and actions will be more smoothly carried out if personnel are familiar with the environment, and if the guidance given is compatible with the surroundings of the event. The execution of these roles and actions will also only be possible as part of a coordinated response including crowd management and control of access and egress routes. Thus it is essential that all parties forming the initial response to a major incident, including medical and crowd safety, prepare and train together to ensure optimal care of casualties.

The exact number of personnel needed to deal with individual casualties and form the initial core response to a major incident is difficult to predict with accuracy, as many factors can influence patients' presentation at a given event. These factors are described below, along with a medical resource model that has been proposed for use in planning for medical cover at events in South Africa.

5.4 Communications

Functional communication networks are essential for a rapid and cohesive medical response. Hand-held radios are often used, with different, prearranged frequencies being used by different parties. It is important to have redundancy built into the system, as communication systems are often compromised in the event of a major incident. It is also important to note that, in events with a lot of noise, such as rock concerts or football matches with vuvuzelas, normal auditory communication devices may be ineffective and other techniques may need to be employed to ensure widespread, accurate communication.

5.5 Equipment and local facilities

Equipment and facilities may be limited, depending on the nature and location of the event, and planning should ensure that they are able to meet the anticipated demands. Each category of staff working in the medical team will have preferred lists of equipment, supplies and facility requirements. However, it is advised that standardised, interchangeable equipment, with which the entire team is familiar, be utilised wherever possible. Planning should also include alternatives for major incident situations, where, by definition, the demand outstrips the supply.

5.6   Access and egress

Access and egress routes should be planned beforehand and be clearly identifiable. Alternative and additional transport routes and methods to be used in the case of a major incident should be identified as part of planning.

5.7   Risk assessment and medical resource deployment

Many risk factors have been described which have a direct impact on the number of persons requiring medical intervention at a mass gathering. Commonly described factors that determine the potential number of patients that may present, and the ability to deal with these patients, at a mass gathering are listed and described below:

- Nature of the event;
- Nature of the venue;
- Seated or unseated;
- Spectator profile;
- Past history of similar events;
- Expected number of spectators;
- Event duration;
- Seasonal considerations;
- Proximity to hospitals;
- Profile of hospitals;
- Additional hazards;
- Additional on-site facilities.

1.   Nature of the event

The nature of the event is an important consideration in predicting medical attendances. For example, a rock concert with a younger group profile and increased potential of alcohol and drug abuse may pose a greater risk than a classical music concert with a similar number of attendees.

2.   Nature of the venue

Venue construction, size and set-up may increase or decrease the risk profile. For example, an event hosted in a purpose-built stadium will pose less of a risk than one in a venue consisting of temporary structures, or an event spread out over a large area. Indoor events have also been shown to have a lower risk profile than similar events held outdoors, where exposure to the elements may increase the risk of illness among the spectators.

3. Seated or unseated

An event allowing for only seated attendees will have a lower risk profile than one allowing for unseated spectators. This may be due to the fact that the capacity of the venue is exceeded when unseated spectators are catered for, which has its own inherent problems.

4. Spectator profile

Profiling of potential spectators is extremely important in planning for a mass gathering. An event in which the attendees are mainly family groups will pose far less of a risk than, say, a rock concert with a predominantly younger audience. While the literature associates events of audiences younger than 35 with the highest risk, it must be remembered that an event that attracts a predominantly elderly profile, such as papal visits, can likewise result in high patient numbers.

5. Past history of similar events

Information regarding previous events, including data pertaining to the type of incidents and medical problems that arose, is extremely important when planning for similar events. It is the responsibility of all medical planners to maintain adequate documentation of events, including risk profiles and patient presentation rates, in order to contribute to future planning of similar events worldwide.

6. Expected number of spectators

This is one of the easier parameters to quantify. Attendance at previous events, in the case of annual or other repeated events, can inform planning. Early consultation with event organisers and the number of pre-booked tickets will aid in determining the numbers expected.

7. Event duration

The duration of the event is another important factor in determining the number of medical staff that will be required to provide cover at a mass gathering. Specifically, events of an extended duration add a number of additional risks that need to be considered. A shift system for medical staff may need to be employed so as to adhere to legislation covering maximum length of time that a medical staff member may be deployed. It is also likely that the number of patients presenting for medical attention will increase the longer the event continues. This is especially pertinent at events where alcohol is on sale, as well as those at which spectators are exposed to environmental elements. The length of time that people are expected to queue to enter a venue should be included in the overall duration of the event.

8. Seasonal considerations

Expected weather conditions are an extremely important factor to take into account, especially when the event is taking place outdoors. In South Africa, higher temperatures are more likely to be a problem than the opposite extreme.

Hot and humid conditions have been associated with higher patient presentation rates, and consideration needs to be given to the fact that medical personnel will potentially also be affected. Planning should thus include a suitable shelter from which medical staff can function.

9 and 10. Hospitals

The distance between the event venue and appropriate hospitals has a direct impact on medical resources planning. The number and category of staff necessary to provide stabilisation before transfer would necessarily increase proportionally with the distance from support facilities. The number of ambulances may also need to be increased, given that, should they be utilised to transfer a patient, they would be lost to the event for longer periods due to longer transport times. If a helicopter service is available for transferring patients, this needs to be incorporated into the medical plan and necessary requirements fulfilled, such as the provision of a landing zone and the requisite aviation approval to operate out of this zone.

11. Presence of additional hazards

Consideration must also be given for any other potential hazards that may be present or associated with the event. This will be based on event intelligence, and it is therefore vital that a complete profile of the event is obtained from the event organisers prior to deciding on the medical resources to be deployed. Table 5.10 highlights some of the potential hazards that may be present.

12. Additional on-site facilities

The capability of on-site medical facilities is a determinant as regards the number and qualification of medical personnel required. The presence of automatic external defibrillators within public areas has become popular over the last few years. These can be found later for at most international airports and other public areas which cater for large numbers of people. These provide the public with rapid access to a life-saving procedure without requiring large numbers of qualified medical personnel. Likewise, any medical facility at the event that may be able to provide a procedure otherwise only performed at a hospital will potentially decrease the number of resources that may have been required to transfer the patients to hospital.

5.8   Medical resource models

There are no universally accepted standards to determine the number of medical staff that should be provided at mass gatherings. A resource often quoted is *A Guide to health, safety and welfare at music and similar events*, which was developed by the UK Health and Safety Executive. This guide has been modified to better suit the South African context and to take into account the limited available medical resources as compared to developed countries.

The calculation of resources needed at a particular event is performed in the following way: within each of the categories listed earlier, the particular risk factors are identified and allocated a score. These are given in Tables 5.1–5.12, with the number of the table corresponding to that of the factor described earlier. Only one score is allocated per category and this will be the highest possible score within that particular category. For example, in Table 5.1 a New Year celebration event may also include a pyrotechnical display. Both these risks are listed under the category of 'Nature of event'. A single score of 7 will be allocated for the New Year celebration as it is higher than the score of 4 allocated to a pyrotechnical display.

Once a score has been allocated for each category the following calculation is done:

Event risk score = (sum of the scores of Tables 5.1 to 5.11) minus the score of Table 5.12

The resultant risk score obtained is then referenced against the medical resource matrix defined in Table 5.13.

Example

An event that scores 43 on the risk profile will require the following medical resources to be deployed at the event:

- 2 ambulances;
- crew members to staff the ambulances;
- 12 BLS (Basic Life Support) providers;
- 1 ILS (Intermediate Life Support) provider;
- 1 ALS (Advanced Life Support) provider;
- 1 doctor;
- 1 medical coordinator.

Validation

A retrospective validation of this model has been performed, showing an acceptable rate of under-prediction of staff. This study was for football and rugby events only. At the time of going to press, a prospective validation was underway using medical and event data from the 2010 FIFA World Cup. An electronic copy of this model is available at www.emssa.org.za

Summary

Mass gatherings have a higher patient presentation rate than that found in normal populations. They also pose an increased risk for major incidents. Planning for these events, including consideration of factors influencing patient presentation rate, is essential for the mitigation and amelioration of these risks.

Tables 5.1–5.12

Table 5.1: Risk score for nature of event

1. Nature of event	Risk score
Classical performance	2
Public exhibition	3
Pop/rock concert	5
Dance event (rave/disco)	8
Agricultural/country show	2
Marine	3
Motorcycle display	3
Aviation	3
Motor sport	4
State occasions	2
VIP visits/summit	3
Music festival	3
International event	3
Bonfire/pyrotechnical display	4
New Year celebrations	7
Demonstrations/marches	5
Sport event with low risk of disorder	2
Sport event with medium risk of disorder	5
Sport event with high risk of disorder	7
Opposing factions involved	9

Table 5.2: Risk score for venue

2. Nature of venue	Risk score
Indoor	1
Stadium	2
Outdoor in confined location, e.g. park	2
Other outdoor, e.g. festival	3
Widespread public location in streets	4 ➲

2. Nature of venue continued	Risk score
Temporary outdoor structures	4
Includes overnight camping	5

Table 5.3: Risk score – seated or standing

3. Seated or unseated	Risk score
Seated	1
Mixed	2
Standing	3

Table 5.4: Risk score for audience profile

4. Spectator profile	Risk score
Full mix, in family groups	2
Full mix, not in family groups	3
Predominately young adults	3
Predominately children and teenagers	4
Predominately elderly	4

Table 5.5: Risk score in relation to intelligence gathered from previous events

5. Past history	Risk score
Good data, low casualty rate previously (less than 0.05%)	-1
Good data, medium casualty rate previously (0.05%–0.2%)	1
Good data, high casualty rate previously (more than 0.2%)	2
First event, no data	2

Table 5.6: Risk score as it relates to attendance number at an event

6. Expected numbers	Risk score
< 1000	1
< 3000	2
< 5000	4

6. Expected numbers	Risk score
< 10 000	8
< 20 000	16
< 30 000	20
< 40 000	24
< 50 000	28
< 60 000	32
< 70 000	36
< 80 000	42
< 90 000	46
< 100 000	50
< 200 000	60
< 300 000	70

Table 5.7: Risk score as related to duration of the event

7. Expected event duration (including queuing from gate open time)	Risk score
Less than 4 hours	1
More than 4, less than 12 hours	2
More than 12 hours	3

Table 5.8: Risk score as it pertains to seasonal variation

8. Seasons (outdoor events)	Risk score
Summer	2
Autumn	1
Winter	1
Spring	1

Table 5.9: Risk score in relation to hospital proximity

9. Proximity to hospitals (nearest suitable emergency centre)	Risk score
Less than 30 min by road	0
More than 30 min by road	2

Table 5.10: Risk score related to the profile of ECs available

10. Profile of hospitals	Risk score
Choice of emergency centres	1
Large emergency centre	2
Small emergency centre	3

Table 5.11: Risk score for additional hazards

11. Additional hazards	Risk score
Carnival	1
Helicopters	1
Parachute display	1
Street theatre	1
Water hazard	1
On-site alcohol use	1

Table 5.12: Event medical facilities as a mitigating factor

12. Additional on-site facilities	Risk score
Suturing and/or plastering	−2
Vending machine for over-the-counter medication	−2
Public access AED	−1
Existing full-time operational medical facilities on-site	−2

Table 5.13: The medical staff resource matrix

Score	Ambulance	BLS*	ILS**	ALS***	Ambulance crew	Doctor	Nurse	Coordinator
<20	0	2			0	0	0	0
21-25	0	4			0	0	0	0
26-30	1	4	1	0	2	0	0	0
31-35	1	6	1	1	2	0	0	visit
36-40	1	8	1	1	2	0	0	visit
41- 45	2	12	1	1	4	1	0	1
46- 50	2	16	2	2	4	1	1	1
51-55	3	20	3	3	6	2	1	1
56-60	3	24	3	3	6	2	2	1
61-65	4	32	4	4	8	2	2	1
66-70	5	40	5	5	10	3	3	1
71-75	6	48	6	6	12	3	3	1
76-80	8	64	8	8	16	4	4	1
81-85	10	80	10	10	20	5	5	2
86+	15	120	15	15	30	6	6	2

*   BLS = Basic life support

** ILS = Intermediate life support

***ALS = Advanced life support

5.9 References

1. Arbon P. Mass-gathering medicine: a review of the evidence and future directions for research. *Prehospital and Disaster Medicine* 2007;22(2):131–5.
2. United Kingdom Health and Safety Executive. *The event safety guide: a guide to health, safety and welfare at music and similar events*. HSG 195. 2nd edition. London: HMSO; 1999.
3. Arbon P, Bridgewater FH, Smith C. Mass-gathering medicine: a predictive model for patient presentation and transport rates. *Prehospital and Disaster Medicine* 2001;16(3):150–8.
4. Milsten AM, Maguire BJ, Bissell RA, Seaman KG. Mass-gathering medical care: a review of the literature. *Prehospital and Disaster Medicine* 2002;17(3):151–62.

6

Disasters

*W Lubinga, N Ford, K Chu, A Argent, T Ligthelm, H Ras, N Kissoon
and T Hardcastle*

Objectives

By the end of this chapter, the reader will:

- know about common types of natural disaster;
- know the problems of dealing with displaced populations;
- understand how to undertake health assessments following disasters;
- understand the principles of medical support post-disaster;
- understand key public health issues following a disaster;
- understand what factors cause children to be at particular risk
  during disasters;
- be able to effectively plan for and deal with children affected by disaster;
- understand how to deal with mass fatalities;
- know the principles of body identification.

6.1   Types of disaster

In this chapter, attention is focused on uncompensated major incidents: disasters. While these may be classified technically as natural or man-made, this text refers mostly to man-made events in the context of major incidents. Man-made disasters include wars and terrorist activities; they are almost always preventable.

Natural disasters

A wide variety of natural phenomena can result in disasters, including earthquakes, tsunamis, volcanoes, floods, avalanches, thunder and lightning storms, tornadoes, hurricanes, pandemics, wildfires, famine, droughts and other severe weather extremes. These natural events result in a multiplicity of secondary effects, including loss of human life, and significant damage to property, the environment and the economy.

As natural phenomena, disasters are usually unpreventable, despite being relatively predictable. Although the actual natural event may be unpreventable, the argument does exist that the effects of such an occurrence can be reduced through planning and other proactive factors. As an example, the effect that the South East Asian tsunami of 2004 had on human mortality and morbidity might have been reduced by means of appropriate early warning systems or by something as simple as planting trees close to coastal settlements. Such plantations have been shown to minimise the effect of the wave surge associated with tsunamis.

Each type of natural disaster has particular relevance and significance in the geographical region in which it is most frequent. In southern Africa, there are more documented occurrences of wildfires, severe storms, flooding and droughts than there are of earthquakes or tsunamis.

Earthquakes

An earthquake is a sudden motion or trembling of the ground produced by the abrupt displacement of rock masses in response to tectonic forces. An earthquake's *focus* is the point at which the motion starts; the *epicentre* is the point on the earth's surface that is directly above the focus. An earthquake's *magnitude* is a measure of its strength as calculated from records made on a calibrated seismograph. In 1935, seismologist Charles Richter first defined magnitude, and the Richter scale is named in his honour. An earthquake's *intensity* is a measure of its effects at a particular place: intensity is determined from observations of the effects on people, structures and the earth's surface.

Southern Africa, due to its extensive and widely distributed mining industry, is predisposed to man-made earthquakes. The region lies on an intra-plate region which has a natural seismic regime characterised by a low level of activity by world standards. In South Africa, seismic events are recorded at least daily, but these do not come to the attention of the public as they are minor (less than 2.0 on the Richter scale) and occur deep below the surface of the earth. The strongest recorded earthquake in South Africa took place in 1969 in Ceres: it was 6.3 on the Richter scale and occurred at a depth of about 33 kilometres. Thirteen people were killed and damage estimated at US$ 24 million was reported.

Table 6.1: Noteworthy earthquakes in the 20th century in South Africa

Date	Time (SAT)	Region	Intensity	Magnitude	Remarks
31 Dec 1932	08h32	Off Cape St. Lucia	VIII	6.0 to 6.5	Poorly constructed buildings badly damaged; one or two collapsed; cracks and fissures in ground reported ⊃

Date	Time (SAT)	Region	Intensity	Magnitude	Remarks
29 Sept 1969	22h03	Ceres, Tulbagh, Wolseley	VIII to IX	6.3	Serious damage to certain buildings in area; damage varied from almost total destruction of both old and poorly constructed buildings, to large cracks in the better-built ones. 12 people were killed and many more injured.
08 Dec 1976	10h38	Welkom	VII	5.2	Extensive damage to many buildings and breaking of windows. The most dramatic was the collapse of a block of flats, six storeys high which took place 75 minutes after the seismic event.
07 March 1992	02h43	Carletonville	VII	4.7	Unusual amount of damage recorded, due to the high population density around the epicentral area. Houses were damaged as far as Pretoria.

Floods

Despite southern Africa being a drought-prone region, it is also prone to flash floods, with several reported flood disasters every year.

Unfortunately, these incidents often affect vulnerable population groups living in informal settlements that have been erected in flood-prone areas. Floods are further compounded by the affected areas suffering secondary incidents, such as fire, breakdown of infrastructure, failure of sanitation and new epidemics of diarrhoeal illnesses, in addition to the population having no suitable accommodation.

Table 6.2: The impact of floods

Impact of floods on public health

- immediate increased risk of death, injury, illness and disability;
- damage to/loss of primary lifelines – water, food, energy, shelter;
- damage to/loss of infrastructure (including hospital itself), utilities, facilities and services;
- displacement of population;
- breakdown in security;
- breakdown in sanitation;
- breakdown in communication networks and information flows;
- exposure to toxic substances;
- possible environmental pollution;
- high levels of stress;
- high risk to be compounded by secondary events, including fires and epidemics.

Health priorities for response

- search and rescue, triage, first aid, medical evacuation, hospital care;
- surveillance and reporting systems to monitor caseload, morbidity and mortality;
- services for the homeless/displaced – water, food, shelter, health, energy, security;
- protect public, staff and facilities;
- stress management (staff and public);
- care of the dead;
- deal with rumours and misinformation;
- deal with the media and international aid.

Elements of recovery

- documentation and analysis;
- access and equity issues;
- health education, public awareness, public information and community involvement;
- social and counselling services for the affected groups – disabled, displaced;
- infrastructure demolition, repair and replacement;
- economic regeneration.

Drought

The effects of drought on health in a region are illustrated in Figure 6.2. Much of the African continent suffers the effects of drought. As a slow-onset disaster, drought is often not covered by the media to the same extent as an acute disaster, and thus does not receive the same amount of international support. The effects, however, can by just as devastating on the population as the more publicised disasters, such as terrorist attacks or major earthquakes.

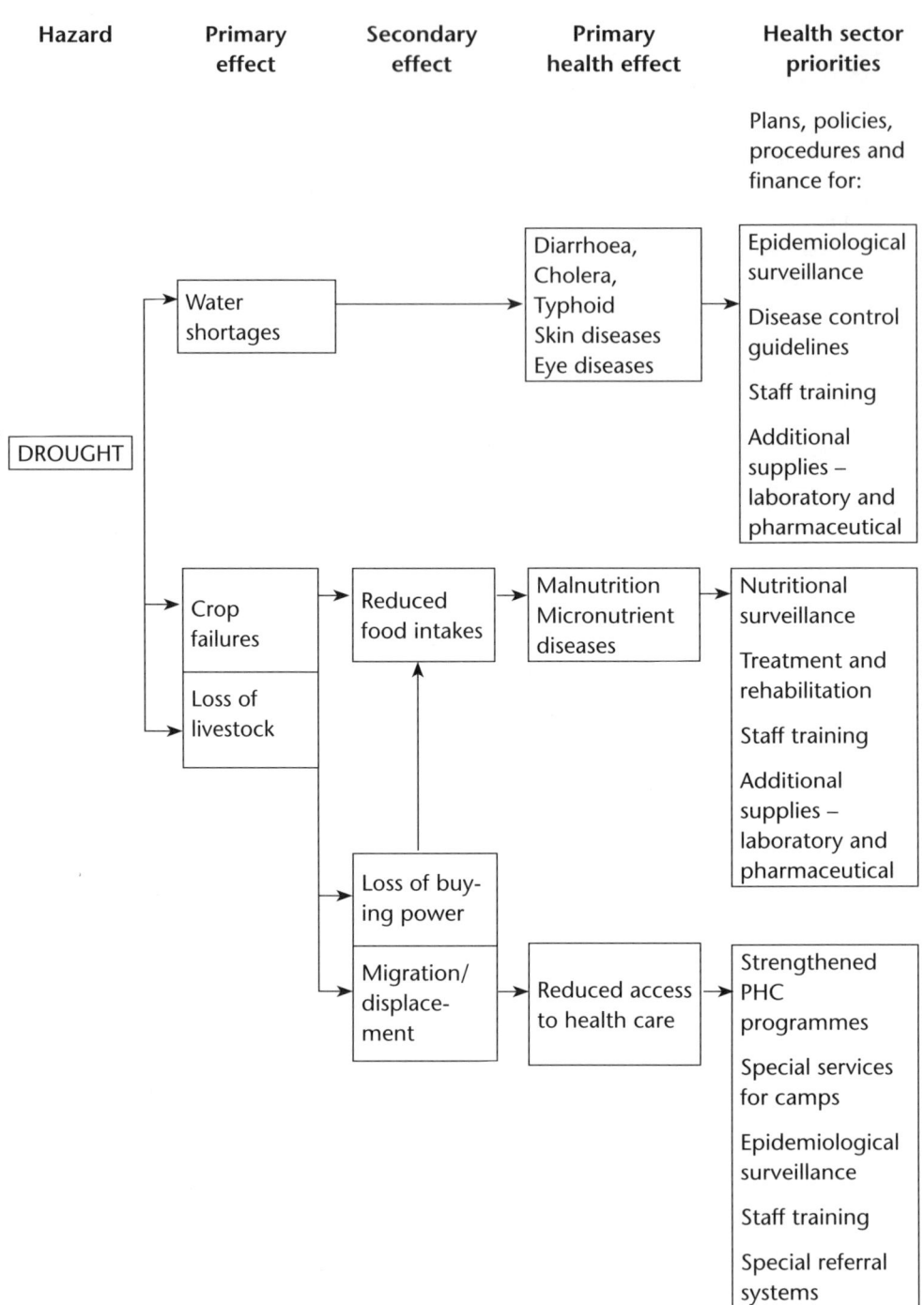

Figure 6.1: The effects of drought

Health effects of natural disasters

The health effects of common types of natural disaster in this region are presented in Table 6.3.

Table 6.3: Natural disasters – health effects and responses

Hazard	Impact on public health	Health priorities for response
• Epidemics; • Environmental pollution	• Immediate increased risk of death, illness and disability; • Risk of infection or contamination for relief personnel; • Exposure (long-term) of public to toxic substances; • Overload of facilities and services; • Rumours; • Diversion of resources	• Confirm the problem; • Identify the cause; • Provide treatment; • Activation of surveillance and monitoring systems to monitor caseload, case fatality rates, morbidity and mortality; • Prevent spread; • Protect staff and facilities; • Care of the dead; • Dealing with the media and international aid
• Storm; • Earthquake; • Volcano; • Flood; • Landslide; • Tsunami; • Fire	• Immediate increased risk of death, illness and disability; • Possible environmental pollution; • Exposure (long-term) of public to toxic substances; • Damage to or loss of essential life support services – water, food, shelter; • Displacement of population; • Breakdown in security; • Breakdown in communication networks and information flows; • Damage to and loss of facilities, services and staff; • High levels of psychosocial stress	• Search and rescue, triage, first aid, medical evacuation, hospital emergency care; • Activation of back-up systems; • Activation of surveillance and monitoring systems; • Special services for the homeless and displaced – water, food, shelter, health, security; • Stress management; • Care of the dead; • Dealing with the media and international aid
• Drought; • Famine; • Pests; • Plagues; • Infestations	• Long-term risk of increased morbidity and mortality; • Breakdown in food security; • Population displacement; • High levels of psychosocial stress; • Exposure to toxic substances (chemical sprays)	• Reinforcement of essential services; • Activation of surveillance and monitoring systems; • Special services for the homeless and displaced – water, food, shelter, health, security; • Stress management; • Care of the dead; • Dealing with the media and international aid

Risk reduction

There are certain steps which can be taken to reduce risk from natural disasters. Key points are presented in Table 6.4.

Table 6.4: Natural disaster risk reduction measures

Hazard/vulnerability reduction	Emergency preparedness
• Demography and land utilisation; • Siting and construction standards of public-sector infrastructure; • Private sector involvement in public issues – housing, infrastructure, environment; • Public health, curative care and mental health programme coverage; • Food safety, communicable disease and vector control programme coverage; • Staff awareness and staff training; • Public awareness and public information programmes.	• Legal mechanisms, policies and procedures; • Technical guidelines; • Staff recruitment and training; • Resource development and resource allocation; • Planning processes and planning objectives; • Buffer stocks and stockpiles; • Early warning systems; • Public health, mental health and hospital programme planning; • Reporting systems; • Public awareness and public information; • Role of international agencies in relief and development; • Services for special groups such as the disabled, displaced; • Contingency planning for: ▪ reception/care of displaced people; ▪ first aid and triage; ▪ emergency transport; ▪ hospitals and health centres; ▪ mass casualty management; ▪ hazardous substances; ▪ injury/disease surveillance; ▪ medical supplies systems; ▪ temporary accommodation.

6.2 Displaced populations

Displaced populations are communities or large groups of persons who have left their habitual place of residence due to an emergency. Disasters resulting in mass displacement can be either natural (hurricane or floods) or man-made (conflict, generalised violence, widespread persecution). When people are displaced within their own borders, they are referred to as 'internally displaced persons' (IDPs); when they are displaced outside of their country of origin, they become refugees.

The 1951 Refugee Convention defines a refugee as someone who, 'owing to a well-founded fear of being persecuted for reasons of race, religion, nationality, membership of a particular social group or political opinion, is outside the country of his nationality, and is unable to, or owing to such fear, is unwilling to avail himself of the protection of that country'. In 2008, there were an estimated 16 million refugees across the world. Major countries of origin included Afghanistan (2.8 million), Iraq (1.9 million) and Palestine.

Formal refugee status is determined for each individual by the host state following a procedure commonly referred to as the asylum process. In situations of mass influx, states may not be able to process claims individually and might decide to offer temporary protection: status determination is frozen and protection from refoulement is granted. (The principle of 'non-refoulement' is an international legal provision to protect refugees from being involuntarily returned to places in which their lives or freedoms are at risk.)

Internally displaced persons are defined as 'persons or groups of persons who have been forced or obliged to flee or to leave their homes or places of habitual residence, in particular as a result of or in order to avoid the effects of armed conflict, situations of generalised violence, violations of human rights or natural or human-made disasters, and who have not crossed an internationally recognised state border'. Displaced populations far outnumber refugees, with an estimated 26 million people internally displaced across 52 countries in 2008. The region with the largest IDP population is Africa, with some 11.6 million in 19 countries. In 2008, large-scale displacement (>200 000 persons) occurred in each of the following countries: Philippines, Sudan, Kenya, Democratic Republic of Congo (DRC), Iraq, Pakistan, Somalia, Colombia, Sri Lanka and India. Sudan's Darfur region alone contains some two million IDPs and is home to the largest IDP camp, sheltering around 130 000 people.

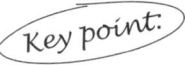 **Internally displaced persons far outnumber refugees in Africa.**

The assignment of refugee status is often contested as it implies different responsibilities to the host country. The rights of refugees are clearly ascribed by the 1951 Refugee Convention and 1967 Protocols, ratified by 144 states. These international laws clearly define who is a refugee, and set out the rights of individuals who are granted asylum and the responsibilities of nations that grant asylum.

Displaced people may have fled their homes for similar reasons as refugees, but because they remain within their own territory they are still subject to the laws of that state (even if that government might be the cause of their displacement). Many countries, particularly in southern Africa, house substantial numbers of foreigners who lack clear legal status, either because they are transients (e.g. migrant labourers) or because the host country is reluctant to provide clear legal status. Mass internal displacement thus may include substantial numbers of foreigners, who are often among the more vulnerable members of the society, and may even become deliberate targets of xenophobic violence. Such was the case in South Africa in 2008, when some 100 000 people were displaced as a result of xenophobic violence. In such situations, human rights law may provide the most useful legal framework for the assignation of people's rights to access and state responsibilities to provide assistance and protection.

Irrespective of their legal status, displaced populations and refugees very often depend on humanitarian assistance for basic survival needs, such as shelter, water, food, sanitation, health care and protection.

Rapid health assessments

A rapid assessment of the major vital needs of a displaced population is essential for planning and delivery of effective assistance during an emergency. By definition, displaced persons are away from their usual resources and have special needs: they have lost access to their land, homes, property and social support, and are vulnerable to physical and sexual violence. Women and children are particularly at risk.

Information on demography, mortality, morbidity and nutritional and immunisation status are required, as well as the availability of food and water resources and basic living conditions. A particularly high incidence of infectious diseases, such as measles and acute watery diarrhoea, afflict these populations living in crowded conditions with often poor sanitation and hygiene. Depending on their origin, special medical needs, such as chronic illnesses (i.e. HIV), should be considered. The psychological trauma of displacement may require the provision of psychosocial support. Population needs will vary according to the type of disaster. Information on demographics, major causes of mortality and morbidity and nutritional status will form part of the initial rapid assessment.

Table 6.5: Main indicators for emergencies

Mortality
- Crude mortality rate ≥ 1 death/10 000/day
- Under 5 mortality rate ≥ 2 deaths/10 000/day

Measles vaccination coverage
- Minimum 95% of children 9 months–15 years vaccinated

Food rations
- Minimum 2 100 kcal/person/day, including 10–12% proteins and minimum 15% fat

Water
- Minimum quantity of clean water of 15–20 litres/person/day
- Minimum 2 water containers of 20 litres per household

Hygiene and sanitation
- 1 latrine per 20 people (separate for men and women)

Shelter and non-food items
- Protection from wind, rain, freezing temperature and sunlight
- Minimum shelter 3.5 m^2/person
- Minimum site area 30 m^2/person

Demographics

The size of the affected population (e.g. number of displaced people) indicates the magnitude of the disaster and provides a denominator for the calculation of rates of mortality and morbidity. Demographic information should include age and sex distributions, as certain interventions (e.g. vaccination) will target certain groups; in some circumstances additional information, such as ethnicity or origin, may be relevant. A census, during which every individual is registered, may not be possible. Other methods including counting habitats and applying an average household size, and deriving data from other activities (e.g. vaccination).

Mortality and morbidity

Mortality is often highest in the first weeks post-emergency. The rapid reduction of excess mortality is the primary objective of humanitarian assistance. Measures include:

- The crude mortality rate (CMR), which is the total number of deaths per 10 000 persons/day;
- The under-5 mortality rate (U5MR) and the proportional mortality, or number of deaths attributed, to a given risk factor.

During the initial phase, sample surveys can estimate mortality rates retrospectively, with heads of household questioned on the number of deaths over a given recall period, together with the main causes of death that can be expected to be reliably ascertained verbally. Prospective surveillance should be established as soon as possible.

Morbidity, as measured by incidence (new cases over a given time period) and prevalence (number of cases at a specific time), can be assessed retrospectively via health registers or household surveys, again pending the establishment of prospective surveillance systems. Vaccination coverage, also amenable to retrospective assessment, can provide a good rapid indication of epidemic risk.

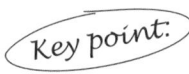 **The rapid reduction of excess mortality is the primary objective of humanitarian assistance.**

Nutritional assessment

There are two manifestations of acute malnutrition: marasmus (fat and muscle depletion; children appear very thin) and kwashiorkor (fat and muscle depletion plus oedema, i.e. body swelling due to fluid loss from tissues). Acute malnutrition has a profound effect on immunity, increasing morbidity and mortality from infectious diseases, especially of diarrhoea and acute respiratory infections. Prevalence of acute malnutrition can be measured through a representative sample survey to assess anthropometic indicators: weight, height, presence of oedema and mid-upper arm circumference (MUAC). The population at greatest risk is children aged 6–59 months. Weight-for-height indices are most often used to assess acute malnutrition, expressed in z-scores and compared to reference curves. In case of extreme emergency, MUAC assessments (<100 mm) provide a rapid way to identify children (height 65–110 cm) at high risk of dying.

6.3 Post-disaster medical support

In a simplified classification system, disaster medicine can be divided into four phases, namely:

- Preparation;
- Response;
- Recovery;
- Mitigation.

Medical support in the recovery phase is just as important as in the acute phase of life support during the response and is an often neglected phase of medical care. Disasters often trigger redevelopment and the establishment of a new balance. This is also applicable to medical response where disasters initiate new development in healthcare facilities. However, this section will deal with medical care post-disaster and will not address the developmental aspects of disaster medicine.

Primary health care

The establishment of a post-disaster comprehensive primary healthcare capability for survivors and the displaced population is a challenging activity. The basic approach must be to provide service to the community at at least the same standard as pre-disaster, while ensuring that the temporary facilities will blend into the future restored health system of the community. A guideline is not to provide routine services which were not available prior to the event, except if it can be maintained through developmental intervention.

Taking the disruption of a disaster event into account, primary healthcare capabilities must be established within reach of the target community. Often, public transport is not functioning and roads are impassable, making it impossible for the survivors to reach facilities. Establishing small decentralised clinics within various temporary accommodation facilities makes the health services more accessible than centralised capabilities. Satellite clinics can also be operational on a rotational basis.

The focus in these clinic facilities lies in managing minor ailments, preventing the spread of communicable diseases, providing medication and giving health education. Survivors often try to recover possessions from ruined buildings, resulting in injuries. The clinic capability must therefore include equipment to treat minor injuries and the means to evacuate more serious injuries.

Preventing the outbreak of communicable diseases is a critical aspect in any displaced persons accommodation facility. This includes health education on a continuous basis to identify cases at an early stage, implementing and supervising isolation and prevention through vaccination. Launching a mass immunisation program requires a detailed analysis of the present vaccination status of the community, the ability to launch and maintain a campaign and the logistical implications associated with immunisation, including cold chain management. Measles remains the most prevalent disease outbreak among displaced populations.

During a disaster, patients often lose their total stock of chronic medication, while records at healthcare facilities may be destroyed as well. This necessitates an active programme by the decentralised clinics to trace survivors on chronic medication and to replenish a basic stock of medication or an acceptable replacement that may be available. This often requires total reassessment of patients' conditions and the start of a new treatment regime based on available drugs. Decentralising visiting specialists' teams to clinics, and then feeding prescriptions to a central pharmacy for issuing of chronic medication, may be the solution. Challenges lie in the psychiatric patient environment, where the dosage of a treatment plan is often only tailored over a period of time. It may be necessary to admit these patients temporarily to a facility (sometimes a temporary established psychiatric capability) before discharge back into the community.

Tracing the diabetic patients and providing insulin kits with syringes are important early post-disaster actions. This is often limited to a basic insulin provision process, to be followed afterwards with the specific type required.

Creating care capability/capabilities for the vulnerable population, especially the paralysed, bedridden elderly, orphaned children and babies, is a logical outflow of establishing a comprehensive post-disaster healthcare capability. These patients need to be traced within the community, registered and monitored by the healthcare personnel. It may be necessary to mobilise community involvement to establish temporary care capabilities within the displaced persons camp, where members of the camp take care of these patients under the guidance and supervision of the healthcare practitioners.

Monitoring the nutritional status of the displaced population, especially the vulnerable, is a critical step to activate nutritional support systems timeously.

Often, patients also lose medical support and aid in the event. This mainly includes eyeglasses, which may cause serious dysfunction. Establishing mobile optical clinics, where a basic assessment is done and an appropriate pair of glasses is issued from a stock of prepared glasses, has proven successful in the past. In less developed parts of the world, welfare organisations often maintain the capability to issue second-hand, tested and classified glasses after a basic eye examination. Bringing such a clinic capability into the disaster area may bring temporary relief until long-term processes can be re-established. Planning a referral system to address lost leg braces, hearing aids and artificial limbs must be an integral part of post-disaster medical planning.

Key point: **Post-disaster medical facilities must aim at providing services aligned with what was available in the community prior to the event, and deliver these in such a way that they can be reabsorbed into the local health system as soon as possible.**

Key point: **Emphasis should be placed on preventing chronically sick patients from developing into acute cases.**

Key point: **Care capabilities for vulnerable groups need to be established, providing temporary care but with an emphasis on optimal reintegration into the community.**

Environmental health

A critical step in the post-disaster medical support is to establish effective environmental health monitoring and measures. Utilising environmental health practitioners early in the relief effort may contribute to the health status of the survivors.

Drinking-water provision is a critical process in disaster relief, but the monitoring of the quality of the water is just as important. Although the emphasis falls on quantity of water available to survivors rather that quality, basic measures to safeguard water are essential. In this respect, the supervision of cleaning of water tankers prior to use and basic chlorination of water are both useful interventions.

Inspection of food storage and mass food preparation facilities are critical environmental health interventions. It may also be useful to use environmental health officers to inspect all fresh food donations prior to distribution. This is a critical step to prevent outbreaks of diarrhoeal diseases, but must be implemented with sensitivity as it often causes unhappiness on the part of donors.

Inspecting and advising on acceptable sanitation facilities is a further function for environmental health management. Monitoring the effectiveness of sanitation measures, and providing health education on the importance of safe sanitation and hygiene, should be part of interventions. In this regard, all clinics, food and water distribution and aid capabilities can be targeted for health education.

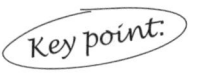 **Environmental health interventions must be implemented as soon as possible after a disaster or major incident to evaluate water and food safety. This includes inspection of all mass feeding schemes.**

Psychosocial support

Comprehensive psychosocial support to all victims and next-of-kin is an integral part of post-disaster medical support. The support measures need to be implemented as early as possible and be integrated into the total health support program.

Using screening teams of social workers, psychologists and culturally acceptable members of the clergy to initially debrief all survivors and to assess the vulnerability for post-traumatic stress is a useful process in manageable numbers of survivors. In large disaster populations, self-reporting and initial group debriefing are options. It is critical that all efforts should be made to reach all the survivors through a basic phychosocial support team and to assess their needs.

In visiting all survivors by a multi-disciplinary support teams, the basic social needs, including serious financial challenges, can be identified. Processes to apply for financial support and insurance claims can be initiated by the social worker, and documentation on deceased relatives can be completed. The psychologist component of such a team can facilitate basic debriefing and assess the need for referral for medium- and long-term counselling. Members of the clergy can assist in establishing a caring paradigm within the community and assess the need for long-term religious support. Adding a nursing component to the team helps to assess the physical health status of the community as well as identify health needs such as chronic medication. Support teams should, on a daily basis, provide feedback reports on all information and findings to a central database. This database then forms the basis for the second phase of intervention, which includes direct intervention and therapy.

A sensitive area for psychosocial support is the support of relatives during identification of bodies. This is a very traumatic experience for relatives, especially when no alternative measures other than identification of corpses are available. Allocating specific social workers to support and debrief relatives during these processes contributes to social support.

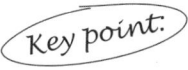 **Multi-disciplinary screening of all survivors is essential, including debriefing and identification of risk cases for referral.**

Donations

Following a disaster, various institutions often want to donate medical equipment, and specifically drugs and medicine. This is a pitfall that often results in truckloads of expired drugs being handed over, with full media coverage, which becomes the problem of the medical coordinator to destroy afterwards! A basic guideline is to establish a logistical coordination section early in the response, to whom all role-players give feedback for needs. All offers for donations are then channelled to the logistical section, which only accepts donations of items required. All other offers are recorded and accepted only if the need for the items arises. All disaster medicine coordinators are able to share the humorous and often frustrating experiences of donations of expired drugs, truckloads of contraceptives, shoe shops donating all their single shoes (either right or left) or crates full of sequin-embroidered evening gowns. Basic guidelines for drug donations are available from the WHO website, while the Pan American Health Organization (PAHO) has issued very useful guidelines on receiving medical equipment donations. In summary, if it is not needed, do not accept it, as each donation needs to be declared and an account given on how it was managed.

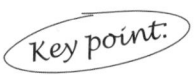 **Offers of donations of medicine and medical equipment post-disaster must be judiciously evaluated and managed with care to prevent dumping of useless drugs.**

Research

Disasters are a very popular field for research and quasi-research, not always with scientific objectives. Especially in a major incident or a smaller disaster situation, the survivors are swamped with researchers who want them to complete questionnaires on various areas of their experience. This is often related to the social sciences, and specifically post-traumatic stress research. As the sample group is often relatively small, the survivors are soon saturated with research efforts. It is recommended that a credible ethical committee is appointed soon after a disaster situation and that all research proposals are vetted by the ethical committee to prevent saturation of the sample group with sometimes useless research efforts.

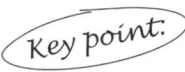 **Ethical aspects of research following a major incident require clear guidelines and scrupulous supervision.**

Re-establishing routine health services

All efforts should be focused on re-establishing routine health services to the responsible authorities. This is often a time-consuming process, especially if large numbers of healthcare practitioners from the region were killed in the event. However, a systematic phasing-in of routine services and phasing-out of *ad hoc* external services should be the target.

A critical aspect is to ensure that all records of the interim *ad hoc* interventions are handed over to the routine health services to ensure a continuation of care.

In summary, post-disaster medical support should focus as comprehensively as possible on the needs of the community and establish in survivors a feeling of being cared for. But role-players should at all times guard against creating a dependent society unable to care for itself. Efforts should focus on re-establishing routine services with the optimum use of donated resources.

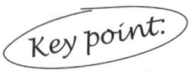 **The philosophy of post-disaster care is to create an environment in which survivors feel cared for.**

Summary

Post-disaster medical planning and interventions are just as important as the rescue interventions in the acute phase, and often have a longer-term impact. Therefore, proper planning is required to address survivors needs in a humane and optimal approach.

6.4 Public health in disasters

A displaced population will have many needs to meet in the acute phase of the disaster (first days and weeks). A rapid needs assessment identifies the specific requirements and the severity of the deficiencies of the population; however, there are a number of basic needs that almost always must be met to avoid excess mortality. These should be addressed in a systematic manner. For example, in July 1994 over half a million Rwandan refugees fled into eastern Congo. The mortality rate in the first month was 10%, mostly due to a cholera epidemic. A *Shigella* outbreak followed, with over 15 000 cases due to inadequate safe drinking water, overcrowded conditions, poor sanitation and food shortages.

The following essential priorities should be considered during the acute phase of a humanitarian crisis:

- Adequate and appropriately spaced and sited shelter;
- Sufficient and safe food;
- Sufficient and safe water;
- Adequate sanitation and waste disposal;
- Mass vaccination, with measles vaccine as a constant concern;
- Control of communicable diseases and public health surveillance;
- Security.

Shelter

Displaced persons are by definition homeless. They have frequently travelled long distances (often by foot) and been exposed to harsh conditions for days or weeks. Establishing adequate shelter quickly is essential for survival, ensuring security, protection against wind, rain, freezing temperatures and direct sunlight, and resistance to poor health and disease. Shelter should provide a minimum of 3.5 m^2 per person, for a total minimum site area of 30 m^2/person. Finally, exposure to risk factors that pose a threat to security should be assessed, including registries for reports of violent events, including sexual violence and robberies. Such data can be derived from clinical records of qualitative surveys (key informant interviews).

A well-planned site must be secure, near a water source, with enough space for all persons. It must be accessible to transport vehicles, be protected from wind and other elements, avoid low-lying/waterlogged areas which can be vector breeding grounds and have ideal land for crop growing. The layout of the site should respect the cultural norms of the population. Involving the IDPs/refugees in the planning is ideal. Families should not be separated. Consideration should be given to security within the camp, particularly for women at night. Each family should be given a shelter kit including plastic sheeting and rope or a tent, and essential non-food items such as a water container (40 litres/family), soap, blankets, mosquito nets, cooking sets, fuel, bedding equipment and clothes.

Sufficient and safe food

Nutrition is one of the top priorities in the emergency phase. The risk of malnutrition is higher in a displaced population because food may have been scarce during the cause and process of the displacement. The minimum energy requirements are 2 100 kcal/person/day with 10–14% from protein and 17–30% from fat. Common vitamin deficiencies include vitamins A, B1, B2, B3, C, iron and iodine. If acute malnutrition is encountered, therapeutic feeding centres may be necessary. Dry rations for home preparation should be provided where possible. Mass feeding (the provision of cooked food for immediate consumption) is usually provided when people do not have the means to cook for themselves, or where security is a concern (potential for repeat displacement, or in situations when food is a valuable commodity). Consideration should also be given to providing sufficient fuel (i.e. firewood) to prepare food.

Sufficient and safe water

Humans cannot live more than 72 hours without water. Water is needed for drinking, cooking and personal hygiene. Access to safe water is essential to prevent the spread of cholera and other waterborne illnesses. Without clean water and appropriate sanitation and waste disposal, the camp can become a breeding ground for enteric pathogens. Watery diarrhoeal outbreaks are common. Clean water sources should be identified and chlorinated. There should be sufficient water supply for at least 15–20 litres/person/day; during a cholera outbreak, as much as 60 litres/person/day should be provided. Water quality can be assessed by measuring the presence of faecal coliforms, with <10/100 ml considered acceptable. If chlorinated, free residual chlorine should be between 0.3 and 0.8 mg/litre depending on pH. Basic information on hygiene and sanitation can be collected through household surveys and by assessing programme distributions. The distribution of water is important: there should be a minimum of one tap per 200–250 persons or one hand pump per 500–750 persons. Water sources should be located no farther than 500 metres from any household and water containers distributed to each family.

Adequate sanitation and waste disposal

Sanitation facilities are important, particularly to prevent the spread of faecal-oral pathogens. Designate an area at least 30 m away from clean water sources for latrines and waste-water disposal. One latrine per 20 users is the minimum standard. The area should be safe at night and, if possible, separate facilities provided for men and women. It is highly recommended to involve the community and other stakeholders in the design and construction of the latrines, and in so doing ensure higher compliance. In situations where the population has not traditionally used toilets, it may be necessary to conduct a concerted education/promotion campaign to encourage their use. An area at least 50 m away from water sources should be fenced off for solid waste disposal.

Mass vaccination

The risk of infectious disease outbreak is high in displaced populations, where overcrowding and poor health is common. Measles is a particular concern due to its high case-fatality rate and rapid spread; it has been reported as the leading cause of death in children in several emergencies. For example, in 1985 a severe epidemic in Sudan resulted in over 2 000 deaths over a four-month period. Immediate mass vaccination of all children under 15 years is recommended by the WHO in the first few days after a major disaster, and one confirmed case in a closed setting should be regarded as an epidemic. The approach should be three-fold:

- A mass vaccination campaign to achieve 100% coverage of children under 15 years;
- Routine selective vaccination of vulnerable populations, including re-vaccination of children under 9 months;
- Screening and treatment of cases.

Measles cases should be isolated, and appropriate therapeutic care provided, including vitamin A supplementation, antibiotics and nutritional supplementation.

Other vaccines to consider in overcrowded conditions include pertussis, meningitis and yellow fever. In situations of prolonged displacement, the provision of vaccines is normally provided under the WHO's Expanded Program on Immunization.

Control of communicable diseases and public health surveillance

Major infectious causes of mortality in the acute emergency phase include measles, diarrhoeal diseases and acute respiratory infections. The incidence of these diseases will be greatly reduced by addressing the other acute priorities of adequate and appropriately spaced and sited shelter, sufficient and safe food and water, adequate sanitation and waste disposal and mass measles vaccination (see Table 6.6).

Table 6.6: Public health impact of selected disasters

Effect	Complex emergencies	Earthquakes	High winds (without flooding)	Floods	Flash floods/ tsunamis
Deaths	Many	Many	Few	Few	Many
Severe injuries	Varies	Many	Moderate	Few	Few
Increased risk of communi-cable diseases	High	Low	Low	Varies	Low
Food scarcity	Common	Rare	Rare	Varies	Common
Major population displacements	Common	Rare	Rare	Common	Varies

In addition to essential vaccination, simple hygiene and sanitation measures are essential to reduce the potential for outbreaks. The risk of diarrhoeal diseases can be substantially reduced by ensuring clean water and food and adequate hygiene, while the provision of shelter, clothing and blankets can limit the risk of acute respiratory infections. To prevent malaria, areas of stagnant water should be eliminated as these are breeding grounds for mosquitoes; mosquito nets should also be provided in malaria-endemic areas.

A public health surveillance system should be implemented to monitor potential epidemics. All agencies providing health care for the population should be included in a surveillance network and informed of the diseases at risk and their standard case definitions. Epidemic definitions and thresholds need to be established, as well as consistent case definitions. Outpatient and inpatient facilities, as well as community health workers, should be involved to ensure rapid notification of any suspected cases. A single case of cholera, measles, yellow fever, *Shigella* or viral haemorrhagic fever is considered an outbreak. The thresholds for other diseases will vary according to what is considered an increase from the normal expected cases for that region. The objective of outbreak control is to lower the number of cases and reduce mortality among cases. Controlling the source or vector is essential to interrupt transmission. Susceptible groups, including children, pregnant women and immuno-compromised people, must be protected.

Security

The population may have been displaced because they were victims of violence or natural disaster. In a conflict, the perpetrators may have followed, so the site may not be secure from further injuries. After a natural disaster, ensure that the new site is away from the risks of the disaster. Ensure that there are enough watchmen/ security guards and a well-defined perimeter. Mental health care should be provided for victims of sexual violence and the war wounded. Healthcare professionals are rarely able to secure the protection of populations, but through advocacy they can highlight the need for this to be addressed by the proper authorities.

6.5   Children in disasters

Children are at particular risk in nearly all forms of disasters; this is reflected in the excess paediatric mortality in events such as earthquakes and tsunamis. They are at risk for a multiplicity of reasons (see Table 6.7), including physiology and anatomy, behavioural stages, organisation of schools and educational facilities, pre-existing problems such as technological dependence or illness, and adult behaviour. Children's vulnerability is compounded by the limited capacity of most health systems to deal with increased numbers of children in need of acute care. Moreover, while acute needs are important, longer-term public health problems are frequently far greater in magnitude with their potential impact on health. As an example, in the earthquake in April 2009 in L'Aquila, Italy, approximately 295 people were killed and 1 000 were injured, but 55 000 people were left homeless. While there is typically a surge in demand for acute medical services, additional resources are required to meet the specific needs of children, including: prevention of infectious diseases; creation of safe environments; dealing with the psychosocial aftermath of the events; and re-creating appropriate educational and training facilities.

Not only are children caught up in general disasters, but they are sometimes specifically involved in tragedies that affect institutions where large numbers of children are grouped together in schools (as happened in the Sichuan earthquake in China in May 2008). Some mass casualty events have even been specifically targeted at children.

Although many disaster plans make provision for the care of vulnerable sectors of the population, relatively few plans are specifically geared for the needs of children, and particularly for children across the full range of developmental stages. Unless these needs are specifically addressed in the planning for, and organisation of, disaster relief, it is inevitable that children will suffer unnecessary harm.

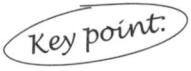 **Children form a vulnerable group that needs to be given particular attention, especially during the planning phase.**

The particular needs of children

Some of the reasons for the vulnerability of children in disasters are outlined in Table 6.7 Children are vulnerable at virtually all phases of disasters, and it is important always to consider both their specific needs and the skills and resources that are required to fulfil these needs at various stages.

Death and injury

In the acute phase of physical disasters, such as tsunamis and earthquakes, children have been particularly vulnerable to death and injury. With limited strength and capacity to flee and/or shelter from danger, mortality has been particularly high in young children in these events.

The care of children in acute disasters may be considerably complicated when parents have been killed or injured, or when children have been separated from their parents. Apart from the psychological trauma of separation, consent for procedures and ongoing care is also problematic.

Infection

In general, children, and especially infants, are more susceptible to infection than adults. Thus children may be afflicted as part of a widespread infective process (possible influenza epidemic), but they may also develop infections in the environment that develop subsequent to a disaster.

Effect of conflicts

There are considerable differences in mortality rates for children following conflicts. In most cases, the rates of death increased sharply, although there have been other situations in which mortality rates dropped, largely related to populations who were displaced as a result of the conflicts.

Psychological concerns

Specific and focused care is required from the time of the disaster onwards to ameliorate the long-term psychological problems for children affected by disasters. Particular attention needs to be focused on the family.

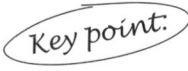 **Children present with unique needs and challenges when they have been victims of a major incident or disaster.**

Table 6.7: Special needs of children

Anatomy and physiology	Consequences	Implications
Cardiovascular physiology: • Low blood volumes and limited cardiac reserve	• More liable to: • Consequences of vomiting and diarrhoea (either infective or chemical); • Consequences of limited water availability; • More susceptible to dehydration and have limited reserve • Very limited reserve for blood loss	• Need for oral rehydration resources • Increased need for intravenous access and therapy • Need for rapid control of haemorrhage ⮕

Anatomy and physiology	Consequences	Implications
Respiratory physiology: • High oxygen consumption, • Limited oxygen reserve • High respiratory rate • Breathe gas at lower levels because of being smaller	• More vulnerable to airborne toxins (sarin or chlorine) or pathogens such as anthrax (in context of chemical or biological attack) • Many toxic gases are heavier than air, so children are more exposed than adults • In nuclear contamination, radioactive material may be at lower levels • Higher susceptibility to CO poisoning	• More services may be required. May need different gas masks and filters • Increased need for environmental ventilation and monitoring • Increased care with heating and power sources after incident
Skin: • High surface area and permeability (particularly infants < 6 months of age) • Rapid heat loss • Relatively poor keratinisation	• High absorbance of toxins (chemical and radioactive) that are absorbed via skin • Rapid heat loss • More liable to abrasion, burns (thermal and chemical)	• Special needs for paediatric decontamination • Increased needs for warming and environmental control
Musculoskeletal: • Limited strength and speed • Softer bone structure	• Limited capacity to escape from danger and harm • Increased damage from falling masonry etc. • Different injuries to adults	• Significant needs for paediatric orthopaedic services • Equipment required for stabilisation and treatment of fracture may be different
Nutrition: • Extremely limited nutritional resources (particularly in small infants) • Different nutritional needs to adults • Require assistance with feeding	• Children cannot cope for long without food and water intake	• Systems required to provide appropriate food supplements for children rapidly

Anatomy and physiology	Consequences	Implications
Pharmacology: • Routes of administration of medication • Susceptibility to toxins	• Smaller children are not able to take tablets • Children may be more susceptible than adults to short-term toxins (e.g. organophosphates) as well as radioactivity	• Medication (e.g. required in nuclear event) must be available in form that can be taken in appropriate dosage by children • Increased attention to protection from toxins
Developmental and psychosocial issues: • Age- and individual-dependent children are often grouped in areas away from parents (schools etc.) • Remain vulnerable to dangers in the environment, including abusive adults	• Limited capacity for self-care in the aftermath of a disaster • Small children may not be able to provide information about identity and place of origin • Psychological consequences of disaster will depend on age and development stage • May investigate dangerous items or areas as part of curiosity and ignorance	• Resources required for basic care and not just medical care • Systems must be in place to identify children and ensure that they are kept together with family or guardians • Appropriate structures required to provide psychological and social support over a period of time • Need to address environmental safety post-incident • Protect from abusive adults
Infection control:	• Children will have limited immunisation	• In mass relocalisation situations, infectious disease interventions (including immunisation programmes) are required to prevent development of epidemics
Children with special needs:	• Dependency on technology which may be affected by the disaster	• Range from nebulizers to ventilators

Resources for care of children in disasters

Not only are children more likely to suffer injury in physical disasters, the facilities available for their care are likely to be more limited than would be the case for adults. The special needs of injured children include: a range of equipment sizes; personnel with special expertise in dealing with children; increased nursing requirements post-intervention, etc.

Particular insight into the needs of children and the availability of specific paediatric resources will be required by any team coordinating both planning for, and response to, any disaster in which significant numbers of children are involved.

Facilities

Even in well-resourced areas, children's services in general have extremely limited capacity to deal with a surge, and there are limited alternatives.

Equipment

The equipment required for the care of children (and particularly small children and infants) is different to that required for adults. The majority of injuries requiring early treatment will be orthopaedic, and hence there is a major need for orthopaedic devices, which may be in short supply, particularly in the countries affected.

Provision of food and pharmaceutical supplies

Children have different food and pharmaceutical requirements to adults. For small infants, breast feeding remains the most important source of nutrition, and should be encouraged if at all possible.

Personnel

There is a need to involve trained paediatric personnel in the disaster management process at all levels. However, these personnel are unlikely to be of significant assistance unless they have gone through some training, as the skills required in an acute disaster are very different from those required in normal paediatric practice.

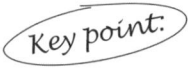 **When planning for children in a disaster situation, cognisance must be given to the fact that their needs are not the same as those of adults.**

Paediatric planning for disasters

Planning for the needs of children is complicated by a number of factors. Children are not a homogeneous group of people. Children of different ages and developmental stages have very different needs (infant foods versus adult nutrition); capacity to respond to situations (adolescents versus infants); vulnerability to infection (infants versus adolescents); needs for parental care, etc. There are also children with specific needs, and in the richer parts of the world there is an ever growing population of children who are dependent on technology such as home ventilators.

Some disasters are completely unexpected, and detailed planning to deal with such events is impossible. However, many disasters are predictable, and with increasing access to geological, meteorological and other data across the world, many regions will have increased capacity to consider and plan for disasters.

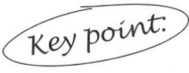 **Planning for children in a disaster goes a long way in mitigating against the effects such an incident will have on mortality and morbidity of children.**

Summary

Planning must address the unique needs of children (immediate and long-term), the context of the likely disaster and the resources available. Planning should involve clinicians, health planners, the public and children. Protocols and processes should be devised *a priori* and should be transparent, taking into consideration the ethical principles of fairness and equitable care.

6.6 Mass fatalities

A mass fatality incident is any event that produces more fatalities than can be handled by using local resources. No minimum number of fatalities constitutes a mass fatality incident, because of the fact that communities vary in size and resources.

Deaths in a mass fatality incident are usually sudden, unexpected, violent and indiscriminate, and the numbers involved are usually staggering. The number of deceased may not create a mass fatality incident, but rather the manner in which the deaths may occur and the conditions of the deceased bodies.

Disasters can be divided into two categories:

- *Open disasters:* unknown individuals with no prior records or descriptive data available – for example, a bomb explosion;
- *Closed disasters:* identifiable group – for example, an aircraft crash.

There are many actions that form part of the response to a mass fatality incident. These actions start after an incident, once life and property have ceased, through to the release of the body and personal effects to those responsible and eligible to direct the disposition of the body and to receive effects.

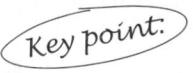 **Mass fatalities are not limited by the number of fatalities and are divided into open or closed disaster incidents**

Storage of the deceased

The deceased are generally the last victims of major incidents to be managed on the scene. They may be found at the incident site (bronze zone) or in the casualty clearing stations or even at the hospitals. The first step in the management of the dead is to confirm and declare death, which is the responsibility of pre-hospital providers of ILS or ALS grading and doctors. An appropriate 'declaration of death' form should be completed for each body, and these may then be removed to the storage area after the police have completed their task of evidence-gathering. Bodies should only be removed after permission of the police has been obtained or if the position of the body is hampering the rescue of survivors.

The storage of the bodies of deceased victims of major incidents requires three main aspects:

- Bodies must be stored in a manner to preserve tissue for identification, ideally at a low ambient temperature around 4 °C.
- Bodies must be stored in a manner that preserves the dignity of the dead: the body must be covered and stored with personal effects in a safe environment, especially at the incident site or in a temporary mortuary.
- Personal effects and clothing are considered as evidentiary items, and these should be suitably marked and linked to the bodies of the deceased for later identification.

Initially, a temporary storage area should be set up, where the bodies can be accommodated prior to removal to formal mortuaries. In South Africa this is a health responsibility, and the forensic pathology services of the provinces provide vehicles and mortuaries for the storage of the bodies of the deceased. This may be as simple as a large tented area with cooling fans to a formal setup such as a refrigerated mobile mortuary.

All the bodies should be moved thereafter to the state mortuary, after suitable documentation of the on-scene evidence. The law in South Africa states that all fatalities after a major incident require a medico-legal postmortem to determine the mechanism of death, before a death certificate is issued.

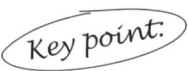 **Death declaration allows for the body to be moved to a mortuary area, and follows clinical and ECG confirmation of death.**

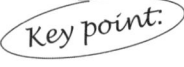 **In mass fatality situations, dignified and safe body holding areas should be arranged until bodies can be moved to a formal mortuary.**

Disaster victim identification

Disaster victim identification (DVI) is all the procedures used to positively identify victims of a multiple fatality.

The most important requirement for victim identification work is the application of international standards. It also forms the common basis for multinational DVI operations. DVI is not, and never will be, a rapid process. There is an absolute need for accurate identification. The prospect of mistaken identity, and returning the wrong victim or body parts to a family, is unthinkable.

All the role-players will be placed under immense pressure to return victims to families at the earliest possible opportunity. The process will be closely scrutinised by the press and foreign embassies in cases where foreign nationals are among the deceased. Additional pressure will also be delivered as a result of faith and cultural demands surrounding attitudes to death and the religious requirements for speedy funeral arrangements.

The victim identification process is in fact the comparison of ante-mortem data, recorded from the families or next of kin of those reported missing, and the postmortem data, recovered during the mortuary process. The primary aim is also to match postmortem data to postmortem data in the case of fragmented bodies, and then to match postmortem data to ante-mortem data to positively identify the victim.

Victims of large-scale fatal incidents are identified on the basis of an assessment of multiple factors. The condition of the bodies will, to a large extent, influence the nature and quality of postmortem and the applicability of specific methods of identification.

It is generally accepted that the only safe way to significantly reduce the chance of misidentification is to deploy forensic techniques as primary identifiers. All the methods used for identification must be scientifically sound and reliable.

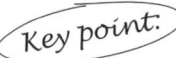 **The primary and most reliable means of identification are:**
- **Fingerprint analysis;**
- **Comparative dental analysis;**
- **DNA analysis.**

Secondary means of identification include personal description and medical findings, as well as evidence and clothing found on the body. These means of identification serve to support identification by other means and are under no circumstances sufficient as a sole means of identification.

Visual identification by means of a photograph or witness may provide an indication of identity but is not sufficient for positive identification of victims, specifically in a large-scale disaster.

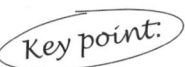 **Identification based solely on photographs is notoriously unreliable and should be avoided.**

The Interpol DVI guide and forms

The International Criminal Police Organization (Interpol) is a significant role-player in crimes that extend across international boundaries. Currently, Interpol is made up of 188 member countries. Through the combined efforts of police, support staff, elected committees and working groups that comprise police officers and scientific consultants, Interpol has moved international collaboration to a high level. Over the last few decades, Interpol and its member countries have played a very prominent role in DVI operations. One of the reasons was assistance to provide closure to family and friends who are missing a loved one, as a result of conflict, disaster or disease.

The first Interpol DVI guide was published in 1984, and since then numerous disasters have occurred throughout the world. As a consequence, the contents of the guide have been re-examined to take into account the lessons learned from various responses to disasters, as well as advancements in victim identification techniques. The latest version of the Interpol DVI guide, which is circulated to all Interpol member countries, is also available for download from the Interpol website (www.interpol.int).

The purpose of the guide is to promulgate good practice in disaster victim identification. The DVI guide cannot address every possible eventuality but can give sound practical advice on all the major issues of disaster victim identification and all the processes involved.

In order to assist with the standardised collection of ante-mortem and postmortem data Interpol have compiled DVI forms to produce a comprehensive selection of data fields to record all the required information. As in the case of the DVI guide, the DVI forms are regularly revised. Typically, the ante-mortem forms are printed on yellow paper and the postmortem forms on pink paper.

The data on the respective forms are compared and potential matches are located – for example, between a found body and a missing person. The final result is normally submitted to an identification board for final verification and, if appropriate, declaration of a result and issuing of a death certificate.

Interpol is currently using the DVI Systems International (Plass Data Software) for comparison of large-scale data. The fields from the DVI forms are incorporated into the software application. Search algorithms within the application are used to generate possible matches, when searches are done against the collaborating database. The application is designed to direct to the most likely matches based on available evidence. The final comparisons must still be done using forensic physical methods.

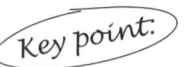 Interpol provides an international disaster victim identification service through its 188 member countries.

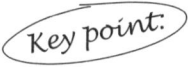 In a mass fatality event, the importance of a collegial and cooperative professional relationship between all the different role-players, whether police, emergency services or medico-legal, can never be overstated.

Summary

Mass fatalities occur as part of a major incident or as an isolated mass fatality incident. It is essential that all the authorities are aware of the systems in place to declare death, safely and professionally store the bodies of the deceased and provide for identification of the deceased in a manner that can assure the family that the body is indeed that of their loved one.

6.7 Resources

New York State Department of Health – Emergency Preparedness Guidelines: www. health.state.ny.us/environmental/emergency/health_care_providers/

Children and disasters – website related to the American Academy of Pediatrics: www.aap.org/disasters/index.cfm

The youngest victims: disaster preparedness to meet children's needs: www.aap.org/disasters/pdf/Youngest-Victims-Final.pdf

Federal Emergency Management Agency (FEMA) website: www.fema.gov

World Health Organization – WHO Health Action in Crises: www.who.int/hac/en/

Centers for Disease Control – Emergency Preparedness and Response: www.bt.cdc.gov/disasters/

Safe Hospitals Bibliography: safehospitals.info/index.php?option=com_newsfeeds &task=view&feedid=11&Itemid=198

The Sphere Project – Humanitarian Charter and Minimum Standards in Disaster Response (2004): www.sphereproject.org/content/view/27/84/lang,english/

6.8 References

1. Allen K. Rainbow nation's outsiders live in fear. BBC, 28 May 2009. Available from: news.bbc.co.uk/2/hi/africa/8070919.stm. Accessed 19 August 2010.

2. Jennings E, Birkeland N. *Internal displacement: global overview of trends and developments in 2008.* Geneva: Norwegian Refugee Council; 2009.

3. Checchi F, Grais R, Mills E. Public health in crisis-affected populations. Available from:www.reliefweb.int/rw/lib.nsf/db900SID/AMMF-7F3FSF?OpenDocument. Accessed 19 August 2010.

4. Depoortere E, Brown V. Rapid health assessment of refugee or displaced populations. MSF/Epicentre, Paris, 2006. Available from: www.refbooks.msf. org/MSF_Docs/en/MSFdocMenu_en.htm. Accessed 19 August 2010.

5. World Heath Organization. Guidelines for Drug Donations. 1999. Available from: whqlibdoc.who.int/hq/1999/who_edm_par_99.4.pdf. Accessed 19 January 2010.

6. World Health Organization and Pan American Health Organization. *WHO-PAHO guidelines for the use of foreign field hospitals in sudden-impact disasters.* Washington, DC: World Health Organization; 2003.

7. Checchi F, Grais R, Mills E. *Public health in crisis-affected populations.* London: Humanitarian Practice Network; 2007.

8. Expanded programme on immunization, 1994. Accelerated measles strategies. *The Weekly Epidemiological Record* 69: 229–34.

9. Goma Epidemiology Group 1995. Public health impact of Rwandan refugee crisis: what happened in Goma, Zaire, in July, 1994? *The Lancet* 345: 339–344.

10. Médecins Sans Frontières (MSF). *Nutrition: situation with displacement of population.* Brussels: Médecins Sans Frontières; 2007.

11. Paquet C. Vaccination in emergencies. *Vaccine* 1999;17(suppl 3):S116–19.

12. Peyrassol S. *The priorities: situation with displaced population.* Brussels: Médecins Sans Frontières; 2007.

13. The Sphere Project. Sphere humanitarian charter and minimum standards in disaster response. Geneva: The Sphere Project; 2004.

14. Seaman J, Maguire S. ABC of conflict and disaster. The special needs of children and women. *British Medical Journal* 2005;331:34–6.

15. Doocy S, Rofi A, Moodie C, *et al.* Tsunami mortality in Aceh Province, Indonesia. *Bulletin of the World Health Organization.* 2007;85:273–8.

16. Guha-Sapir D, Panhuis WG. Conflict-related mortality: an analysis of 37 datasets. *Disasters* 2004;28:418–28.

17. Toole MJ, Waldman RJ. Prevention of excess mortality in refugee and displaced populations in developing countries. *Journal of the American Medical Association* 1990;263:3296–302.

18. Task Force on Community Preventive Services. Recommendations to reduce psychological harm from traumatic events among children and adolescents. *American Journal of Preventative Medicine.* 2008;35:314–16.

19. Proctor LJ, Fauchier A, Oliver PH, Ramos MC, Rios MA, Margolin G. Family context and young children's responses to earthquake. *Journal of Child Psychology and Psychiatry* 2007;48:941–9.

20. International Criminal Police Organization (Interpol). Interpol fact sheet. Disaster victim identification. Com/FS/2009-06/FS. Available from: www.interpol.int. Accessed 19 August 2010.

21. Jensen RA. *Mass fatality and casualty incidents – a field guide.* Boca Raton, FL: CRC Press LCC; 1999.

22. US Department of Homeland Security. Joint field office activation and operations: interagency integrated standard operating procedure. Version 8.3, April 2006. Washington, DC: Department of Homeland Security; 2006.

7

Challenges

T Ligthelm and W Smith

Objectives

By the end of this chapter, the reader will be able to:

- optimise the value of dignitary visits to a hospital during a major incident through pre-planning and a structured approach;
- maintain effective external and internal communication during a major incident;
- appreciate the use of resuscitation, primary health care and field hospital facilities in a major incident;
- help to ensure cooperation between the military and civilian role-players in a major incident;
- effectively evacuate large numbers of casualties using different modes of mass transport.

7.1 VIP visits

Visits by various levels of dignitaries and community leaders are an integral occurrence after any major incident or disaster. The reasons for these visits to the impact sites and care facilities vary from role-player to role-player. It is essential to try to establish the reason(s) for the visit to be able to accommodate the needs in advance.

Such visits are often supportive in nature, to show support to the victims, their next-of-kin and the community. These visitors would like to meet victims and relatives and have an opportunity to talk to them personally and often in private.

VIP visits may also be evaluative, where responsible political leaders visit the site of an event to evaluate the effectiveness of the response. These visitors often prefer to visit the command centre(s) and then talk to some survivors to evaluate the response.

However, some visitors' purpose is purely to gain advantage of the situation and to be seen. These visitors are often the most difficult to accommodate as they want to be filmed while trying to assist in the rescue, often disrupting the real rescue efforts.

Whatever the reasons for a visit, it is important for command or management to plan in advance for these visits.

VIP liaison officer

The first step is to appoint a senior ranking person as the VIP liaison officer as soon as possible, if such a person was not identified in advance. It is important that the identified manager is senior enough to liaise effectively with the leaders, but is not required to make decisions during a visit. This should not be the commander/manager himself, because every visit will then paralyse command's decision-making function. The VIP liaison officer should, however, liaise very closely with the command structure to ensure that the visit is optimised and objectives achieved.

All liaison for VIP visits must then be channelled directly to the VIP liaison officer and a programme/roster established for visits. This is especially important for political leaders, who hardly ever want to arrive simultaneously with a member of the opposition!

VIP reception point

Identify a central point for all visits to start. This makes it easy to plan the programme, and it becomes routine to arrange parking for VIP convoys or the landing of helicopters. Establish a simple routine that all VIPs are met at the same point. Confirm in advance with all VIPs that protocol will be adhered to, but no special honours will be paid to visiting dignitaries. Ensure efficient security at the arrival point, and keep media and the public at a safe distance.

Introductory briefing

Plan a short briefing to all VIPs on the event, and the response, directly after their arrival. Highlight in the briefing what has been achieved, but also what challenges are being experienced. The commanders should be introduced to the VIPs in such a way that they can withdraw without offending the VIP.

Clarify in advance with the VIP where and when the media will be present. As a guide, the media can be allowed to record the arrival of the VIP, but should not be present during the initial briefing. This allows the VIP manager to share openly the appropriate information with the VIP and sketch challenges that are experienced. Compile a short summary in writing of the event, with basic data such as time of the event, some technical data on the event, number of victims and numbers of responders busy addressing the situation, and make this available to each VIP on arrival. Within a hospital setting, specify the number of patients treated, admitted, surgeries and deceased. This ensures that the VIP has the correct facts when answering media questions.

Depending on the situation, refreshments can be served during this briefing, but be very sensitive about the nature of the incident and the type of refreshments served. A useful guideline is to accompany the VIPs to the staff resting and refreshment area and serve them together with the staff.

Site tours

Normally, the VIP requires a tour through the site or through the facility. This tour needs to be planned in advance and the route pre-determined. It is recommended that a limited number of media representatives and photographers are allowed to accompany the VIP. A guide is to register all media representatives and then to allow a different local, regional and international representative to accompany each VIP visit group. If patients are to be visited, this should be arranged in advance and identifiable permission from the patient needs to be obtained. VIP visitors normally want to be photographed while shaking hands with a patient. Arrange this type of picture in advance, and plan which members of the medical staff will flank the VIP.

Allow a short private session for the VIP to ask questions or raise concerns. Often the VIP wants to clarify issues they saw before they answer questions from the media. Make sure the VIP has the facts bulletin handy, with the most up-to-date figures and numbers.

Media statement

Conclude the visit with either a media statement by the VIP or a media conference where questions can be addressed to the VIP. It is sometimes required that the commander/manager joins the VIP at this point. Ensure that an appropriate area is identified for the media briefing. It is recommended to position the VIPs behind a table to allow them to use notes inconspicuously. It is also advised that the VIP manager be positioned next to the VIP to assist with questions.

Use the opportunity to guide the VIP to thank all responders or staff members.

Summary

VIP visits occur frequently and monotonously after a major incident. By keeping to a standard programme, such visits become easier and less challenging to organise and to execute.

7.2   Dealing with the media

The modern media can reach any incident site or healthcare facility, anywhere in the world, very soon after an event and sometimes even before the rescue teams! It is therefore essential for commanders to plan in advance on how to deal with the media and to ensure effective public information.

Media liaison officer

Depending on policy within the service or facility, a specific media liaison officer needs to be appointed as soon as possible after the event and provided with formal guidelines. The most important aspect of media relations is to provide the media with sufficient appropriate information in a reliable and structured way, or they will find what they think is appropriate information themselves!

A three-phase approach is recommended. These phases are as follows:

- Issue structured media releases or statements on a regular basis;
- Conduct regular media briefings;
- Allow adequate media tours to obtain images of the event or the response.

Media statements

As soon as is realistic after an event, a formal media release or statement should be compiled. Such a statement should include basic information on the event, including accurate times and basic technical data that is *available* and *confirmed* at that moment in time. It is not recommended that specific numbers of casualties or diseases be mentioned (as these are most often unconfirmed, and when changed drastically lead to continuous enquiries). The statement should indicate what responses are presently taking place, as well as any positive information that is confirmed at that moment. This statement is issued in writing. Guidelines include using a formal structure and formal letterhead and indicating a person to handle enquiries. The statement should also indicate when the next statement will be issued.

As the situation develops, more comprehensive statements may be issued, providing more detail and, as soon as it is confirmed, specific numbers of survivors received at the facility. As soon as possible, a specific information point for relatives should be established, and its location and telephone numbers issued in a statement. All enquiries about individual survivors are then channelled to this information point. The detail of such a point should be included in each subsequent statement.

Structured media statements are also the ideal channel to communicate specific information to the public. The type of information will vary according to the event. Basic preventative health education information may be included in the event of an outbreak of a communicable disease. A call for blood donors may be issued in a trauma event, while a hospital may require volunteers to help with cleaning during strike action. Whatever the event, the information included in the media statement must be *clarified* and *confirmed* at the appropriate level before it is released. In particular, information of a technical/clinical nature must be checked and clarified by appropriate subject experts prior to release. The moment wrong or inaccurate information is released in a statement, the system loses its credibility and the media start searching for other sources.

Do not try to hide the truth from the media; they will uncover it! Do not use phrases such as 'no comment' or 'off the record', and never speculate in any media releases.

As the situation develops and response gets more structured, the statements are expanded and become more detailed. As the situation stabilises, the frequency of statements can be scaled down, for example, to a daily statement only.

Modern technology makes it possible to issue a comprehensive statement, with appropriate pictures, to the media very early after an event. Continuing with the service ensures that the media is used optimally as an integral component of the response.

Media conference

Depending on the policy of the specific service, a structured system of media conferences may be appropriate. In a multi-system response, it is recommended that the highest authority involved convene the media conference and involve the other role-players, instead of every individual hospital calling a media conference. It is essential that adequate information is available to justify a media conference. Consolidate the information in a structured media statement that is released simultaneously with the conference.

A specific spokesperson must be appointed to present the briefing during the media conference. It is important to select a spokesperson who has the appropriate skills and can present the professional image the institutions wish to project. An appropriate location and background for filming should also be planned for the briefing.

On completion of the briefing. a structured opportunity for questions by the media is allowed. This needs to be controlled, and only official released information should be used when answering media questions.

The media conference is concluded with a clear indication of when and where the next conference will take place.

Photo opportunities

The modern media require images of the event, and the response taking place, to enhance their coverage. If no structured opportunities are made available, they will use *any* means to gain access to the event or the hospital, and to photograph uncontrolled situations.

It is recommended that a photo opportunity be arranged following the media conference. This can be a structured walkabout through the hospital, a tour through the site on a specific vehicle or an arranged overflight by helicopter.

Whatever the format, photographers should be briefed in advance on what is allowed to be filmed and what not. The main principle stays the same: if you don't want to see something in a newspaper, put it where they can't see it. They are then accompanied and allowed to take pictures from the angles they prefer. It is, however, important to control ethical issues such as bodies, identifiable patients or personal particulars.

Public information

A structured public information or enquiry system is critical in any major incident or disaster response. This is a specific identified point where information can be obtained on individual victims, survivors or diseased, and needs to be established centrally as soon as possible following an event.

If numerous hospitals are used to receive casualties, the information must be fed through to a central point where relatives can enquire about the whereabouts of their loved ones. Such information may include pictures of unknown patients that can be displayed centrally and electronically to enhance identification.

A public information point should be equipped with adequate means of communication, preferably not on the same telephone system as the hospital or facility, as that system is often overwhelmed with calls. This must include telephone and electronic mailing capabilities, especially in an event where international enquiries can be expected. The centre should be staffed by trained personnel, such as social workers, able to communicate with stressed relatives. Translation capabilities or multi-language skills must be planned, especially if victims include foreigners speaking a different language.

Accessibility to the relatives, with adequate parking, catering facilities and space for religious counselling should be considered when selecting a site for an information centre. The centre must, however, be away from the disaster site and arrival points for casualties must not be within view. Separate facilities in which next-of-kin of the deceased can be informed in private must be planned. Relatives should be protected against inquisitive public or the media. A counselling or support service to relatives is an integral part of the centre.

Communicating effectively to the media and the public is a critical element of the effective management of a disaster or major incident.

Internal communication

It is essential to inform staff members of the situation on a continuous basis. This will discourage staff members from speculating. Often, inappropriate statements in the media are the result of an uninformed staff member coming into contact with the media. This can only be countered by efficient internal communication.

It is also very important to identify a staff member to monitor what is reported in the media This should include the non-formal media such as Twitter and Facebook, as this may influence staff morale as well as the public image of the institution.

7.3   Field treatment facilities

The need for the establishment of temporary on-site treatment facilities after a major incident must be fully appreciated before a decision to establish such facilities is taken. Field treatment facilities can vary from a casualty clearing station in the open, a temporary resuscitation and treatment capability or a primary healthcare facility for addressing minor ailments to a sophisticated field hospital with surgical facilities and a holding capability for hospitalised patients.

The nature of the event must be analysed before taking a decision on the need for a treatment facility. A short-duration event, such as a bus incident in an urban area, is unlikely to justify the need for a full treatment capability, whereas an extensive earthquake that has destroyed all existing infrastructure may justify the deployment of several field hospitals. The longer the duration of the response, the more likely a treatment capability should be considered.

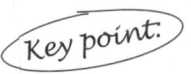 **The decision to establish a field treatment capability needs to be fully appreciated by considering all factors and evaluating the advantages and disadvantages fully.**

Casualty clearing station

The function of a casualty clearing station is to assemble patients at a central point, to re-triage and to perform life-saving interventions. These interventions are normally limited to Priority 1 patients and patients are not discharged from the facility.

The establishment of a casualty clearing station is a standard procedure in any major incident, and is discussed in detail in Chapter 2.

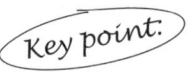 **A casualty clearing station is established to consolidate the casualties and to coordinate the transport of casualties.**

Patient treatment and resuscitation capability

The function of a treatment facility escalates from a casualty clearing station as definitive treatment is administered and patients may be treated and discharged from the capability.

In appreciating the feasibility for the establishment of such a facility, it is necessary to analyse the total treatment chain for patients, from the site of the event to definitive care need. If an on-site treatment capability will contribute to the logical flow of patients, will alleviate the transport of unnecessary patients to the already overburdened hospital and alleviate the load on other hospitals, the capability should be considered. If the facility only duplicates the capabilities of the available hospitals that can cope with the load, such a facility becomes a time-wasting stop that may be detrimental to the outcome of the casualties.

If a field resuscitation and treatment facility is indicated, it needs proper planning to be effective:

- Positioning must be within the logical direction of evacuation of casualties.
- To be effective, the facility must be fully operational on site within 24 hours after the impact.
- An appropriate venue or space needs to be identified. If existing buildings are to be used, these need to be inspected for safety and stability by an engineer, especially after a natural event such as an earthquake or hurricane. Other considerations are as follows:
  - access roads that will be able to handle an increase in vehicles even if the weather deteriorates;
  - adequate parking for vehicles to off-load patients, with preferably a circle flow to the entrance;
  - wide enough entrance to allow stretchers to be carried into the venue;
  - adequate space to manage the expected number of casualties and be able to expand should the need arise;
  - logical flow from entrance to triage to treatment to transfer or discharge must be possible;
  - exit from which discharged patients can leave the facility without interfering with the inflow of new patients;
  - adequate lighting to accommodate functioning after dark;

- access to drinking water and adequate ablution facilities. If treatment is envisaged, hand wash or hand decontamination facilities must be planned;
- adequate ablution for the planned staff as well as the expected patients needs to be planned;
- an even floor level, with a washable floor surface, would be a recommendation;
- protection against changes in the weather. After a major disaster this may be a luxury, but protection against the elements needs to be considered in selecting a venue.

- If tented facilities are to be used, the same basic principles apply; however, ground surface and water drainage is critical for tented facilities. Often, a hard surface such as a parking area looks ideal, but it may be impossible to pitch tents on the concrete surface. Tented facilities must be properly anchored to protect against wind storms. A grass sports field with floodlights and existing ablution facilities is a very useful solution.
- The facility must be totally self-sufficient for at least the first 48 hours.
- Power supply needs to be planned. This may include power supply to equipment as well as diagnostic apparatus.
- The equipment must be appropriate for use in field conditions. It is recommended that the equipment lists for a field treatment facility be planned well in advance. It is not always possible to stockpile such equipment, but if the needs are predetermined, it is possible to identify in advance from whence such equipment can be collected when required:
  - plan for the basic needs;
  - stick to the type of equipment that is used regularly by the staff who will be using the facility;
  - ensure compatibility of supply systems such as power and oxygen;
  - plan a service of comparable standards of care that was available in the affected area prior to the event.
- Plan appropriate communication to link the facility with the response to the disaster as well as to the hospitals receiving patients transferred from the facility.
- Plan security for the facility, including access control.

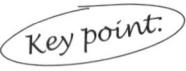 **A treatment facility is only established if it integrates into the logical flow of patient evacuation, contributes to limit unnecessary transport of casualties and alleviates the pressure on already overburdened hospitals.**

Primary healthcare facilities

The need for the deployment of primary healthcare capabilities after a disaster must be appreciated in detail. The guiding questions should be: what was available in the region prior to the event, and what is still functioning at that moment? It is critical to consider an exit strategy before establishing such a facility. If no clinic existed prior to the event and the need is now visible, it is unlikely that it will be possible to close the facility after a week or two. It must then be approached from a developmental perspective, and a plan must be made for the long-term needs of the community.

It is often necessary to establish a primary healthcare clinic temporarily after a disaster, until such time that the health and transport systems of the community can resume normal functioning. It may be necessary to establish this type of facility close to sites where survivors are accommodated, as transport to existing clinics may not be functioning.

It is ideal that the clinic be planned in such a way that it can blend into the existing health system after a period of time, and that a continuum of care is established. This makes it ideal to use some of the healthcare providers in the area to assist at the temporary facility, as it will accommodate the transition to a long-term system and the transfer of patient records to the long-term system.

Such a capability can also provide mental health and debriefing support as an integral part of the response.

The World Health Organization (WHO) has an excellent publication on the equipment and medicine required to establish such a clinic facility. This publication can be downloaded from the WHO website (www.who.int).

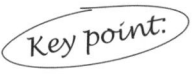 **Primary healthcare capability is established to provide a clinic-level service in an area until such time that routine health services can be re-established.**

Field hospital facilities

Field hospitals are larger, more permanent facilities, with the capability to admit and treat a specific number of casualties. As these facilities are often designed for military operations, they are predominantly equipped for trauma and the treatment of adults.

The need to deploy a field hospital facility must be very accurately appreciated by a team of knowledgeable experts with experience in the deployment of such facilities. This appreciation must be based on sound disaster medicine principles and not on political, publicity or emotional reasons. As these facilities take time to be mobilised and deployed to an area, they often arrive at a time when they are no longer needed.

Field hospitals are designed in different ways, and consist of various designs. These vary from re-deployable, semi-permanent buildings and container-designed facilities to full canvas (tented) facilities or combinations of these systems. Each of these systems has a different lead time to deploy and erect the facility on the appropriate site.

Often, these systems are modular, which makes it possible to deploy only those elements of the field hospital that may be required, often in support of an existing partially functioning or overloaded hospital. For example, mobile surgical theatres may be deployed to supplement the facilities at a community hospital to manage a large number of trauma cases.

The need for such a facility needs to be analysed accurately, as it is often more effective to evacuate a large number of patients to an existing functioning hospital with substantial resources than to transport a single operating theatre to a small rural hospital. It is critical to understand that these facilities are normally large units with between 60 and 120 beds, theatre capabilities, high-care units and a full support element of diagnostic, logistical and catering facilities. In requesting a field hospital, the size of what is requested needs to be understood. Often role-players request a 'field hospital' when they mean a single treatment tent! A field hospital is often transported in more than 20 large containers.

Although field hospitals designed specifically for disaster relief operations do exist at an international level, in the southern African region these assets are all under military control.

When planning for a field hospital deployment, various factors need to be considered:

- *Timeliness:* will it be possible to deploy the facility to the impact area within effective timelines to make a difference in the outcome for patients? This includes the time to mobilise the equipment and staff, transport the entire component to the impact area, deploy it to the appropriate site and getting the facility operational. Depending on the system, a standard military field hospital will take between 3 and 14 days from activation to readiness to receive casualties. In an international deployment this can even be longer to accommodate customs, visas, professional registration of practitioners and over-flight rights. The target timeline for a field hospital is that it must be fully operational within 3 to 5 days post-impact.
- *Appropriateness:* are the field hospital's facilities appropriate for the needs? Military field hospitals are designed to manage mainly trauma of adult (mostly male) casualties for relatively short periods of time until casualties are transferred back to the home country and standard hospital facilities. In a disaster, it is often women and children that are in need of care, often not with penetrative trauma and often for an extensive period of time until local facilities can be rebuilt. Is the required level of specialities available? This may include obstetrics, paediatrics, neurosurgery or communicable disease expertise, aspects that are not normally addressed in a military field hospital.
- *Efficiency:* will the field hospital be able to deliver an efficient service to the affected population? The hospital is not a stand-alone capability, but must fit into the overall treatment plan for patient care. Will the evacuation lines be able to deliver patients to the hospital, and will transfer from the hospital to the next level of care be possible? Will the transport system be able to move and off-load the hospital should it arrive by air or rail?
- *Absorptive capacity:* is there the capacity in the impact area to absorb and support such a facility should it be deployed? The existence of an effective command structure is essential to accommodate the facility and to ensure that it is utilised optimally within the treatment plan.
- *Sustainment:* will sustainment of the hospital be possible once it is operational? This includes the availability of basic services such as water and the outflow of sewage to the need for oxygen, blood, food and medicine. This is especially important when the logistical supply lines stretch over borders. Any deployed capability must be self-sufficient for at least the first 48 hours after arriving.
- *Cost:* although cost is often moved to the back in large humanitarian operations, it is essential to consider the cost-effectiveness of deploying the facility versus other possible solutions.

- *Effectiveness:* this is an overarching principle that needs to be appreciated prior to a decision to deploy a field hospital. It is essential to determine what other solutions there may be for the needs of the affected population, and to ensure that the field hospital is the most appropriate solution. Beware of the donation of drugs, as these are often expired drugs dumped on the disaster situation from warehouses. The WHO has published very useful guidelines on accepting drug donations.

If the appreciation indicates that the field hospital is the most appropriate solution, basic guidelines will assist in deploying the facility:

- Plan the appropriate mode of transport. These capabilities can be moved by ship, rail or large transport aircraft. Each mode of transport has its own requirements at the receiving end.
- Plan for appropriate off-loading capabilities. Off-loading the equipment normally requires large fork-lift trucks or cranes and it cannot be done by hand only.
- Identify the appropriate site for the hospital:
  - large enough to accommodate the facility – as a guide two sports fields (rugby or soccer size fields);
  - access and road surface for large heavy trucks to move/transport the equipment;
  - ground surface that is secure, has good drainage and is capable of supporting trenches for piping and cables (a tarred parking area may be ideal if surface piping and cables are to be used);
  - adequate electrical supply of the correct voltage will be a recommendation – if not generators must be deployed;
  - feeding into a sewage capability. The hospital normally has its own ablution capabilities, but the sewage must either be piped into an existing functional network that can accommodate the volume, or septic tanks/bladders must be used and emptied daily with suction trucks;
  - access for ambulances to deliver or collect patients;
  - landing space for helicopters, especially large military helicopters.
- Additional site factors to consider include:
  - access to the hospital by the community, including visitors;
  - access control and security – a fenced facility is strongly advised;
  - culturally acceptable outlay and processes;
  - feeding into higher levels of care for patients not managed at the level and transferred to a higher level of care, often in another region or even another country;
  - management of corpses to be planned for.
- Plan the sustainment of the hospital from local resources. This normally includes fresh food, blood, oxygen and other medical gases, medical waste removal, refuse removal and fuel for generators.
- In an international situation:
  - status of foreign healthcare practitioners practising in the country to be clarified;
  - authorisation to bring drugs into the country through customs to be clarified;

■ availability of local support staff, especially cleaning and laundry staff, needs to be considered.

The International Committee of the Red Cross (ICRC) has published an excellent publication on establishing field hospitals (available from http://www.icrc.org).

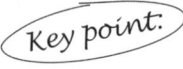 **The deployment of a field hospital is a major undertaking that is the result of clearly identified needs. It requires adequate pre-deployment planning, transport capabilities and support services to function. It takes time to deploy and requires substantial manpower and space.**

Summary

The deployment of temporary treatment capabilities require a detailed appreciation and a needs analysis, and must contribute to patient care. Various types of facilities may be deployed, but the choice must contribute to the local health system. An exit strategy must be decided upon prior to deployment. Deploying a field hospital is a time-consuming logistical operation that requires considerable human and other resources and space.

7.4 Civil–military cooperation

In a disaster or major incident, various resources available to the authorities are often mobilised in the relief effort. This may include military capabilities, forcing civilian and military counterparts to work together to save lives and alleviate suffering.

The primary function of a defence force is to defend the territorial integrity of a country and to maintain peace. However, many countries also use their defence capability in support of the people. It is in this humanitarian role that the military is often used in disaster relief operations.

To ensure mutual cooperation between civilian organisations and the military structure, it is necessary for the different role-players to respect and understand one another's capabilities. The military has certain strong points, such as command and logistical support, while the civilian structures often have more experience in disaster relief and a more consensus-based approach. These different capabilities can be synergetic in achieving the goal.

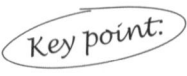 **Mutual cooperation between civilian organisations and military structures is possible through mutual respect and understanding.**

Organisational culture

Every military force has a specific and often unique organisational culture under which it operates. Not understanding such a culture often leads to serious misunderstandings and frustrations for civilians, especially non-governmental organisations (NGOs) working with the military.

Chain of command

A military organisation is always strictly hierarchical, with clear lines of command. This determines the authority to issue orders and to instruct subordinates to execute specific tasks. In working or liasing with the military, it is essential to determine who is in command and to respect the command line. On the opposite side, the military would like to liaise with the civilian command, meaning that within the civilian environment the 'commander' needs to be identified for healthy interaction. This is not always that easy, as especially NGOs and volunteer groups often function on consensus approaches, with no formal appointed leader. Turf wars between NGOs often cause serious malfunction, resulting in the military taking an authoritarian approach and assuming command. However, this is not necessary if civilian counterparts are harnessed into a team and the most logical leader takes the lead, be it civilian or military.

Hierarchical approach

A military structure is always hierarchical, meaning that every soldier has a rank above him until you reach the pinnacle of the commander in chief, who is normally the head of state of the country. This requires the soldier to obtain authority for requested action from a higher authority. This is often interpreted as an inability to take decisions, but is a logical command process. Respecting the military approach – that they will request authority to execute a function – leads to healthy cooperation, and ensures that a support action is not suddenly stopped when higher authority becomes aware of it.

The most visible aspect of the hierarchical structure is the rank structure of the military. Civilians are often overwhelmed by the sea of stars and stripes that suddenly appear, and try to address every member of the military according to his or her envisaged rank, which can cause even more chaos. As a basic concept, the military is structured into two main groupings: the officer grouping, who are mainly involved in planning and decision-making; and the non-commissioned officer grouping, who are mainly responsible for the execution of the orders from the officers. Officers are mostly identifiable by insignia worn on the shoulder; non-commissioned officers are generally identifiable by insignia worn on the upper arm. (This is not always the case in all military organisations, and the naval environment in particular has different types of rank markings.) For civilian counterparts who are not familiar with a specific country's system of rank insignia, it is recommended to avoid using specific ranks to address military members, and to use a neutral courtesy approach.

Meetings

The military is used to structured meetings, resulting in clear decisions on what will happen next and ending with orders to the soldiers. In a civilian environment, especially the humanitarian philanthropic groupings, this is often not the situation. This can result in misunderstanding, as the military interprets these everlasting discussions to try to reach consensus as a lack of leadership and decisiveness. The solution is normally to ensure that all meetings have a structured agenda, and that all decisions are clearly recorded.

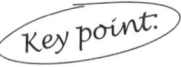 The military has a strict hierarchical chain of command. Individual members should be addressed through neutral courtesy terminology rather than by trying to address every member according to rank.

Military processes

Within the civilian/military cooperation environment, following specific sequential processes often contributes to synergetic cooperation.

Requests for military cooperation

It is essential for civilian organisations to know their military counterparts, especially at a local and regional level, in order to feed requests for assistance into the military system at the appropriate level. When government departments or agencies request military cooperation, this is normally done at the head-of-department level, and may even go to the political level with ministerial interaction. As a guideline, channelling formal requests to the command level, rather than liaising with a local uniformed friend, often leads to a healthy start for cooperation.

As part of the planning to manage a major incident or disaster, it is recommended that channels for requests for military support should be clarified in advance.

Liaison officer

As soon as a formal request is received and approved/or preliminarily approved, a liaison officer is identified to liaise with the civilian counterparts. This officer is not necessarily going to be in charge of the operation, but is the contact person for all follow-up liaison. To prevent confusion, it is essential for both the military interaction as well as civilian liaison to flow through the identified liaison officer.

Mission

For every operation, a specific mission or tasking is identified, clarifying the boundaries for which the specific officer has the authority to issue orders and to specifically guide the appointed commander into what is expected from him/her to execute. This is normally the result of the request received for help and/or an appreciation process to identify the needs.

It is essential for good cooperation that a clear mission for the military's role in an operation is identified, as it will prevent future misunderstandings or expectations. Military commanders are very sensitive to 'mission creep', where the tasking escalates or expands slowly into more and more areas of the situation, often resulting in conflict between role-players.

Rules of engagement

Each military operation will have rules of engagement, which delineate the circumstances and limitation under which the military will initiate and continue in an engagement. This will have a significant impact on the operation, logistics, movement and liaison with the various role-players. This is especially visible when a military force is mobilised to support a foreign country in a humanitarian relief operation.

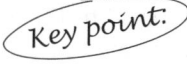 **Requests for military support need to be formal and guided to the appropriate command level, and may require ministerial-level liaison. A military liaison officer may be appointed to liaise with civilian counterparts to identify specific needs. The military will support a specific mission with specified rules of engagement guiding the actions.**

Military response

Depending on the situation, the military normally responds to a humanitarian operation with a Joint Task Force. This refers to a grouping of the various capabilities of the military combined in an orderly way to execute the mission.

Command

The first question that normally arises in a civil/military operation is: who is in charge? The simple answer, except if specific legislation dictates differently, is nobody! The military normally remains in command of its own resources, while the civilian organisation controls its own capabilities. This is, however, brought together in a joint operation centre or structure where the different role-players agree on actions.

It has happened, with good results, that specific military officers are appointed to command a specific function, while military assets have been placed under the leadership of an NGO expert. It is strongly recommended that, as soon as cooperation starts, the command and control aspects are clarified through an open discussion and then communicated down both lines to ensure everybody knows who controls what.

A Joint Task Force commander is officially appointed and all the resources allocated are placed under this officer's command to use within the rules of engagement to execute the mission.

Military resources

The military has three services, namely:

- *Army:* responsible for landward defence and specific resources used on land. These include capabilities such as trucks for transport, human resources for search and rescue operations, water purification capabilities and emergency lighting.
- *Air Force:* controls all the airborne capabilities. These include helicopters and cargo planes, airfield control capabilities and air reconnaissance capabilities.
- *Navy:* controls the maritime environment (where applicable in sea-bordering countries), which includes ships and boats and, in some countries, also the maritime helicopter capabilities.

In some countries, such as South Africa, the health-related capability is grouped in a separate service, such as a military medical or military health service. This will include all medical assets, emergency medical teams, deployable hospital capabilities and the resources needed to take care of patients during air or sea evacuation.

Various other disaster-related capabilities are embedded in the basic military structures, and include assets such as military police, mass catering capabilities, intelligence and map and photo creation capabilities, etc.

Medical or health capabilities

Military medical capabilities include numerous resources which can be utilised in disaster or major incident operations, over and above the support resources of transport and manpower.

The basic capability is to render emergency care to the wounded soldier. This entails skilled emergency medical capabilities, with equipment to render advance life support. Many of these members have rescue and extrication capabilities and can be deployed by foot, vehicle, parachute or boat operations. Most military health organisations train their emergency care staff to at least the same standards as their civilian counterparts.

Ambulance transport capabilities include large numbers of ambulances capable of transporting lying and sitting patients with the required equipment to maintain care in evacuation. This can often be expanded to include air and boat evacuation capabilities, up to mass evacuation capabilities.

Deployable capabilities include field resuscitation facilities designed to render advanced life support in a static position before evacuation. This is often supported by field surgical capabilities, which can be deployed to a disaster site to provide damage control, such as surgical interventions under general anaesthesia. Facilities to be erected in the refugee or displaced person environment to provide primary health care capabilities are often the most needed capability that can be provided by the military. All these capabilities are staffed by medical officers, nursing officers and other healthcare practitioners.

Larger capabilities include field hospitals to provide comprehensive hospitalisation, theatres and after-care capabilities. Some countries can also deploy capabilities such as hospital ships – such as the USNS *Mercy* and *Comfort* of the United States Navy or the RFA *Argus* of the Royal Navy – which can provide a complete floating hospital with up to 1 000 beds. This capability was used in the Haiti earthquake in January 2010.

The psychosocial support capability of the military is an aspect often forgotten. This includes large numbers of social workers, psychologists and members of the clergy, who are used to working together as a team. This capability is a valuable asset to address post-traumatic stress screening and intervention.

Military pharmacists are experienced in controlling bulk drugs and medical equipment, and are a valuable asset in managing drug donations and distribution.

The environmental health capabilities of the military include environmental health assessment, inspection of donated or emergency food resources, water testing to advise on the erection of refugee camps and inspection of refugee facilities and sanitation.

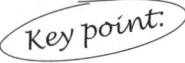 A specific command line will be established and a commander appointed. The military commander remains in command of the military resources at all times. Various resources are available within the different services of a defence force. The military health or medical service is staffed by healthcare practitioners with the equivalent training and experience as their civilian counterparts.

Summary

In summary, civilian/military cooperation is possible with synergetic results based on good communication, understanding and mutual respect for experience and capabilities. The military can provide resources that can be integrated in an effective response to a major incident.

7.5 Mass patient evacuations

Various events may necessitate the movement of large numbers of lying or sitting patients to alternative locations. This may be pre-event – for example, when patients from care facilities are moved to safer areas as a hurricane is moving towards a low-lying area – or post-event, when casualties may need evacuation to care facilities after an earthquake has destroyed all hospital facilities in a region. Examples of the mass evacuation of patients include the evacuation of hospitals in New Orleans after Hurricane Katrina in 2005, the evacuation of casualties back to Australia after the Bali bombing incident in October 2002 or the total evacuation of the city of Darwin on Christmas Day 1974 after Cyclone Tracy.

In such an event, various modes of mass transport can be used to evacuate patients, but in a desperate situation all forms of available transport may be used. This can include all forms of road transport, large air transport capabilities, various forms of rail transport and the use of ships on navigable waterways. Whatever mode of transport is used in mass evacuation, proper planning, proper command and continuous care are the cornerstones of a successful operation.

Mass patient evacuation is defined as moving large groups of patients to facilities for continuation of care; in contrast, mass evacuation is where large groups of people are moved to a safer position. A large group is defined as 20 or more patients moved simultaneously.

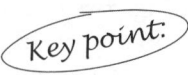 Proper planning, proper command and continuous in-transport care are the cornerstones of mass patient evacuation.

Needs for mass patient evacuation

It is essential to verify the need to move large groups of patients from one location to another. The need may also directly influence the mode of transport. If the need is to get patients to higher ground due to approaching flood water, there will be no time to wait for a special mode of transport to arrive, and all available resources must be used. However these types of situations are the exceptions, and usually there is some time for planning.

The reason is often associated with a risk or perceived risk. Patients are removed from a danger area due to the negative effect the risk may have if an event occurs. A hospital below the expected flood line may be evacuated prior to a cyclone moving into the area.

Post-event evacuation may include the evacuation of relatively stable patients from partially collapsed and un-functional hospitals after an earthquake, or the movement of large numbers of rescued casualties from the affected area to hospital facilities in an unaffected area of the country.

In specific situations, large numbers of patients with specialised needs – for example, burn patients – may be moved to centres of excellence or, due to the intensity of the care they require, be distributed to various centres.

It is essential, in the planning phase, to analyse the reason for the planned evacuation and to confirm the necessity for it. Mass patient evacuations are not without risks, and the reasoning for the evacuation should justify the risk.

The reason may also have an influence on the mode of transport that will be used, which may be influenced by the diagnosis of the casualties. Various modes of transport have different physiological effects on the body; for example, it would not be recommended to transport specific communicable diseases in an open-plan military aircraft where decontamination would be very difficult afterwards.

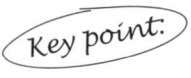 **The need for the mass evacuation needs to be analysed critically to determine the feasibility for the evacuation and to guide the evacuation process.**

Pre-planning

Whatever the reason for a mass patient evacuation, proper pre-planning must be done and proper command established. Safety of staff and patients should be analysed and measures implemented to provide optimum safety.

The primary step is to determine how many patients need to be transported from point A to point B. This will be the source for a thorough appreciation of what transport capability, or combination of capabilities, can be used to move the patients. This includes an analysis of the condition of infrastructure available, such as road conditions, the availability and serviceability of the rail network and the serviceability and length of available runways. Other factors that may influence the evacuation need to be analysed in detail, including present and predicted weather conditions, timelines (including timelines coupled to the risks) and daylight hours available. A factor often driving timelines is the quality of present care facilities for patients: for example, patients lying in the open for the second day after an earthquake will dictate different timelines versus patients being cared for in a hospital but in need of transport to another hospital.

It is difficult to make informed decisions before details of the patients who need to be moved is available. The availability of this information will be directly influenced by the situation and the communication available. It may vary from a rough estimate of numbers of casualties to a detailed name list with all clinical data.

As soon as possible, the clinical conditions of the patients need to be analysed in detail. A standard starting point is to number all patients and to ensure that these numbers are attached to the patient using a basic hospital identification tag. If time permits, it is beneficial to use a team to assess all patients and to compile the data. It is recommended that a basic spreadsheet be compiled with numbers, names, age, diagnosis, present conditions, care required during transport, special needs, present location and destination. If computerised, this data can be manipulated into detailed patient lists for various purposes.

Firstly, patients need to be triaged and the priorities recorded. Secondly, patients are evaluated to determine the ideal method of transport required. Distinguishing between those who can be transported in a sitting position and those who need to lie down during movement and transport is the basic analysis. These groups are then subdivided into those sitting patients who may be able to walk to the mode of transport versus those who will require a wheelchair. The lying patients are subdivided into those who can be moved by wheelchair to the mode of transport versus those who require a stretcher from bed to bed. A simple code system can be used for these subgroups, in combination with the triage priority, giving a clear overview of the operation ahead: for example, 9 x Priority 3 stretcher and 5 x Priority 3 chair patients. This information is captured in the database.

Only after such a detailed analysis, which does not necessarily need to take days, will the full need be visible, allowing the planning of evacuation modes.

With the information on infrastructure, resources and patient needs available, detailed planning can commence. The total process, from present position of the patient to the admission at the destination, needs to be planned in detail.

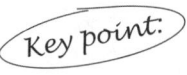 **The support systems available for a mass evacuation need to be appreciated in full, such as length and condition of runways and serviceability of railway lines. A comprehensive data sheet must be built up of patients, their triage priority, diagnosis and mode of transport required (i.e. sitting or lying).**

Modes of evacuation

Road transport

Road transport is often the easiest and most available mode of transport. Vehicles may vary from basic ambulances and school buses for sitting patients to trucks for large groups of stretcher patients. Road transport is often also used in combination with other modes of transport – for example, as the feeder transport to an aeroplane or train.

In using vehicles, the optimum use of all vehicles must be planned, including using available seats in an ambulance for sitting patients. The use of larger vehicles decreases the speed of transfer, but allows for more economical use of staff to care for patients. Buses can be used to transport lying patients by placing stretchers over the backrest of the standard benches; however, loading is often challenging. It is recommended to pre-position stretchers in the bus; patients can then be brought into the bus on scoop stretchers and un-scooped onto the pre-positioned stretchers. Another alternative is to use large transport trucks, such as furniture removal trucks, to move a group of stretcher patients together with a staff complement, but take air-flow into account.

In planning to use road transport, it is essential to evaluate the road conditions for the full route to be used for the evacuation. Ensure that the type of vehicles planned will be able to travel all the way from point A to point B. Often after a disaster, this type of information is not available or is unreliable, and may require scouting of the route prior to movement, to prevent a convoy of patients becoming stuck – for example, at a washed-away bridge.

It is recommended to move groups of vehicles in a structured convoy under a structured command, as it makes sustainment, recovery of broken vehicles and support between vehicles easier. In planning the convoy, staff must be allocated to vehicles based on the condition of the patients being transported.

Planning for refuelling points is essential, and it is necessary to confirm that the type and volume of fuel required will be available. Sustenance, such as food for patients and staff, replenishment of supplies, especially oxygen, and disposal of waste, must be planned at pre-determined intervals.

In a mass evacuation, or when using road vehicles to feed patients to other modes of transport, a circle system is often used: after unloading, vehicles return to collect the next wave of patients. In such a system, the decontamination of vehicles prior to reloading must be considered, to prevent cross-contamination or the transmission of communicable diseases.

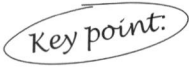 **Road transport is often used in conjunction with other modes of transport, such as air or rail. The full route that will be used needs to be assessed, and, if indicated, scouted. Fuelling along the route must be planned.**

Rail transport

Rail is often a forgotten mode of transport for patient evacuation. The advantage of rail is that a large number of patients can be evacuated in relative comfort with the ability of a small group of staff to move between the different coaches.

Standard rolling stock can be used effectively to move patients. Sitting coaches are ideal for mobile patients, while standard sleeper coaches can be used to transport stable lying patients. Parcel vans (or brake coaches) normally have large sliding doors, making them ideal to transport stretchers and more critical patients. If open-plan parcel vans are used, patients need to be positioned longitudinally facing the direction the train is moving to minimise motion sickness. Some of the brake coaches are equipped with toilet facilities; alternatively, caravan-type chemical toilets must be planned.

A standard sleeper coach can accommodate 39 lying patients, while a parcel van can easily accommodate 24–28 stretchers. A sitting coach can transport approximately 74 sitting patients.

The total railway line must be pre-assessed to ensure that the train will be able to reach the destination. Equipment must be pre-positioned in the different carriages to speed up the loading and departure of the train(s).

Loading a train is a time-consuming and labour-intensive operation. When a platform is available, patients can be carried directly into parcel vans, while sitting patients can be moved into the train with stretcher chairs with ease. Loading lying patients into sleeper compartments is more difficult, as doors and corridors are too narrow for stretchers. It is recommended that teams be positioned inside and outside the train and that patients be passed through the windows into the compartments on spine boards or scoop stretchers. Patients can then be transferred to the bunks inside the individual compartments. The use of a standard industrial forklift to lift lying patients to the level of the windows eases the loading process, especially when a platform is not available. The patient on a spine board is placed on the forks of the fork-lift, lifted to window level and then pulled into the compartment.

A reception and triage area must be established on the platform or close to the train. On arrival, patients are checked against the data lists and re-triaged. Patients need to be placed in the train based on their triage priority. It is not possible to provide efficient care to patients on the top bunks of compartments; therefore, patients requiring continuous care during transport must be placed on the lower levels, while stable patients are positioned on the upper levels.

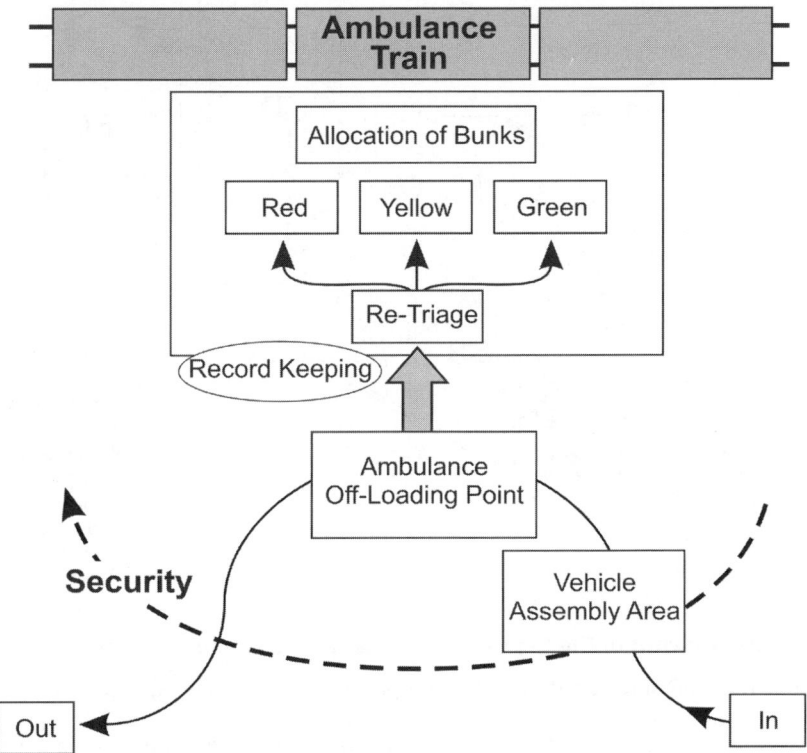

Figure 7.1: Basic layout of a loading point

(Note: The same principles can be used for loading aircraft or ships.)

Planning for adequate water and food is essential, while additional water to keep the sewage system functioning may be necessary. An important aspect is that trains do not have 220 v AC power outlets available, requiring planning for the self-sustainment for power needs.

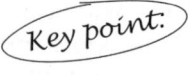 Standard rolling stock can be used to establish evacuation trains. Rail transport has the capability to move large groups of patients in comfort with few members of staff taking care of them. Loading a train is a relatively time-consuming activity.

Air transport

Air transport (both rotor-driven and fixed-wing craft) is often considered the fastest mode of transport. However, pre-flight activities and loading may be very time-consuming, making the consideration of other modes of transport an option.

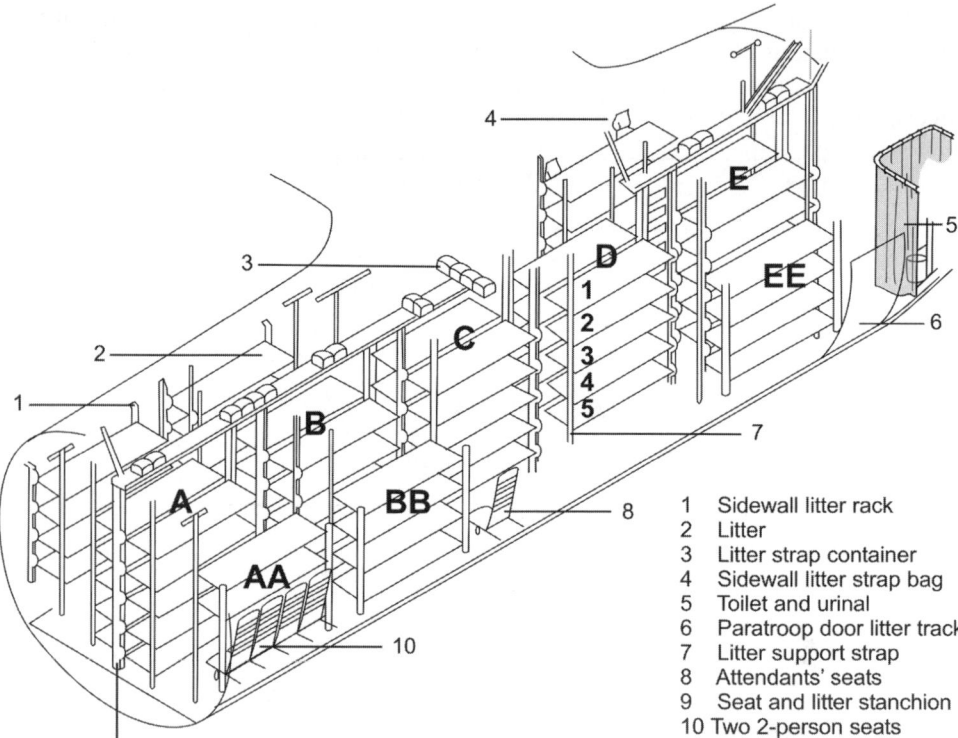

1 Sidewall litter rack
2 Litter
3 Litter strap container
4 Sidewall litter strap bag
5 Toilet and urinal
6 Paratroop door litter track
7 Litter support strap
8 Attendants' seats
9 Seat and litter stanchion
10 Two 2-person seats

Figure 7.2: Basic layout of the C-130 Hercules cargo aeroplane for mass air evacuation

(Note the numbering of rows and stretchers for pre-planning positioning of patients.)

In a mass evacuation by air, the only resource readily available is large military transport planes. These planes have the capability to transport large numbers of stretcher patients with relative ease due to large loading doors and substantial space inside. The use of smaller aircrafts for transporting individual critical patients remains an option.

Military transport planes include the widely used C-130 Hercules, which can load up to 72 stretchers; the Russian-built Antonov range of transport planes includes the An-26, which can accommodate 24 stretchers, while the huge An-124 can transport 288 stretchers. The Puma/Oryx helicopter can carry 6–8 stretcher patients, while the twin-engine Chinook helicopter can transport 24 stretchers.

To use air evacuation, it is necessary for a specialist to evaluate the length of the runway or landing zones to ensure that the size of aircraft to be used can land and take off with the load. The runway surface, landing lights or improvised landing lights all require specialist advice. This information needs to be confirmed as there is no margin for error. The runway length determines the size of aircraft which can be used.

The weather predicted for the time of evacuation and the journey to the destination must be analysed. A sudden change in the weather could jeopardise the entire operation and force a postponement to a later time.

It is essential to adhere to the capacity and design of the aircraft, and to secure all items, including stretchers, placed inside the plane. A large number of unrestrained stretchers on the floor is an extremely dangerous situation, and should be avoided at all costs. Most transport planes have special harnesses from which to hang standard NATO military-type canvas stretchers. If these are not available, stretchers must be secured to the floor safely using ratchet straps or even rope.

A feeder system must be planned to transport patients to the airfield. At the airfield, strict control over ambulance movement is essential, and ambulances must be allowed to approach only after the plane has parked and switched off its engines, and only after it has been confirmed that no other planes are going to land or take off. Ambulances should be guided to a pre-designated receiving area to off-load patients. No ambulances should be allowed to drive directly to the cargo doors without proper supervision, as high vehicles or antennas on the roofs of ambulances can damage the plane.

Loading a large transport plane is very labour-intensive and requires the manhandling of stretchers to the various positions in the plane. Patients need to be placed in the plane based on their triage priority. In some planes, up to 5 patients are hung above one another, making it nearly impossible to reach the top two stretchers in flight. Unstable patients must therefore be placed on the lower levels, with stable patients placed on top. The plane must be loaded and all stretchers must be filled from the front, as it is nearly impossible to carry stretchers in the narrow aisles between rows of stretchers. Positioning patients in the plane requires clinical judgment to evaluate the effect of G-forces during takeoff and landing, especially with head-injury patients.

Patients need to be prepared for air evacuation with special attention paid to the influence of the gas laws on the body.

Key point: **Moving large numbers of casualties by air requires specialist clinical knowledge to assess casualties prior to transport as well as specialist knowledge on runways and weight distribution. An adequate feeder system needs to be planned to transport casualties to and from the airfield.**

Sea or water evacuation

Using ships or boats to evacuate large numbers of patients is often the solution to a disaster situation in the maritime environment. This will obviously be determined by the available navigable water.

Water evacuation is relatively slow in comparison to other modes of transport, and is also influenced by prevailing weather conditions. However, the use of boats provides space for care during transport.

Loading large numbers of stretcher patients onboard a large vessel is labour-intensive. It is challenging to carry stretchers on board via a gangplank. If cargo vessels are used, cranes can be used to hoist platforms with several stretchers on board.

Although cargo vessels or ferries often have adequate space to transport a large number of stretchers on vehicle decks or in cargo bays, the ventilation in these areas is often problematic. It is essential to assess the airflow to determine suitability for patient care, and such areas often require measures, such as the provision of large fans, to create airflow. Sanitation capabilities on cargo vessels are also inadequate for a large number of patients, and need to be substituted with additional chemical toilets.

Patients positioned on the longtitudal axis of the vessel, facing forward, experience less motion sickness.

When loading patients on board, safety measures need to be addressed, and if at all possible all patients should be fitted with a flotation device while aboard. Flotation devices or lifejackets should be used for patients during loading, and especially during hoisting.

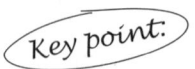 **Placing casualties on board ship requires a proper assessment of space, airflow and sanitation capabilities.**

Preparing for evacuation

As soon as planning is finalised, a detailed name list must be compiled from the database. If more than one vehicle or craft is to be used, a list of planned patients per craft or vehicle must be compiled. These lists should also be forwarded in advance to the destination(s) to ensure that the receiving facilities are aware of, and prepared for, arriving patients.

Patients are numbered and transported to the craft, train or ship for evacuation. As a guide, patients are moved to the craft in reverse triage order, meaning that the Priority 1 patients remain until last in the care facility and are then moved to the craft. On arrival, they are off-loaded first to limit the 'out of hospital' time to the minimum.

All clinical notes and diagnostic studies available should accompany patients. A useful method is to use a large envelope for all the documentation, which is then attached with string to the patient's body. Often, a quantity of luggage needs to accompany the patients. These are best managed as separate items that are marked with the patient's particulars and then transported under secure circumstances to the craft or plane and loaded prior to loading the patients. The volume and weight of luggage need to be taken into consideration during planning.

Patients need to be stabilised and resuscitated as far as possible prior to evacuation. However, this may not be possible in certain unstable disaster situations. If possible, each patient's airway should be secured, and if compromised the patient should be intubated to ensure a definitive airway. At least one functional intravenous line is recommended, and adequate fluid should be available to sustain the line for the duration of evacuation. A urinary catheter is recommended for all lying patients, especially for long-duration evacuations. A naso-gastric tube must be inserted prior to air evacuation.

Specific loading areas must be planned with adequate lighting and resources to manhandle stretchers, with a circle flow for vehicles. Patients are individually checked against name lists and clinical conditions are re-assessed for triage priority.

Staff allocation to the various vehicles or craft need to be carefully planned based on the condition of the patients. Staff are then allocated on the basis of available resources, as well as space on the vehicle or craft. Personal protective clothing needs to be available to all staff.

At the destination, a dispersion point needs to be planned. On arrival, each patient is again checked against the name list and all personal belongings and documentation are loaded with the patient before transport to the admission facility.

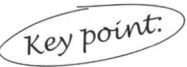 **Patients need to be optimally stabilised prior to transport.**

Logistics and equipment

Equipment for care during the journey needs to be planned and positioned for use during evacuation. The equipment will differ vastly based on available resources, condition of patients and skill levels of staff. As a basic guide, a full set of resuscitation equipment should be available in each vehicle or craft, as patient condition may deteriorate during evacuation.

Additional intravenous fluid, oxygen, sanitation equipment, blankets and dressings should be available.

Command and communication

A key element for a mass evacuation is the establishment of clear command channels to control loading, moving and transport during the operation. Each convoy, train or ship needs a clearly identifiable medical commander, who liaises directly with the crew, driver or ship captain. This needs to be supported by effective communication, which is ideally maintained during the entire movement to the destination to ensure that the destination team knows the time of arrival and any changes in the condition of patients during evacuation.

Mass evacuation of patients is a challenging operation, requiring optimal planning within the timelines available, and must be executed with military precision and proper command. This planning should take note of the need to:

- plan space for patients dying en route;
- plan resuscitation criteria, futility criteria and level of care;

- plan the triage of which patients are evacuated and which remain behind because of various considerations;
- plan for the need to transport without oxygen present, as is often the case in major disasters;
- plan for the possibility of a downgrade in medical care with its consequences.

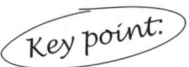 **Mass patient transport requires adequate planning and efficient command and communication to execute.**

Summary

All modes of transport can be used to evacuate patients. All modes require proper planning and a detailed assessment from point A to point B, and may require scouting of the route. Adequate resources are required to load the modes of transport, equipment must be pre-planned and in-transport care must be planned.

7.6 References

1. Advanced Life Support Group. *Major incident medical management and support.* 2nd ed. London: BMJ Books; 2002.
2. Noltkamper DF. Media relations. In: Ciottone GR. *Disaster medicine.* 3rd edition. Philadelphia: Mosby Elsevier; 2006.
3. World Health Organization. *Rapid health assessment protocols for emergencies.* Geneva: World Health Organization; 1999.
4. World Health Organization and Pan American Health Organization. *WHO-PAHO guidelines for the use of foreign field hospitals in sudden-impact disasters.* Washington, DC: World Health Organization; 2003.
6. Hayward-Karlson J, Jeffery S, Kerr A, Schmidt H. *Hospitals for war-wounded.* Geneva: International Commitee of the Red Cross; 1998.
7. World Heath Organization. Guidelines for drug donations. 1999. Available from: whqlibdoc.who.int/hq/1999/who_edm_par_99.4.pdf. Accessed 19 January 2010.
8. Pan American Health Organization, World Health Organization, ICRC. *Management of dead bodies after disasters.* Washington, DC: Pan American Health Organization; 2006.
9. Cabot S. Disaster field hospitals: triage and treatment in time of crisis. Available from: www.blu-med.com/pdf/sandra_cabot.pdf. Accessed 19 January 2010.
10. Mothershead J, Yeskey K, Brewster P. Selected federal disaster response agencies and capabilities. In: Giottone G (ed.). *Disaster medicine.* Philadelphia: Mosby Elsevier; 2006. pp. 95–101.
11. USAID. *Field operation guide for disaster assessment and response.* 3rd edition. Washington: USAID; 1998.
12. Tran MD, Garner AA, Morrison I, Sharley PH, Griggs WM, Xavier C. The Bali bombing: civilian aeromedical evacuation. 2003. Available from: www.mja.com.au/public/issues/179_07_061003/tra10048_fm.html. Accessed 19 August 2010.

13. Chai J. Treatment strategies for mass burn patients. *Chinese Medical Journal* March 2009;122(5).
14. Emergency Rail Concepts. Hospital evacuation trains. Available from: www. emergencyrailconcepts.org/medical.htm. Accessed 19 August 2010.
15. Hatfill S. Disaster trains. Available from: cryptome.org/disaster-train.htm. Accessed 19 August 2010.
16. US Department of Health & Human Services, Agency for Healthcare Research and Quality. Recommendations for a national mass patient and evacuee movement, regulating, and tracking system. Appendix F: resource requirements models. Available from: www.ahrq.gov/prep/natlsystem/natlsysapf.htm. Accessed 19 August 2010.

8

Special Incidents

M Stander, T Ligthelm, T Hardcastle, B Steyn, N Ford, K Chu, L Blumberg, J Frean, R Swanepoel and M Mendelson

Objectives

By the end of this chapter, the reader will be able to:

- appreciate the process of burns triage during a major incident;
- describe the challenges unique to creating burns surge capacity;
- understand the aspects of terrorism that make these special incidents;
- understand the medical aspects associated with blast injury;
- understand how major incident management should be modified to manage nuclear risk;
- understand the requirements for modification of personal protective equipment (PPE), and the limitations of working in such equipment;
- understand the requirements for evacuation and care of the nuclear-contaminated patient;
- know what a 'biological agent' is, and the range of possible biological agents encompassed in a bio-threat;
- know how to approach the management of a bio-threat, including 'white powder' incidents;
- know about the important viral haemorrhagic fevers (VHFs) in Africa;
- have an understanding of the approach to healthcare provider post-exposure prophylaxis (PEP) for potential body-fluid pathogens;
- know the current approach to the emergency management of suspected cholera cases;
- understand the procedures and the role of emergency care personnel during the management of hazardous chemical incidents;
- be aware of the importance of correct scene management;
- know about the important toxic industrial chemicals;
- have an approach to the treatment of casualties from a hazardous chemical incident;
- understand the needs of vulnerable groups in major incidents, including the elderly and disabled.

8.1 Burns incidents

Burns major incidents are uncommon events, but, when they occur, demand a unique and dedicated response. The incidence of burns major incidents in South Africa is currently unknown, although it is estimated that 3.2% of South Africa's population are burnt annually. The majority of patients affected are less than 20 years old, and it is generally a problem of low socio-economic status. Only 0.2% are classified as severe burns. The average mortality for adults is 10.2%, and 4.1% for children.

There are several obstacles that have been identified in the provision of optimal burn care in low-income countries, including:

- Limited number of specialised burns units;
- Financial constraints;
- Lack of dedicated infrastructure in burns units;
- Close link to low socio-economic status;
- Despite low technology, major burn surgery is a very expensive service;
- Nationwide shortage of ICU facilities;
- Shortage of dedicated theatre time;
- Decreasing number of trained nursing staff;
- Impact of AIDS pandemic;
- Lack of dedicated private sector facilities for burn care.

Against this background, it can be appreciated that the provision of adequate burn care in the event of a major incident will be challenging. These patients utilise extensive resources, supplies, personnel and time, and often their recovery and rehabilitation take much longer than other subsets of patients.

With limited resources in each geographic area of a country, capacity may be created for burns major incidents by the creation of a national burns major incident plan; extra capacity may even be found across international borders.

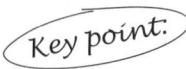 **The provision of specialised burns care to patients remains a challenge.**

Burns triage

The concepts of triage have been covered in detail in Chapters 2 and 3. It is accepted that triage in major incidents provides a unique challenge with limited resources; however, failure to triage adequately compromises the response and patient outcomes.

There is currently no international gold standard for the triage of burns patients during a major incident. Certain parameters, including burn size, patient age and the presence of inhalational injury, are known to predict mortality and have been utilised for this situation. Assessment of burn severity is a critical step in the triage process. Accurate triage by healthcare providers who have burns expertise helps to minimise the requirement for scarce burn facilities. Accurate estimation of injury at the disaster site under suboptimal conditions is difficult, especially with respect to burns patients. Even in developed countries, inappropriate under-triaging of patients still occurs.

Certain criteria will influence the triage and treatment process, such as additional injuries, treatment facilities, transportation capacity and the availability of specialised burn centre beds. Because total body surface area (TBSA) involved is an important prognostic factor, it cannot be completely ignored on-site.

There are two aspects of current accepted triage practice which makes the application to burns patients controversial: modern burn survival rates have dramatically improved due to innovations in treatment; and it is difficult to withdraw clinical care from patients who would otherwise survive in a non-major incident situation.

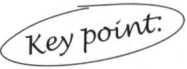 **Primary triage of disaster burns patients needs to be conducted as accurately as possible on-site.**

Burns surge capacity

In developing countries, there are too few dedicated ward and ICU beds for burns patients, and too few specialised burns centres. The result is a day-to-day shortage in burn bed capacity, and many patients need to be treated and managed at non-specialised centres. A burns major incident will prove to be challenging in terms of increasing capacity for these patients.

Alternatives to conventional ward beds need to be considered, such as the Dallas Convention Center Medical Unit, which was established as an alternative site for medical care in the aftermath of Hurricane Katrina. Many sites rely heavily on their trauma centres to create surge capacity, supported by the creation of robust outpatient capacity (as the majority of patients will not be severely burnt but will need to be followed up). Collaboration between all role-players, including EMS, hospitals and specialised centres, is also important.

Creating in-hospital surge capacity follows standard principles, as described in Chapter 4: as in other situations, the limiting factor tends to be the provision of adequately trained staff.

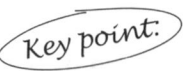 **Hospital major incident planners need to consider the creation of extra capacity for burns patients.**

8.2 Terrorism

Terrorism is defined as the calculated used of weapons and violence to attempt to instil fear and panic into communities, with the intention of the furtherance of a religious, political or social agenda. Health service providers are not immune from the effects of terrorism. Typically, terrorists operate in clandestine, cellular organisations that are impatient with society and have a tendency to increase the level of violence as pressures on the group mount.

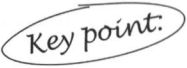 **Terrorism is violence intended to create fear and panic in society, out of a desire to further a religious, political or social agenda.**

Recent terrorist activity

Table 8.1: Recent terror attacks

Date	City	Mechanism	Number injured	Number killed
Sept 2001	New York	Hijacked commercial aircraft intentionally crashed into targeted major buildings	>2000	>2800
Oct 2002	Bali	Multiple explosions	196	>200
Nov 2003	Istanbul	Improvised explosive devices	>750	>60
Feb 2004	Moscow	Bomb explosion in the underground railway system	130	40
Mar 2004	Madrid	Bombs on commuter trains	>1400	>180
Jul 2005	London	Bombs in underground trains and a city bus	>700	>50
Jul 2005	Sharm el-Sheik	Car bombs	>110	>80
Oct 2005	Bali	Bomb blasts	>100	>20

In addition to the events listed in Table 8.1, the ongoing, almost daily bomb blasts in Afghanistan and Iraq have killed and maimed many innocent civilians and international military personnel.

Terrorist methods of injury

The prime aim of terrorism is to maim, injuring physically and psychologically, and to overwhelm the healthcare resources, leading to maximal morbidity and mortality.

The means used include commercial and industrial explosives, stolen military hardware, chemical and biological warfare and the ever-present risk of radio-nuclear devices. These can take the form of bombs planted in vehicles, in structures or carried on the person of suicide bombers (which carry the additional risk of human tissue missiles). Conventional weapons use on civilian non-combatants are also considered in this category.

For the purposes of this section, the focus will be on blast-related injuries, as the other forms of terrorism are discussed later in this chapter.

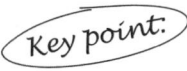 **There are numerous methods of terrorist activity.**

Why are these special incidents?

Terrorist attacks are considered special incidents because there is a requirement for effective command and control to be established rapidly and early, involving multiple services, including the military. Other safety factors to be considered include the possibility of secondary devices, multiple dispersed devices or the risk of 'dirty bombs'. Responder safety factors must rate highly before entering the scene. Communication may be difficult due to the risk of radios and cellular phones being used as activator devices for secondary explosives. Access and egress may be difficult due to debris, and the ability to access victims may require prolonged extrication, with the attendant risks of crush injury and renal failure.

Medical aspects of terrorism: blast injury

Blast injury is a syndrome of injuries caused by the effects of explosion. It is generally divided into four stages/phases:

- *Primary blast injury* is due to the direct blast-pressure effects, with rupture of tympanic membranes, lung tissue and hollow viscera as the most lethal injuries in this category. This is the most lethal phase. During this phase, those victims close to the blast may be dismembered and others suffer traumatic amputations.
- *Secondary blast injury* is the commonly noted penetrating wounds caused by missile particles, flying debris, shrapnel or home-made projectiles. In patients distant from the explosion, these injuries are the most severe.
- *Tertiary injuries* are caused by the blast wind (sometimes called the blast overpressure) which can disintegrate bodies and items close to the blast, but commonly causes the structural instability of buildings, with subsequent collapse or the flinging of the patient against solid objects, leading to crush, blunt and penetrating injuries. This is the group of injuries with the high risk for crush-myonephropathic syndrome and renal dysfunction.
- Finally, the miscellaneous *quaternary effects* include the effects of burns, toxic gases and other contaminants. These lead to respiratory problems and may be easily overlooked in casualties who may have deceptively few external injuries.

Most commonly, a combination of effects is noted. These effects depend on the type of ballistic device, such that mines and similar devices are smaller in effect, with the object of amputating limbs and causing sepsis.

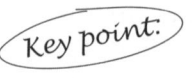 **There are four phases traditionally described with blast injuries, and these may be found to a lesser or greater extent in any patient.**

Summary

Civilian major incidents involving explosives are mostly not due to terrorism; however with the ever-present risk of terrorism, vigilance and preparation are essential. The main risk to providers of emergency care is a secondary device, while the chief pathology is the four types of blast injury. Conventional approaches to major incidents should be modified to mitigate the risk of additional injury.

8.3 Nuclear incidents

Southern Africa has been relatively shielded from exposure to the risk of nuclear major incidents, due to the lack of major nuclear sites. It is important to note, however, that smaller radioactive stores are found in many hospitals and industrial sites and that the risk of there being a radio-nuclear component to a major incident is not impossible. Additionally, there are regularly vehicles transporting radioactive cargo on our roads. Three case reports of single or small group incidents have been recorded since 1977, involving a total of about 12 patients.

To date, there has not been any major nuclear incident in the history of southern Africa; however, the Chernobyl disaster and similar international events are fixed in memory. During civilian incidents, radiological and other CBRNe (Chemical, Biological, Radiological, Nuclear) threats are often overlooked.

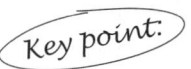 **Nuclear incidents are most likely to be civilian rather than military in nature.**

Radio-nuclear risk

The challenge of radio-nuclear incidents is in the manner in which radioactive materials affect the body. Material released into the air or soil can affect humans directly through crop and animal contamination, with the subsequent spread of radiation in milk or meat products. All these can have short-term and long-term effects on the human physiology.

Table 8.2: Types of radiation and protection methods

Alpha
- Shielded by paper, first layer of skin
- Threat is inhalation or absorption of alpha emitter in wounds
- Internal hazard

Beta
- Three-metre range in air
- Shielded by plastic safety glasses or thin metal
- Skin and eye hazards
- Internal and external hazards with wounding/ingestion

Gamma
- Similar to X-rays, very penetrating in tissue and lighter materials; long range
- Shielded by lead, steel, concrete
- External and internal hazards

Radiation incidents can contaminate the patient in a number of ways. There may be whole-body or partial-body external radiation, wound contamination with radioactive material during trauma and blast incidents, or there may be ingestion through normal bodily orifices. Combinations of these mechanisms can occur, with eventual incorporation of the radioactive substances into internal organ systems.

Managing nuclear incidents

The initial management of a major incident applies to radio-nuclear incidents in all their forms. Early assessment of hazards will identify the risk of radiation injury, and the appropriate safety measures to prevent escalation of the incident should be instituted. The general management of these incidents will fall under the command of the police and fire/rescue services, with emergency medical services ideally entering a decontaminated zone or treating outside the bronze zone once the patients have been evacuated and decontaminated.

Radiation physicists and other experts should be consulted on the overall incident management. Patients will be either exposed or contaminated, with the latter having ingested, inhaled or touched the radioactive substances, while the former have simply been in proximity to the incident. Water is adequate for decontamination of gross soiling from radio-nuclear incidents. Staff should position themselves upwind of the incident, about 20 metres away from the bronze area. Standard precautions apply to personnel. Clothing should be removed and a complete wash-down should follow. No special effort needs to be made to contain the runoff.

Key point: **Water is adequate for decontamination.**

Key point: **Standard precautions are adequate protection.**

Personal protective equipment for nuclear hazards

Personal protective equipment (PPE) to prevent skin contamination of particulates is very effective against particulate-borne radiation hazards (i.e. alpha and beta particles). Typical firefighter 'turn-out' gear, including a self-contained breathing apparatus (SCBA), is generally adequate for this purpose. The use of turn-out gear, or any disposable protective clothing suitable for particulate exposure, should be followed by appropriate decontamination of personnel and equipment. Generally level D protective gear is adequate for radio-nuclear incidents when dealing with the casualties outside the bronze zone.

Protection of internal organs from inhalation of radioactive particulates can be provided by wearing an appropriate particulate respirator. The SCBAs will provide the highest level of protection. Responders should utilise at least a full-face air-purifying respirator with an N95, P-100 or HEPA filter, as appropriate.

The limitation for the emergency service providers is that most of the CBRNe personal protective gear allow for bronze zone times of between 15 and 30 minutes before staff rotation is required.

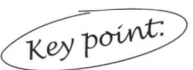 **Adequate PPE is a level D suit with air-purifying respirator.**

Evacuation and treatment of the patient

Tygerberg Hospital in South Africa has a special facility for dealing with radiation incidents, and is the civilian reference resource for the country. Specially equipped ambulances are not required, although lining the vehicle with plastic sheet and the wearing of protective clothing, including eyewear, by EMS personnel, is recommended. Secondary decontamination of the patient follows after immediate triage and resuscitation, using a radio-dosing device to determine the levels of contamination present. Particular attention is paid to the mouth, nose, eyes and ears, as well as any open wounds.

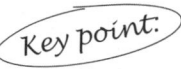 **Adequate decontamination is determined by use of a radio-dosimeter.**

Hospital care of the patient

The risk to hospital providers of care is very low indeed, once gross contamination is removed. Signs and symptoms of radiation injury include nausea and vomiting, cutaneous burns and other wounds, headache, fever and diarrhoea. Evidence of bone-marrow depletion follows over the next few days to weeks. Long-term effects include an increased risk for malignancies and genetic malformations. Exposure to 30 Gray or more is usually fatal.

Further care may include the use of medications and surgical procedures for cases with internal contamination. This includes the use of: enteral absorption blockade (e.g. barium, aluminium or magnesium salts, Prussian blue or activated charcoal); blockade of end-organ uptake (e.g. potassium or calcium salts, renal bicarbonate flushing); dilutional agents such as phosphorus by mouth; and chelating agents (Penicillamine or DTPA).

Excision of wounds may be required. Extensive debridement and limb sacrifice is not usually justified. Provided the hospital physicist is satisfied with the decontamination efforts, wounds may be closed primarily; however, if there is any residual on the dosimeter, delayed closure is advised.

The main aspect of hospital care is the long-term monitoring of the patient for the complications of radiation exposure, namely malignancies and similar disorders. This will be performed by clinicians with training in haematology, oncology, nuclear medicine and radiotherapy.

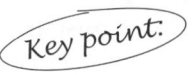 **The decontaminated exposed patient presents no risk to hospital staff.**

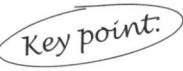 **Acute radiation syndrome and chronic radiation effects will be the main problems for the hospital services to manage.**

Summary

To date, southern Africa has been fortunate not to experience the effects of a major incident with radio-nuclear agents. However, the brief guidelines presented will enable a rational and panic-free response to such an incident. Water decontamination is the most important early intervention and long-term surveillance of the exposed persons is essential.

8.4 Biological incidents

Bioterrorism is the use, or the threat of use, of biological agents against civilians, with the aim of intimidating, creating mass panic among, or otherwise influencing, an audience. Biological agents are living organisms, or material or toxins derived from them, which are intended to cause disease or death in humans, animals or plants. From a terrorist's point of view, bio-weapons are inherently appealing:

- They are relatively easily produced and transported.
- They are difficult to detect, at least in initial deployment; per kilogram of weapon, they may approach the effectiveness of nuclear weapons.
- Some have already been extensively researched, produced and stockpiled.

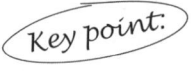 **Biological agents are living organisms, or material or toxins derived from them, which can be used as weapons, often with a delayed onset.**

Bioterrorism scenarios

There are two main bioterrorism scenarios: first, the use of recognised, 'weaponised' bio-warfare agents, such as anthrax; second, the use of common pathogens as weapons, e.g. *Salmonella* or *Shigella* species. While about 30 disease-causing pathogens have bio-warfare/bioterrorism potential, there are some that are particularly suited for this role, such as the agents of anthrax, smallpox, brucellosis, botulism, tularaemia, plague and certain haemorrhagic fever viruses. These are known as Class 'A' agents.

In principle at least, bio-engineering can produce resistance to antibiotics or vaccines, enhance stability and genetically modify benign organisms to produce toxins or virulence factors.

Recent bioterrorism experience

In October 2001, bioterrorist attacks using anthrax began in the USA, resulting in 23 confirmed or suspected cases (one of which was laboratory-acquired) and five deaths. Immediately following these reports, many countries, including South Africa, experienced a spate of bioterrorism threats. Although these 'white powder incidents' invariably turned out to be deliberate hoaxes or to involve mistaken benign material, emergency and medical services were obliged to handle them as potentially genuine threats, and they caused major public disruption. Although the incidence of bioterrorism hoaxes has dwindled, the potential for a real attack has not.

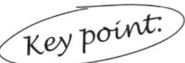 **Most 'white powder incidents' actually turn out to be hoaxes.**

Healthcare workers as 'first responders'

The overt release of biological agents, whether genuine or hoax, will invariably involve traditional first responders (such as firemen). Covert release of biological agents will mean that first responders will be doctors, nurses and civilians. It is obvious that adequate bioterrorism preparedness training, which encompasses surveillance, detection and response, needs to be aimed at health professionals and the public, as well as the traditional first responders.

Table 8.3: Clues to the occurrence of a covert bio-attack

- An outbreak of a rare or novel disease.
- An outbreak of disease in a non-endemic area.
- A seasonal disease in off-season time.
- A known pathogen, but unusual resistance profile or epidemiological features.
- An unusual clinical presentation, or age distribution, of a known disease.
- The emergence of genetically identical pathogens in different areas.

Anthrax

Anthrax is endemic in southern Africa; although human cases are rare, it is useful for clinicians to know about the clinical presentation following either conventional or bioterrorism exposure.

Suspected bioterrorism, including 'white-powder incidents'

In South Africa, the first responder is the South African Police Service (SAPS), in its capacity as primary manager of all suspicious package investigations. Substances or articles suspected of being of biological hazard are secured, then passed to the Chemical and Biological Unit of the SA Military Health Service, who are responsible, after rendering items safe to transport, for delivering the material to a military-contracted laboratory for the identification of anthrax.

As far as human contacts are concerned, a simple algorithm can be applied in the majority of incidents.

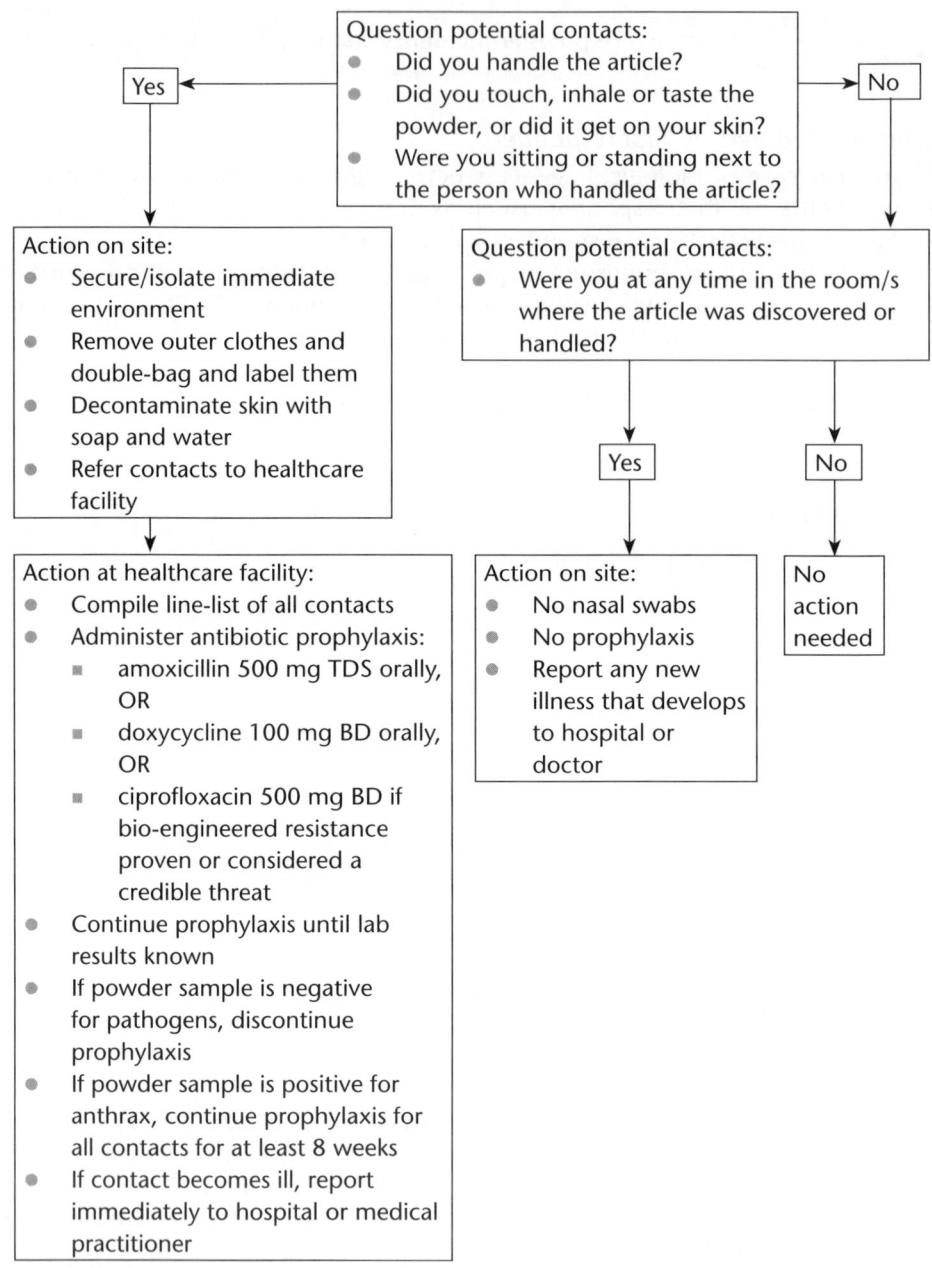

Figure 8.1. Algorithm for suspected deliberate anthrax exposure

Conventional exposure

The common scenario for anthrax in southern Africa is exposure to domestic stock that die suddenly for no apparent reason. The animals are often butchered and eaten, thereby exposing people to cutaneous and gastrointestinal anthrax, whereas accidental inhalational anthrax in humans is usually a result of occupational exposure, e.g. animal hide, hair or wool processing, and this is extremely uncommon.

Clinical features of anthrax

Cutaneous anthrax

Table 8.4: Differential diagnosis of cutaneous anthrax

- Furuncle
- Orf
- Vaccinia
- Glanders
- Syphilitic chancre
- Erysipelas
- Ecthyma
- Tick bite or spider bite (simple forms)
- Orbital cellulites or dacrocystitis
- Deep tissue infection
- Necrotising streptococcal or staphylococcal cellulites (more severe forms).

Table 8.5: Clinical course of cutaneous anthrax

Incubation period: usually 2–7 days (range 9 hours–2 weeks)	
Day 0:	*B. anthracis* enters skin via lesion;
Day 2–3:	Papule appears;
Day 3–4:	Vesicles appear around papule; fluid exudes; oedema, typically massive, starts. No pus or pain, may find lymphadenitis in regional LNs;
Day 5–7:	Original papule ulcerates: eschar;
Day 10:	Resolution begins, may take 6 weeks, minimal scarring results;
	Occasionally develop bacteraemia. Without antibiotic treatment: 5–20% mortality.

Gastrointestinal anthrax

There are two main forms:

- *Intestinal:* nausea, vomiting, fever, abdominal pain, haematemesis, bloody diarrhoea, massive ascites, toxaemia, shock and death.
- *Oropharyngeal:* sore throat, dysphagia, fever, neck lymphadenopathy, toxaemia; 50% mortality even if treated.

Table 8.6: Differential diagnosis of gastrointestinal anthrax

Intestinal form
- Food poisoning
- Acute abdomen
- Haemorrhagic gastroenteritis
- Necrotising enteritis due to *C. perfringens*

Oropharyngeal form
- Streptococcal pharyngitis
- Vincent's or Ludwig's angina
- Parapharyngeal abscess
- Deep-tissue infection of neck

Pulmonary or inhalational anthrax

Clinical presentation is typically as follows:

- Headache, muscle ache, chills, fever, cough;
- Minority have chest pain;
- Sudden development of dyspnoea, cyanosis, disorientation, coma, death in <24 hours unless rapidly diagnosed and aggressively treated with antibiotics;
- X-rays may show a widened mediastinum with or without lung parenchymal changes or pleural effusion;
- Pathology: haemorrhagic mediastinitis; necrotising lung lesion in a few.

Management

Patients need not be isolated (person-to-person spread is not normally a risk). Swabs or aspirates should be taken from under the edge of the eschar, to ensure an adequate sample. Smears should be made of such material on glass slides. Place swabs in transport medium if possible. Blood cultures and respiratory samples should be taken if systemic anthrax is suspected.

Cutaneous lesions should be covered and standard precautions taken with blood, secretions and other body fluids. Antibiotic of choice remains penicillin G or amoxicillin, outside the bioterrorism scenario. In penicillin-allergic persons, quinolones, erythromycin, doxycycline or chloramphenicol are suitable. Intravenous penicillin G, 18–24 million units/day, or IV amoxycillin is used in inhalational anthrax.

Inhalation anthrax is often fatal, unless diagnosed and treated early and aggressively.

Because of concerns about bioterrorism and the possibility of antibiotic resistance-engineered organisms, quinolones or doxycycline are recommended when persons are exposed in credible bioterrorism incidents.

Intravenous hydrocortisone may be life-saving in cases with massive oedema threatening airway obstruction; in cutaneous anthrax, corticosteroids may help to control excessive oedema.

Notification of local health authorities must take place.

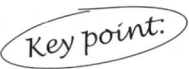 **Most cases of anthrax are conventional exposure and can be treated with conventional antimicrobials.**

Laboratory investigation

Specimens from humans are referred to medical diagnostic laboratories, particularly those of the National Health Laboratory Service (NHLS); some private medical laboratories may be competent and prepared to screen specimens.

Most laboratories, both public and private, refer suspected anthrax exposure-related specimens to the Special Bacterial Pathogens Reference Unit (SBPRU) Laboratory. This is a high-security facility that deals mainly with plague and anthrax diagnosis and is located at the National Institute for Communicable Diseases in Sandringham, Johannesburg.

Specimens should be double-bagged and clearly addressed and labelled '*anthrax*'. Include contact details of the sender for return of laboratory results. Before sending any specimens, notify the NICD Hotline (27(0) 82 883 9920).

8.5 Communicable diseases

This section does not aim to replace a standard infectious diseases text. However, it aims to provide the healthcare provider dealing with major incidents with guidelines to identify and manage communicable diseases of public health importance. Malaria and meningococcal disease are both highly prevalent; the reader is referred to any standard infectious diseases text for details.

Viral haemorrhagic fevers

There are many causes of fever or a haemorrhagic state. It is important to distinguish these conditions from viral haemorrhagic fevers (VHFs) caused by the formidable so-called Class 4 viruses. While the former are more common and do require specific, often life-saving, treatment, the VHFs have a propensity for person-to-person spread and high mortality rates, which necessitate instituting special infection control measures (barrier nursing). Fatal nosocomial infections of CCHf, Marburg, Ebola and the newly identified arenavirus, the Lujo virus, have occurred in South African hospitals in the past.

Many parts of the world have endemic VHFs, and modern travel has made it possible for introduced cases to occur almost anywhere. Many patients from areas in which VHFs are known to occur are transferred for care to urban medical centres, and VHFs need to be considered part of the differential diagnosis.

Healthcare workers should maintain high standards of infection control and biosafety awareness, and all patient care facilities should institute contingency plans for dealing with VHF patients. Certain hospitals are designated for the referral of VHF patients, but transfer of patients is not always possible.

A detailed and accurate history of geographical area of residence or travel, occupational history and possible exposures is key in highlighting the possibility of VHF. While the presentation of fever and bleeding in these patients may suggest the possibility of VHF, *not all patients with VHF will bleed*. The possibility of a VHF must still be considered even in the absence of bleeding in a febrile patient with a compatible history of exposure and travel, and especially, but not exclusively, if there is multi-organ disease with thrombocytopenia and deranged hepatic function.

Table 8.7: Caveats in VHF

- Rare for diagnosis of VHF to be confirmed pre-transfer
- Many treatable infections can have similar clinical picture
- Clinical presentation of VHF varies, and bleeding is not always present
- Frequently limited historical information on exposure
- Limited or incorrect laboratory results on presentation to the emergency unit

Table 8.8: Diagnostic assessment

Any person who presents with any form of haemorrhage should be asked for a travel, exposure and occupational history.
CCHF has frequently been misdiagnosed as local GIT pathology in hunters, abattoir workers and veterinarians presenting with haematemesis.

Key history points
- Age, sex and place of residence of the patient
- Chronic medical conditions and medication, including recent drug and dosage adjustments
- History of the current illness, including results of prior medical and laboratory investigations
- Occupation of the patient and possible exposure to infection as in:
  1. healthcare and laboratory workers who tended, or processed specimens from, patients with confirmed or suspected VHF or undiagnosed fever compatible with VHF (**relatively minor exposures to blood and tissue may not be noticed or reported**)
  2. contact with animals or animal tissues by abattoir workers, veterinarians, farm workers, hunters, taxidermists or persons who work with hides and skins
- Non-occupational contact with known or suspected cases of VHF, or undiagnosed fever
- Non-occupational contacts with animals or their tissues, including blood
- Residence in, or recent travel to, tropical or rural environments
- Handling, or being bitten by, ticks or mosquitoes
- Recent travel to a country known or likely to be endemic for VHF, particularly involving rural environments and contact with animals or insects – but remember that some rodent-associated and mosquito-borne VHF viruses can occur in urban environments
- The date/s of potential exposure/s to infection
- The date of onset of illness (incubation periods are <1 week for arbovirus infections, including Congo fever, but up to 3 weeks for arenavirus, Marburg and Ebola infections) ➲

Presentation of VHF – acute onset of

- Fever

- Fever and acute abdomen and GIT symptoms (frequently misdiagnosed as a surgical cause)

- Fever and rash (petechial, morbilliform)

- Fever and bleeding **but not all patients with VHF will bleed**

- Fever and organ failure

Laboratory results supportive of a diagnosis of VHF

- Thrombocytopenia

- Deranged liver function tests, notably elevated aspartate (AST) and alanine transaminases (ALT)

- Leucopenia typical but not invariable, normal count common, a leucocytosis may suggest an alternative diagnosis but may also present in the course of VHF disease, e.g. Ebola

- **While not all patients with a VHF will bleed, and the platelet count may be normal in Lassa fever-infected persons, the absence of thrombocytopenia in the presence of normal hepatic transaminases levels in symptomatic persons would render the diagnosis of CCHF, Ebola and Marburg disease unlikely**

Differential diagnosis of fever and bleeding

VHFs occur quite rarely in comparison to many other causes of fever, with or without organ damage and bleeding. It is therefore critical to consider a broad differential diagnosis in these patients, both infectious and non-infectious, and to administer empiric treatment while taking the appropriate infection control precautions and awaiting definitive results.

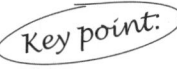 **VHFs occur quite rarely in comparison to many other causes of fever.**

Table 8.9: Differential diagnosis – VHF

- Tick bite fever

- Bacterial sepsis (particularly meningococcal)

- Malaria

- Herpes simplex hepatitis

- **Other bacterial, viral and parasitic causes include:** typhoid, Q fever, hepatitis A, hepatitis B, HIV with opportunistic infections and East African trypanosomiasis

- **Non-infectious conditions:** warfarin overdoses, snake envenomation, e.g. boomslang, heatstroke and haematological malignancies can mimic these signs and symptoms

When the diagnosis of a VHF is suspected, appropriate infection control precautions must be put in place immediately in the emergency centre even before the diagnosis is confirmed. Nosocomial transmission is through direct contact with the blood and body fluids of infected patients through needle stick injuries, splashes onto mucous membranes and skin abrasions. Respiratory transmission through close contact with aerosols is a concern with the arenaviruses. The proper use of personal protective equipment, especially safe removal and disposal of these by the wearer, and safe disposal of the patient's body fluids is critical. At a minimum, healthcare workers caring for suspected VHF cases should wear double gloves, a visor (especially if the patient is actively bleeding) and an impermeable gown and/or apron. An N95 mask should be worn if available, particularly when performing procedures that cause small droplet aerosols, e.g. intubation or suction. If unavailable, a surgeon's mask should be used instead. The patient should be managed in a separate area in the emergency centre until transferred to an isolation unit.

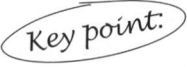 **Isolation of the suspected case of VHF is essential.**

Table 8.10: Diagnostic testing

- Notify the laboratory of a suspected VHF

- Do full blood count, liver enzymes and malaria stains

- Any further testing for other aetiological agents should ideally be delayed until a more intensive assessment of the patient has been made and the diagnosis of a VHF has been excluded

Empiric treatment with a broad-spectrum antibiotic to treat bacterial causes of a similar clinical presentation (especially possible meningococcal disease) should be urgently administered. Cover for tick bite fever, a common mimicker of VHF in Africa, is also appropriate.

Specialist advice and support should be sought from the infection control nurse, as well as the Special Pathogens Unit at the National Institute for Communicable Diseases in Johannesburg, which will also provide specialised laboratory testing for VHFs (tel. 24 hours: 27 (0) 82 883 9920).

VHFs are notifiable to the local authority. Contact tracing and active monitoring for fever and symptoms will be required if a VHF is confirmed.

Crimean-Congo haemorrhagic fever (CCHf or Congo fever)

The disease is seen most frequently in South Africa in the Northern Cape, Free State and North West provinces. However, cases may occur anywhere in the country: abattoir workers have developed the disease within big cities. The tick vectors are widely distributed in Africa. Humans acquire infection from tick bites (genus *Hyalomma*, the bont-legged tick with distinctive brown and white bands on its legs) or from contact of broken skin with fresh infected blood and tissues of livestock (sheep, cattle, ostriches) or through nosocomial transmission.

Clinical features include an incubation period of 1–3 days after tick bite to 5–6 days after contact with infected blood or other tissues. A necrotic eschar at the bite site is more suggestive of tick bite fever (rickettsiosis). Onset is usually very sudden, with severe headache, fever and chills followed rapidly by myalgia with intense backache.

The majority of patients with CCHf are symptomatic and present with some haemorrhage 3–5 days after symptom onset.

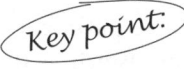 **The findings of thrombocytopenia and raised AST and ALT in the presence of a history of exposure to ticks or blood or tissues of livestock or ostriches or a visit or residence in a rural area should prompt the diagnosis of CCHF.**

Rift Valley fever (RVF)

RVF is a mosquito-borne virus disease of livestock in Africa. Humans acquire infection from contact with infected tissues of farm animals, or less frequently from mosquito bites. Most patients experience benign illness with fever, some with ocular sequelae and <0.5% develop fatal haemorrhagic disease, hepatitis or encephalitis. While human-to-human transmission is not a feature, infection control precautions should be observed in patients who bleed, as other causes of VHF, e.g. CCHf, overlap in terms of geographical distribution, exposures and clinical syndromes.

Marburg (MBG) and Ebola (EBO)

In Africa, Marburg and Ebola viruses appear to be endemic in the tropical region roughly within the area enclosed by Zimbabwe, Angola, Ivory Coast and Kenya: Marburg outbreaks are known to have originated in Uganda, Kenya, DRC, Zimbabwe and Angola, while outbreaks caused by the Sudan, Zaire and Ivory Coast sub-types of Ebola virus have occurred in Sudan, DRC, Uganda, Gabon, Democratic Republic of Congo and Ivory Coast. Bats have been proposed as reservoirs. Poor infection control practices in hospitals have been associated with major outbreaks.

Arenaviruses

Lassa fever is confined to West Africa (Nigeria, Sierra Leone, Guinea and Liberia are particularly affected). There is characteristic pharyngeal and tonsillar inflammation with vesicular or ulcerative lesions and whitish or yellowish exudates, facial oedema and a macular papular rash.

Lujo virus is a newly diagnosed arenavirus, with probable origin in Zambia, that caused a nosocomial outbreak with high mortality in Johannesburg, South Africa, in 2008. No further human cases have been confirmed since the outbreak. The clinical and laboratory features included a prodromal febrile illness, followed by tonsillar pharyngeal ulcerative lesions, facial oedema and a macular papular rash. Bleeding was not a major feature. Thrombocytopeania and pronounced increases in AST and ALT were prominent.

Yellow fever (YF) is a well known mosquito-borne virus which causes outbreaks of fatal disease with necrotic hepatitis in South America, West Africa and, less frequently, East Africa, but it has never been recorded south of Angola.

Dengue (DEN) is a mosquito-borne virus which causes massive outbreaks of disease with fever and joint and muscle pains, and frequently a rash, throughout the tropics in South America, the Caribbean, East and West Africa, Indian Ocean islands, India and South East Asia. A small proportion of patients may develop haemorrhagic disease or shock syndrome.

Post-exposure prophylaxis

Post-exposure prophylaxis (PEP) is provided for selected blood-borne pathogens following occupational or non-occupational injury. This section focuses primarily on exposure to HIV.

Hepatitis B

Healthcare workers (HCW) should be fully immunised against hepatitis B. If not vaccinated, or antibody response is unknown, give hepatitis B immunoglobulin with or without a full accelerated course of hepatitis B vaccination following an at-risk exposure.

HIV

Antiretroviral PEP is indicated for all risk exposures with blood or other potentially infectious material from an HIV-infected source. In areas of high HIV seroprevalence, all exposures involving an unknown source should be regarded as HIV-infected until proven otherwise.

Following occupational exposure, antiretroviral therapy (ART) must be started within 24 hours and continued for 28 days to reduce the risk of significant viral transmission. Percutaneous injury carries a higher risk than mucocutaneous exposure. Accordingly, PEP for percutaneous exposures should comprise triple ART (see Table 8.11). Dual ART with 2 nucleoside reverse transcriptase inhibitors is recommended for at-risk mucocutaneous exposure.

Before prescribing PEP, the recipient should have an HIV test. If HIV-infected, they should be referred to their local HIV clinic, but PEP should not be started.

Counsel and treat common gastrointestinal ART side effects with meto-clopramide and loperamide (if a protease inhibitor is used).

Follow-up with an appropriate clinic must be arranged to support the HCW on PEP.

PEP following sexual intercourse should be started within 72 hours of exposure, be continued for 28 days and made available to patients irrespective of the circumstances of exposure, i.e. assault or consensual.

Intensive counselling and support are required to avoid poor compliance and high rates of loss to follow-up following sexual assault.

Triple ART is generally recommended following sexual assault. Dual therapy is an acceptable alternative if compliance is an issue.

Attention to prophylaxis against pregnancy and sexually transmitted infections other than HIV may be required.

Table 8.11: Selecting patients for PEP intervention

	Status of source		
	HIV-infected	**Unknown**	**HIV-seronegative**
Percutaneous exposure to blood or PIM*	Triple therapy		No PEP
Mucocutaneous exposure or contact with an open wound with blood or PIM	Dual therapy		No PEP
Percutaneous or muco-cutaneous exposure to non-infectious bodily fluids	No PEP	No PEP	No PEP
Antiretrovirals	Dual therapy backbone: TDF or D4T or AZT + 3TC or FTC 3rd drug: lopinavir/rtv or atazanavir/rtv, saquinavir/rtv or efavirenz AVOID – nevirapine, abacavir and indinavir		

TDF – tenofovir, D4T – stavudine, AZT – zidovudine, 3TC – lamivudine, FTC – emtricitabine

* Ascites, breast milk, cerebrospinal fluid, embryonic liquor, pericardial or pleural fluid, wound secretions and sexual fluids including vaginal secretions, penile pre-ejaculate and semen.

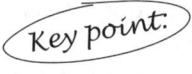 **PEP for healthcare workers is an essential component of comprehensive care during major incidents, where the risk of injuries is higher due to stress and fatigue**

Cholera

Recognition and management of cholera

Cholera is acute diarrhoea due to toxigenic strains of *Vibrio cholerae*-O1 or O-139, which is transmitted from contaminated drinking water or foods (shellfish, fish). Ninety-nine per cent of cholera cases reported to the WHO come from Africa, although over 50 countries reported cases in 2008 with an overall case-fatality rate of 2.7%. Epidemics continue to occur, and cholera should be considered in returning travellers from countries reporting cholera.

Although infection may be asymptomatic, the classical presentation of cholera with acute onset of profuse watery diarrhoea that looks like 'rice-water' should alert the clinician. Volume depletion compounded by vomiting may progress to hypovolaemic shock and death if not corrected rapidly. Muscle cramps are a common sign of potassium depletion.

Cholera can be confirmed by culture of stool or a rectal swab, but treatment should never be delayed. Rapid rehydration and correction of electrolyte losses and acidosis is key. Unlike other diarrhoeal disease, patients may pass large amounts of watery stools and dehydrate within hours. Adequate therapy with appropriate fluids and frequent reassessment is life-saving.

Mild to moderate dehydration is common, and 80–90% may be rehydrated via oral rehydration solution (ORS). A nasogastric tube is a good option if the patient cannot drink but intravenous therapy is not available at the facility. Severe dehydration will require intravenous volume replacement using Ringer's lactate solution or half-Darrow's solution. If Ringer's lactate solution is not available then normal saline solution can be used.

- *If not dehydrated:* discharge with ORS to be taken after each loose stool (<2 years 50–100 ml; 2–9 years 100–200 ml; >10 years as much as wanted).
- *In mild-moderate dehydration:* aim for 2.2–4 *l* ORS in the first 4 hours for patients >15 years or weighing >30 kg. Children aged 5–14 years weighing 16–30 kg should receive 1.2–2.2 *l*. Monitor frequently and reassess level of hydration every 4 hours. Once rehydration has been achieved, replace ongoing losses with ORS as per for patients with no dehydration present.
- *Severe dehydration* is managed with aggressive intravenous fluid replacement with Ringer's lactate solution, half-Darrow's solution or normal saline if neither is available:
- *For patients >1 year age:* give 30 ml/kg as rapidly as possible (within 30 min) followed by 70 ml/kg in the next 2.5 hours.
- *For patients <1 year age:* give 30 ml/kg over 60 min followed by 70 ml/kg over the next 5 hours.

While intravenous rehydration is ongoing, start ORS when the patient is able to take fluids (~5 ml/kg/hour). If still severely dehydrated after intravenous infusion (IVI) replacement, continue with parenteral replacement until signs of severe dehydration have resolved. Continue oral rehydration as for mild-moderate dehydration or replacing losses once rehydration has been achieved.

Antibiotic therapy may reduce the duration and severity of diarrhoea but has little impact on mortality. It is reserved for patients with severe dehydration only.

There is increasing antibiotic resistance in *V. cholerae* strains, particularly to ampicillin, trimethoprim-sulphamethoxazole and doxycycline as well as to nalidixic acid, which may infer poor response to fluoroquinolones. Single-dose azithromycin is a recognised alternative (1 g po stat or 20 mg/kg stat in children). During an outbreak, susceptibility patterns of the organism are important to confirm.

Cholera is nationally reportable. A suspected or laboratory-confirmed case requires immediate telephonic notification to the local authority so that an urgent outbreak response can be effected to determine the source, detect other cases and limit spread.

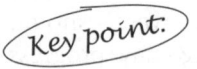 **Cholera may be rapidly fatal due to dehydration – early rehydration is essential.**

8.6 Chemical and hazardous materials

The term 'hazardous materials' (abbreviation Hazmat or HazMat) refers to hazardous chemicals, biological materials and radioactive materials. Since biological and radioactive materials have been discussed earlier in the chapter, this section will concentrate on hazardous chemicals only. The subject is too extensive to cover in detail; therefore, only those aspects that are essential for healthcare providers to function properly in pre-hospital and hospital environments will be provided.

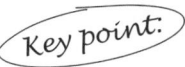 **Hazardous materials include chemical, biological as well as radiological agents.**

Incident management

Incidents involving hazardous materials are managed in the same manner irrespective of the type of hazard or the cause of the incident, although some details may differ according to the situation.

Incidents of this nature will always be managed by more than one department, depending on the scale of the incident. The primary role players in these incidents will always be the fire and rescue services and the SAPS, and one of these will be in command, depending on the nature of the incident. EMS and other departments such as the South African National Defence Force will always play a supporting role.

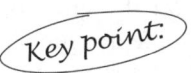 **The fire brigade and police services will most commonly take on the role of incident command.**

Activities upon arrival on scene

Any member of the emergency services that arrives first on a scene is automatically the first responder. The first responder on the scene should follow the guidelines below, but must still work strictly to own agency emergency response plans and procedures.

If there is any uncertainty regarding the presence of a hazardous material, or the type of material present, or if the presence of a specific hazardous material (e.g. radioactive material) has been confirmed visually (label) or by measurement, the relevant agencies and specialists/advisors should be notified, the area secured and controlled at a safe distance and no further action taken.

The following agencies/emergency centres may have to be notified and put on stand-by if necessary according to the local emergency response plan:

- Police;
- Local, metropolitan/district, provincial or national disaster management agency – depending on the level of the incident and the level of coordination required;
- Hospitals – when casualties are present or expected. Notification must include the possibility of contaminated casualties;
- Department of Transport – when roads and airports are involved;
- Environmental health services – in case of potential environmental contamination;
- Department of Defence – if such support is contemplated;
- National nuclear emergency body (for example, the nuclear emergency centre of the Nuclear Energy Corporation of South Africa) – in case of incidents that involve radioactive material.

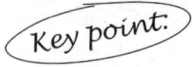 If the presence of a hazardous material is suspected, the relevant specialist authority needs to be informed immediately.

The approach to a Hazmat incident

When approaching an incident, remember that there are hazardous substances that have no distinctive smell or taste:

- Determine the wind direction;
- Always try to approach from upwind and uphill. If it is not possible to approach from upwind and uphill, at least try to approach from upwind;
- Ensure that vehicle windows are kept closed;
- Air conditioners must be turned off;
- Inform other vehicle users;
- Consider best routes, hydrant locations and water supply;
- Evaluate wind speed, direction and impact on contamination;
- If possible, look for labels/placards or other visual signs that indicate the presence of a hazardous substance, such as dead animals or birds lying on the ground, people staggering, gasping or coughing or lack of people or animal life in general;
- Stop at a safe distance (at least 150 m upwind and uphill) from the scene and conduct a scene assessment.

Upon arrival at an established scene, report to the incident command post, which will be marked by a flashing red/blue light or a road cone on the roof of a vehicle.

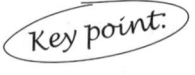 On arrival on scene, one needs to be aware that the threat may not be readily apparent and certain safety steps need to be followed.

Incident layout

After the scene has been surveyed (sized-up), safety zones are established in order to keep control of the scene and for personnel and public safety. In order to execute control on scene, it is divided into three zones: hot zone, warm zone, cold zone. This system applies only to Hazmat scenes, but still corresponds to the bronze, silver and gold system (see Chapter 2) as used throughout this text. Access to zones is restricted to personnel who actually need to be working in a specific zone – this includes officials who are not performing responder duties. Entry and exit registers must be kept for the warm and hot zone.

Hot zone

The hot zone is the area at the centre of the incident, where a detectable vapour or other hazards exist. The perimeter of the hot zone is determined by means of monitoring and includes the downwind hazard area, where hazardous vapours, gas, mists or dusts are detectable. The hot zone may only be entered for specific functions conducted by trained personnel dressed in appropriate protective ensemble. There is no need for EMS personnel to enter the hot zone. Access to this zone is controlled and recorded.

Warm zone

The warm zone is utilised for decontamination of personnel, casualties and equipment and samples, where applicable, that come from the hot zone. It also serves as a safety barrier between the hot zone and the cold zone. Only personnel dressed in applicable protective ensemble, as determined by the incident commander, may enter the warm zone. All personnel must be decontaminated before exiting the warm zone. Access to this zone is controlled and recorded.

The hot and warm zones make up the bronze area.

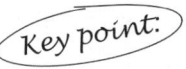 **In Hazmat incidents, the bronze area consists of a hot and a warm zone.**

Cold zone

The area outside the perimeter of the warm zone is the cold zone. The cold zone is the zone that contains the command and support elements. The initial EMS treatment position is situated in the cold zone, next to the exit from the casualty decontamination station. The cold zone is the silver area.

The medical team provides triage, advanced care and stabilisation until the patients are transported to an appropriate medical facility. With large numbers of patients, the area usually is further divided into immediate and delayed treatment zones to help determine priorities in patient transportation.

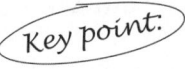 **In Hazmat incidents, the silver area is also known as the cold zone.**

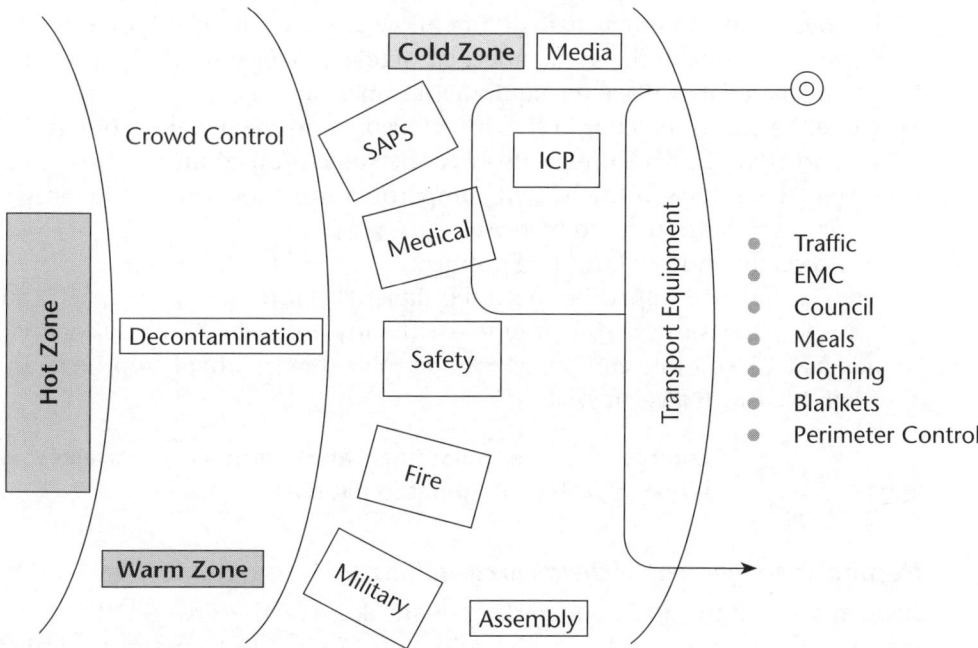

Figure 8.2: Hazmat incident management layout

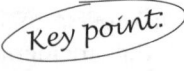 Hazardous chemical incidents are managed by multi-disciplinary teams, of which EMS is an integral part.

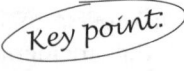 EMS personnel primarily function in the cold zone and, if required, in the warm zone. They hardly ever will have to enter the hot zone.

Transportation of contaminated casualties

A contaminated casualty is a person who has any toxic substance of chemical, biological or radioactive nature on his/her skin or clothes in a quantity that poses a toxic threat to the person, others in close proximity and the environment. The person may suffer from the effects of the substance, other injuries or both.

It is best not to transport a contaminated patient if at all possible. Ambulance crew should try to have casualties decontaminated before loading, although this may not always be possible.

When a contaminated patient has to be transported, the following measures should be implemented to protect personnel and equipment:

- If possible, determine the nature of the contamination.
- All personnel working with the patient or in close proximity to the patient must don proper airway protection (respirator with carbon containing filter), but skin protection in the form of thick gloves and protective clothing may also be necessary.
- Cover the patient in non-permeable material: space blankets provide good protection, but thick plastic material will also be sufficient. The patient must be covered in a manner that will not allow any secondary evaporation.
- Cover the inside of the ambulance, particularly all electronic equipment, with plastic material or place the equipment in plastic bags.
- Close the partition between the driver's cabin and the patient cabin. If there is no partition, the driver must also wear personal protection.
- Open all windows in the patient compartment to allow vapours to escape and prevent concentrations to increase.
- The receiving hospital must be notified.
- The ambulance must be decontaminated before other patients can be transported. Washing the interior with any hypochlorite solution will be adequate. Electronic equipment can be rubbed with a hypochlorite swab and then dried with a clean swab.

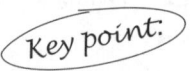 Emergency care personnel must protect themselves when working with contaminated patients

Hospital management of chemical casualties

Incidents involving toxic industrial chemicals pose the greatest threat to the population, followed by illegal dissemination of toxic industrial chemicals. The potential for exposure to pure chemical warfare agents is quite low.

It is impossible to discuss all the relevant toxic industrial chemicals in detail; therefore, only some important aspects of certain toxic industrial chemicals will be discussed.

Toxic industrial chemicals

In order to affect larger numbers of people, it is necessary that the chemical be in gaseous form or a volatile liquid that spreads through secondary evaporation.

The relevant toxic industrial chemicals, with the exception of the organophosphate pesticides, are usually not persistent and may dissipate quite quickly.

There are no antidotes or specific treatment available for most toxic industrial chemicals. The organophosphate pesticides and hydrogen cyanide are the two exceptions. Their treatment will be discussed later.

Classification of toxic industrial chemicals

The toxic industrial chemicals can be classified in the following groups:

- Irritants;
- Ammonia;
- Blood agents;
- Cyanide;
- Systemic agents;
- Arsine;
- Nerve agents;
- Organophosphates;
- Choking agents;
- Chlorine;
- Phosgene.

Ammonia

The largest and most significant use of ammonia and ammonium compounds is in the manufacture of agricultural fertilisers, explosives, plastics, synthetic fibres and resins and pharmaceuticals, as well as the production of various chemical intermediates.

The primary and most immediate effect of ammonia exposure is burns to the skin, eyes and respiratory tract. Nasal and pharyngeal irritation with less tracheal irritation suggests that ammonia is retained in the upper respiratory tract.

Skin and eyes are extremely sensitive to airborne ammonia or ammonium in water. Burns, blisters and lesions of the skin have been reported.

Exposure to highly concentrated aerosols of ammonium compounds can produce burns of the lips, oral cavity and pharynx, along with oedema of these areas.

Acute exposure may cause hypertension, bradycardia and cardiac arrest in humans.

Treatment consists of decontamination as soon as possible, and symptomatic treatment.

Hydrogen cyanide

Hydrogen cyanide produces its effects by interfering with oxygen utilisation at the cellular level. The cyanide ion forms a reversible complex with the cytochrome oxidase enzyme, which is essential for the oxidative process within cells. This results in impairment of cellular oxygen utilisation. The central nervous system, particularly the respiratory centre, is especially susceptible to this effect, and respiratory failure is usually the cause of death.

Table 8.12: Blood concentrations of cyanide and associated clinical effects

Cyanide concentration (μg/ml)	Signs and symptoms
0.2–0.5	None
0.5–1.0	Flushing Tachycardia
1.0–2.5	CNS suppression
2.5–3.0	Coma
>3.0	Death

Successful treatment for acute cyanide poisoning depends on rapid fixation of the cyanide ion, either by methaemoglobin (MetHb) formation or by fixation with cobalt compounds. Any casualty who is fully conscious and breathing normally more than 5 minutes after presumed exposure to cyanide agents has ceased, will recover spontaneously and does not require treatment – the cyanide has been rapidly detoxified by the body. Artificial resuscitation, though possible, is not likely to be helpful in the absence of drug treatment.

Two major treatment approaches are involved in treating cyanide poisoning:

- Provision of alternative binding sites than cytochrome oxidase, for the cyanide ions. Binding sites may be provided by drugs such as dicobalt edentate or hydroxycobalamin, or by the production of MetHb in the blood. MetHb avidly binds to cyanide ions and can be produced by compounds such as sodium nitrite, amyl nitrite and dimethylaminophenol.
- Provision of additional sulphur groups to enhance the detoxification of cyanide to thiocyanate by the enzyme rhodonase. This is accomplished by giving sodium thiosulphate.

It is generally agreed that binding cyanide ions is the first priority of treatment, but that thiosulphate must be provided to permit conversion of the cyanide ions to thiocyanate.

Oxygen should be given, if available. The cardiac rhythm should be maintained, with CPR if necessary. Intravenous sodium bicarbonate should be administered to treat any lactic acidosis. Hyperbaric oxygen therapy is still controversial.

Organophosphates

Organophosphates bind to acetyl cholinesterase, preventing the phosphorylation and deactivation of acetylcholine. The subsequent accumulation of acetylcholine at the neural synapse causes an initial over-stimulation, followed by eventual exhaustion and disruption of postsynaptic neural transmission in the central nervous system (CNS) and peripheral nervous systems (PNS). If the organo-phosphate/cholinesterase bond is not broken by pharmacological intervention within 24 hours, large amounts of cholinesterase are destroyed, causing long-term morbidity or death.

The nicotinic (sympathomimetic) effects from accumulation of acetylcholine at motor endplates cause persistent depolarisation of skeletal muscles, resulting in fasciculations, muscle weakness, hypertension and tachycardia.

Muscarinic effects from potentiation of postganglionic parasympathetic activity of smooth muscles may cause smooth muscle contractions in all organs (e.g. lung, GI, eye, bladder, secretory glands) and reduction of sinus node and AV conduction, causing Brady arrhythmias or resultant ventricular dysrhythmias.

CNS effects may cause excessive stimulation (e.g. seizure), leading to depression and coma and central respiratory depression. Actual signs and symptoms depend on the balance between muscarinic and nicotinic receptors.

Common presenting symptoms include headache, diffuse muscle cramping, weakness, depressed tendon reflexes, excessive secretions, nausea, vomiting and diarrhoea. The condition may progress to seizure, coma, paralysis, respiratory failure and fatality. Eventual resolution of the acute symptoms often occurs, although residual neurologic symptoms may persist if not treated acutely.

Respiratory failure is the most common cause of death.

Treatment involves Atropine to antagonise acetylcholine effects (e.g. bronchoconstriction, bronchorrhoea, excessive secretions). Oximes such as Obidoxime can be used to prevent the organophosphate/cholinesterase bond from becoming permanent. Diazepam is the drug of choice to treat seizures.

Supportive care, including airway control, oxygenation, ventilation and seizure management, is the most important treatment for patients with organophosphate poisoning.

Chlorine

An almost characteristic initial complaint of chlorine exposure is that of suffocation: the inability to get air. Typically, low exposures produce rapid-onset ocular irritation with nasal irritation, followed shortly by spasmodic coughing and a rapidly increasing choking sensation. Substernal tightness is noted early. Intense toxic inhalant exposure may cause pulmonary oedema within 30 to 60 minutes. The sudden death that occurs with massive toxic inhalant exposure is thought to be secondary to laryngeal spasm.

There is no chemically specific prophylactic or post-exposure therapy for chlorine inhalation; therefore, post-exposure therapy is directed toward treating the observed physiological signs and symptoms. Most deaths occur within the first 24 hours due to respiratory failure.

247

Phosgene

Phosgene causes damage to the bronchiolar epithelium, the development of patchy areas of emphysema, partial atelectasis and oedema of the perivascular connective tissue with resultant increased permeability of the alveolar capillaries, causing pulmonary oedema. The trachea and bronchi are usually not affected. The lungs are large, oedematous and darkly congested.

During and immediately after exposure, there is likely to be coughing, choking, a feeling of tightness in the chest, nausea and occasionally vomiting, headache and lacrimation. The presence or absence of these symptoms is of little value in immediate prognosis. Some patients with severe coughs fail to develop serious lung injury, while others with only signs of early respiratory tract irritation develop fatal pulmonary oedema.

A period follows during which abnormal chest signs are absent and the patient may be symptom-free. This interval lasts between 2 and 24 hours, but may be shorter. The patient may recover without further complications; however, the condition may deteriorate and pulmonary oedema may develop. This process begins with coughing (occasionally substernal and painful), dyspnoea, rapid shallow breathing and cyanosis.

Treatment involves initial resuscitation as required. Establishing an airway is especially crucial in a patient exhibiting hoarseness or stridor; such individuals may face impending laryngeal spasm and require intubation.

Pulmonary oedema is the most serious consequence of phosgene exposure and begins with few, if any, clinical signs. Consequently, early diagnosis of pulmonary oedema depends on careful monitoring for dyspnoea or chest tightness. The presence of these symptoms in a case of possible inhalant exposure requires chest X-ray and arterial blood gas analysis. If these investigations are normal, they all must be repeated 4 to 6 hours after the suspected exposure; only then can an individual be discharged. Abnormality of any one of those investigations, in the absence of any other explanation, should prompt institution of therapy for non-cardiac pulmonary oedema.

Even minimal physical exertion may shorten the clinical latent period and increase the severity of respiratory symptoms and signs. Strict limitation of activity (forced bed rest) and litter evacuation are mandatory for patients suspected of having inhaled any of the choking agents.

Pulmonary oedema is managed in the same manner as ARDS.

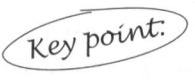 **There is no specific treatment of antidotes for most toxic industrial chemicals; hydrogen cyanide and organophosphates are the exclusions.**

8.7 Vulnerable groups

In addition to the general minimal requirements for any major incident affected population, certain groups of people have specific needs and vulnerabilities that should be considered in the planning and provision of assistance. The groups most frequently at risk in disasters are women, children, older people, the disabled and people living with HIV/AIDS (PLWH/A). Although this list is not exhaustive, these groups generally have reduced abilities to cope with a disaster and may face physical, social or cultural barriers to accessing services and support. In addition, complex emergencies, such as displacement due to xenophobic or political violence, may increase the vulnerability of certain ethnic, religious or political groups, as they may be deliberate targets for violence and displacement, and their ability to access assistance may be limited.

Table 8.13: Considerations for vulnerable groups

- **Health care:** certain groups may require additional medical care, in particular chronic disease management for the elderly and antiretroviral medicines and medicines for opportunistic infections for people living with HIV/AIDS

- **Hygiene promotion:** the provision of safe access to water, sanitary facilities, health care and waste disposal should take into account the specific needs of vulnerable groups

- **Nutritional support:** nutritional planning should, in particular, consider the specific needs of young children, older people, disabled people, people living with HIV/AIDS and pregnant and breastfeeding mothers

- **Social needs:** all members of the affected population should have access to social facilities, including schools, places of worship, meeting points and recreational areas

- **Washing facilities:** the number, location, appropriateness and convenience of facilities should be taken into account to meet the needs of women, adolescent girls and any disabled people

- **Clothing:** adequate consideration needs to be given to the fact that children and adults, males and females, all have different clothing needs

- **Pregnant women:** pregnant and breastfeeding women should receive daily supplements of iron and folic acid

Children

Children, defined by the United Nations Convention on the Rights of the Child as anyone below the age of 18 years, are often excluded from decision-making and often have a limited voice to express their needs. Relief workers should also pay particular attention to the specific needs of children; depending on their age, they may require medical support (vaccination), nutritional support (particularly infants), hygiene materials (washable nappies or diapers) and educational support. Particular attention must also be given to issues of protection from exploitation, including sexual violence.

Older people

Older people are defined by the United Nations as anyone over 60 years, although this definition varies according to cultural and social norms. Vulnerabilities may include chronic health and mobility problems and mental deficiencies, and these are exacerbated by isolation. Specific needs include clothing, medication (in particular for chronic diseases) and additional protein and micronutrient requirements. If supported, older people can, through their knowledge and experience, act as an important source of support, as care providers, resource managers, income generators and community leaders.

Disabled people

In any major incident, disabled people – persons with physical, sensory or emotional impairments or learning difficulties – are particularly vulnerable and often need an enabling social support network. This may be provided by the family (who have heightened needs themselves) but may require additional attention, particularly during periods of displacement and separation. Disabled people may face a range of nutritional challenges, including difficulties in chewing and swallowing, leading to reduced food intake and choking; reduced mobility, affecting food access; discrimination, affecting food access; and constipation. Specific medical support may also be required, such as hearing and visual aids or psychiatric drugs.

Gender

Women and men have the same entitlement to humanitarian assistance, respect for dignity and acknowledgement of equal capacities. Ensuring such entitlements are achieved involves a gender analysis of needs and assistance, which should be sensitive not only to equality in access to assistance, but also to gender-specific needs, such as sanitary materials and family planning for women, and the specific nutritional, medical and hygiene needs of pregnant and breastfeeding women. Specific vulnerabilities of men also need to be considered. For cultural and social reasons, men may be less likely to seek care, and to stay in care, compared to women. In conflict settings, men have been deliberately targeted for violence.

People living with HIV/AIDS

People living with HIV/AIDS often suffer from discrimination, and confidentiality must be strictly adhered to, and protection made available, when needed. Depending on immune status, people living with HIV/AIDS may also have greater needs in terms of nutritional support and medications for chronic and infectious diseases, including antiretroviral medicines.

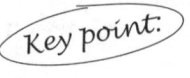 **Large sections of the population are vulnerable following major incidents. Planning and response must take account of these groups' particular needs.**

8.8   References

1.   Barillo DJ. Burn disasters and mass casualty incidents. *Journal of Burn Care and Rehabilitation* March/April 2005;26(2):107–8.

2. Yurt RW, Bessey PQ, Alden NE, *et al*. Burn-injured patients in a disaster: September 11th revisited. *Journal of Burn Care and Research* September/October 2006:635–41.
3. Goh S, Tiah L, Lim H, *et al*. Disaster preparedness: experience from a smoke inhalation mass casualty event. *European Journal of Emergency Medicine* 2006;13(6):330–4.
4. Van Harten SM, Welling L, Perez SGM, *et al*. Management of multiple burn casualties from the Volendam disaster in the emergency departments of general hospitals. *European Journal of Emergency Medicine* 2005;12(6):270–4.
5. Cairns BA, Stiffler A, Price F, *et al*. Managing a combined burn trauma disaster in the post-9/11 world: lessons learned from the 2003 West Pharmaceutical Plant explosion. *Journal of Burn Care and Rehabilitation* 2005;26(2):144–9.
6. Mozingo D, Barillo DJ, Holcomb JB. The Pope Air Force Base aircraft crash and burn disaster. *Journal of Burn Care and Rehabilitation* March/April 2005;26(2):132–40.
7. Harrington DT, Biffl WL, Cioffi WG. The Station nightclub fire. *Journal of Burn Care and Rehabilitation* March/April 2005;26(2):141–3.
8. Tekin A, Namias N, O'Keefee T, *et al*. A burn mass casualty event due to boiler room explosion on a cruise ship: preparedness and outcomes. *The American Surgeon* March 2005;71(3)210–15.
9. Mahoney EJ, Harrington DT, Biffl WL, *et al*. Lessons learned from a nightclub fire: institutional disaster preparedness. *The Journal of Trauma, Injury, Infection and Critical Care* March 2005;58(3):487–91.
10. Leslie CL, Cushman M, McDonald GS, *et al*. Management of multiple burn casualties in a high volume ED without a verified burn unit. *American Journal of Emergency Medicine* October 2001;19(6):469–73.
11. Republic of South Africa. Department of Health. Modernisation of burns services. Available from: www.doh.gov.za/mts/reports/*burns*.html. Accessed 2 January 2009.
12. Barillo D. Burn disasters and mass casualty incidents. *Journal of Burn Care and Rehabilitation* March/April 2005;26(2):107–8.
13. Saffle J, Gibran N, Jordan M. Defining the ratio of outcomes to resources for triage of burn patients in mass casualties. *Journal of Burn Care and Rehabilitation* November/December 2005;26(6):478–82.
14. Yurt RW, Lazar EJ, Leahy NE, *et al*. Burn disaster response planning: an urban region's approach. *Journal of Burn Care and Research* January/February 2008;29(1):158–65.
15. Haberal M. Guidelines for dealing with disasters involving large numbers of extensive burns. *Burns* 2006;32:933–9.
16. Mackie DP, Koning HM. Fate of mass burn casualties: implications for disaster planning. *Burns* 1990;16(3):203–6.
17. Magliacani G, Masellis M. Guidelines for fire disaster medical management in the Mediterranean countries. *Annals of Burns and Fire Disasters* 1999;12:44–7.
18. Berkebile BL, Goldfarb IW, Slater H. Comparison of burn size estimates between prehospital reports and burn centre evaluations. *Journal of Burn Care and Rehabilitation* 1986;7:411–12.

19. Berry CC, Wachtel T, Frank HA. Differences in burn size estimates between community hospitals and a burn centre. *Journal of Burn Care and Rehabilitation* 1982;3:176–7.

20. Wachtel TL, Berry CC, Wachtel EE, *et al*. The inter-rater reliability of estimating the size of burns from various burn area chart drawings. *Burns* 2000;26:156–70.

21. Hammond JS, Ward CG. Transfer from the emergency room to burn centre: errors in burn size estimate. *Journal of Trauma* 1987;27:1161–5.

22. Welling L, Van Harten SM, Henny CP, *et al*. Reliability of the primary triage process after the Volendam fire disaster. *The Journal of Emergency Medicine* 2008;35(2):181–7.

23. Allison K. The UK pre-hospital management of burns patients: current practice and the need for a standard approach. *Burns* 2002;28:135–42.

24. Ashworth HL, Cubison TC, Gilbert PM, *et al*. Treatment before transfer: the patient with burns. *Emergency Medicine Journal* 2001;18:349–51.

25. Eastman AL, Rinnert KJ, Nemeth IR, *et al*. Alternate site surge capacity in times of public health disaster maintains trauma centre and emergency department integrity: Hurricane Katrina. *Journal of Trauma, Injury, Infection and Critical Care* August 2007;63(2):253–7.

26. Vandenberg V, Amara R, Crabtree J, *et al*. Burn surge for Los Angeles County, California. *Journal of Trauma, Injury, Infection and Critical Care* August supplement 2009;67(2):S143–S146.

27. Barillo DJ, Jordan MH, Joez RJ, *et al*. Tracking the daily availability of burn beds for national emergencies. *Journal of Burn Care and Rehabilitation* March/April 2005;26(2):174–82.

28. Giannou C, Baldan M. *War surgery*. Vol 1. Geneva: International Committee of the Red Cross; 2009.

29. Knobel DP. Trauma from bombs, explosives and limpet mines. *Trauma – The Journal of Accident and Emergency medicine* (SA) 1984;1(1):10–14.

30. Coetzer PWW, Smith FCA, Van der Merwe CJ, Becker PJ, Meyer PJ. The epidemiology of terrorism (part 1). *Trauma – The Journal of Accident and Emergency Medicine* (SA) 1987;4(3):15–22.

31. Coetzer PWW, Smith FCA, Van der Merwe CJ, Becker PJ, Meyer PJ. The epidemiology of terrorism (part 2). *Trauma – The Journal of Accident and Emergency Medicine* (SA) 1987;4(4):2–8.

32. Mayo A, Kluger Y. Terrorism bombing. *World Journal of Emergency Surgery* 2006;1:33.

33. Vassallo DJ, Graham PJK, Gupta G, Alempijevic DJ. Bomb explosion on the NS Express – Lessons from a Major Incident, Kosovo 16 Feb 2001. *Journal of the Royal Army Medical Corps* 2005;151:19–29.

34. Rosenfeld J, Fitzgerald M, Kossman T, Pierce A, Joseph A, *et al*. Is the Australian hospital system adequately prepared for terrorism? *Medical Journal of Australia* 2005;183:567–70.

35. Johnston's Archive. Radiation accidents and other events causing radiation casualties-tabulated data. Available from: www.johnstonsarchive.net/nuclear/radevents/radaccidents.html. Accessed 10 June 2010.

36. Ball L. The Royal London Hospital major incident imaging response on 7th July 2005. Available from: www.nordictraumarad.com. Accessed 10 June 2010.

37. Steyn B. CBRNE Teaching series. South African Military Health Service. Department of Health KZN Intranet Accessed 10 June 2010.

38. Alexander DA, Klein S. The challenge of preparation for a chemical, biological, radiological or nuclear terrorist attack. *Journal of Postgraduate Medcine* 2006;52:126–31.

39. Weingart SD, Maltz BR. CBRNE Nuclear and radiologic decontamination. Updated version 9 March 2009. Available from: www.emedicine.com. Accessed 10 June 2010.

40. Van Rensburg LCJ, De Villiers B, Van Zyl CJ. Possible radiation injury at Koeberg nuclear power station. *South African Medical Journal* 1986;70:487–89.

41. US Department of Energy (DOE). Radiological emergency response health and safety manual. US Department of Energy (DOE) Report DOE/NV/11718-440, May 2001.

42. Mayo Clinic Staff. Radiation sickness: symptoms. 9 May 2008. Available from: www.mayoclinic.com/health/radiation-sickness/DS00432/DSECTION= symptoms. Accessed 10 June 2010.

43. Bland SA. Management of the irradiated casualty. *Journal of the Royal Army Medical Corps* 2004;150:5–9.

44. Bland SA. Mass casualty management for radiological and nuclear incidents. *Journal of the Royal Army Medical Corps* 2004;150:27–34.

45. Spencer RC, Lightfoot NF. Containing and combating bioterrorism. *Hospital Medicine* 2002;63:516–18.

46. Spencer RC, Lightfoot NF. Preparedness and response to bioterrorism. *Journal of Infection* 2001;43:104–10

47. Miller JM. Agents of bioterrorism. *Infectious Diseases Clinics of North America* 2001;15:1127–56.

48. Centers for Disease Control and Prevention. Update: investigation of anthrax associated with intentional exposure and interim public health guidelines. October 2001. *Morbidity and Mortality Weekly Report* 2001;50:889–97.

49. Jernigan JA, Stephens DS, Ashford DA, *et al*. Bioterrorism-related inhalational anthrax: the first 10 cases reported in the United States. *Emerging Infectious Diseases* 2001;7:933–44.

50. Bates J. Anthrax: an update for Australia. *Australian Journal of Medical Science* 2002;23:92–101.

51. Polyak CS, Macy JT, Irizarry-De La Cruz M, Lai JE, McAuliffe JF, Popovic C, *et al*. Bioterrorism-related anthrax: international response by the Centers for Disease Control and Prevention. *Emerging Infectious Diseases* 2002;8. Available from: www.cdc.gov/ncidod/EID/vol8no10/02-0345.htm. Accessed 19 August 2010.

52. Frean JA, Arntzen L. Response to the anthrax bioterrorism threat in South Africa. *Annals of the Australasian College of Tropical Medicine* 2002;3:17–19.

53. Miller JM. Bioterrorism – a perspective for the community hospital. *Clinical Microbiological News* 2001;23:179–85.

54. World Health Organization. *Anthrax in humans and animals*. 4th edition. Geneva: WHO; 2008.

55. Swanepoel R. (ed.) *National guidelines for the management of persons with suspected viral haemorrhagic fevers. South Africa 2010.* In press.
56. Paweska JT, Sewlall NH, Ksiazek TG, Blumberg LH, Hale MJ, Lipkin WI, *et al.* Nosocomial outbreak of novel arenavirus infection, southern Africa. *Emerging Infectious Diseases* 2009;15(10):1598–1602.
57. Swanepoel R, Gill DE, Shepherd AJ, Leman PA, Mynhardt JH, Harvey S. The clinical pathology of Crimean-Congo hemorrhagic fever. *Review of Infectious Diseases* 1989;11(suppl 4):S794–800.
58. Van Eeden PJ, Van Eeden SF, Joubert JR, King JB, Van de Wal BW, Michell WL. A nosocomial outbreak of Crimean-Congo haemorrhagic fever at Tygerberg Hospital. Part II. Management of patients. *South African Medical Journal* 1985;9(10):718–21.
59. Republic of South Africa. Department of Provincial and Local Government. Manual: joint management of incidents involving chemical or biological agents and radioactive materials. 3 Feb 2006 (Government Notice 143/3 Feb 06). *Government Gazette* 28437.
60. Marrs TC, Maynard RL, Siddel FR. *Chemical warfare agents: toxicology and treatment.* 2nd edition. Chichester: Wiley and Sons, 2007.
61. Vale JA, Meredith, TJ. Cyanide poisoning. *Medicine International* 1989: 2508–12.
62. Siddel FR (ed.), Takafuji ET (ed.), Franz DR. *Medical aspects of chemical and biological warfare.* Washington, DC: Office of the Surgeon General, Dept of the Army; 1997.
63. Marrs TC, Maynard RL, Siddel FR. *Chemical warfare agents: toxicology and treatment.* 2nd edition. Chichester: Wiley and Sons, 2007.
64. The Sphere Project. Sphere humanitarian charter and minimum standards in disaster response. Geneva: The Sphere Project; 2004. Available from: www.sphereproject.org/content/view/27/84/lang,english/. Accessed 19 August 2010.

9

Equipment Requirements

V Wessels, K Barnes and W Smith

Objectives

By the end of this chapter, the reader will:

- understand the importance of early planning in terms of ensuring that incidents can be managed in a safe and efficient manner;
- realise that equipment requirements vary, depending on the mission to be undertaken;
- understand the importance of correct packaging of equipment;
- realise the importance of maintenance of equipment and adequate stock management.

9.1 Introduction

Equipment requirements for a major incident response can be a daunting issue. Planning such requirements in advance can make a major difference in being able to safely and effectively manage the incident.

Equipment needs should be tailored to the expected environment in which a major incident will be managed. Incidents managed within the usual healthcare facility, for example, are less dependent on the packing arrangements, whereas mobile medical teams require equipment to be specially packed.

The type of major incident can also demand different equipment requirements: for example, structural collapse with multiple trauma cases necessitates limited pre-hospital care, compared to a post-earthquake displaced community which requires emergency and routine healthcare services, in temporary healthcare environments, over an extended period of time.

As a minimum, responders should have sufficient stock of what they normally use, to allow for a sudden increase in demand caused by a major incident or disaster, without being reliant on external sources during the initial phase. This can be accomplished by increasing the routine stock levels to at least 30 days of normal use.

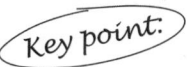 **Equipment needs are often mission-specific, and early planning is essential.**

9.2   Equipment categories

Various lists of equipment required to manage major incidents and disasters have been recommended. It is essential, however, that staff involved in setting up response plans consider the appropriateness of these lists within their own environment before merely adopting these lists. In particular the following must be considered:

- Availability of the equipment, including procurement mechanisms;
- Familiarity of equipment to the staff that will need to use it;
- Cost of the equipment;
- Ease of maintenance;
- Appropriateness of equipment – what may be appropriate in a single-case incident may not necessarily be the case in a major incident.

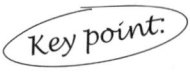 **Rather than adopting existing equipment lists, planners should ensure that the equipment to be deployed is familiar to the responders**

Administrative and command supplies

- Stationery (pens, permanent markers, notepads);
- Triage tags (and patient report forms where appropriate);
- Major incident contingency plan (including action cards);
- Two-way radios;
- Loud-hailer;
- Whistles;
- Whiteboard (magnetic);
- Clipboards;
- Role identification vests;
- Torches (preferably headlight style to allow hands-free use).

Personal protective equipment

This category includes all items required for the healthcare worker to be adequately protected from hazards, either from the patients to be treated or the environment in which they will operate. Users must be familiar with the equipment, especially with regard to the limitations of such equipment.

Routine universal precautions include:

- Examination gloves (note possible latex allergy);
- Eye protection (spectacles or shield);
- Appropriate clothing (e.g. apron, gown).

Special hazards

- Head protection (e.g. helmet designed for the hazard);
- Respiratory protection (communicable diseases vs. environmental hazards, e.g. dust);
- Appropriate clothing (e.g. fire-resistant jacket);
- Foot protection (e.g. steel shank and toecap boots);

- Additional hand protection (e.g. leather gloves);
- Ear protection.

Personal equipment

These items are usually provided by the individual and include items to allow for extended work and stay-over periods, e.g. toiletries, clothes, food. However it is advisable to keep certain 'personal' items as part of the central stock, e.g. toilet paper and drinking water.

Medical supplies

Airway and breathing

This would include items required to open and maintain an airway, e.g. oropharyngeal (and nasopharyngeal) airways, endotracheal tubes, laryngoscope(s), Magill's forceps, introducing stylets, lubrication gel, fixation device or tape (e.g. trachytape), alternative airway device, e.g. laryngeal mask, cricothyrotomy equipment.

- Manual resuscitator with mask, suction device (manual in addition to battery) oxygen masks (high concentration and nebulizer).

Bandages and dressings

- Wound dressings, bandages to secure dressings and support soft tissue injuries and splinting supplies.

Intravenous supplies

- Fluids: isotonic crystalloids (e.g. Ringer's lactate), non-calcium containing fluid for medication administration, colloid solution (e.g. Voluven);
- Administration sets, IV cannulise, fixation items (transparent dressings or tape);
- Diagnostic equipment and instruments:
  - Aneroid sphygmomanometer(s);
  - Stethoscope(s);
  - Torch;
  - Thermometer (preferably NOT mercury-containing glass type);
  - Diagnostic set (auroscope and ophthalmoscope);
  - Rescue scissors;
- Electronic equipment (monitoring, defibrillation, pumps etc):
  - Defibrillator/monitor;
  - Pulse dosimetre.

Surgical supplies

Dependent on skills and experience of staff, but can include suturing supplies, thoracostomy set (IC drain), emergency thoracotomy set.

257

Pharmaceuticals
- Emergency medication (mainly injectables);
- Analgesics (including NSAID, Paracetamol and injectables);
- Anti-emetics, anti-diarrhoeals, antacids;
- Anti-consultants;
- Anti-hypertensive;
- Anaesthetic agents (dependent on available skills).

Rescue equipment
The type and amount of specialised rescue equipment that needs to be deployed is dependent on the nature of the incident.

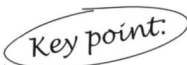 **Type and quantity of equipment is very often mission-specific.**

Patient packaging, immobilisation and transport supplies
- Spine board;
- Foldable stretchers (NATO type);
- Blanket(s);
- Head immobilisers;
- Securing straps/spider harness;
- Traction splint(s);
- Container(s) for vomit or body fluids.

Food and water
Besides bottled water, it is generally easier to obtain food from a supplier at the time of the incident than try to stockpile food items, provided that the supplier is identified prior to the incident occurring.

Sterilising facilities
- Antiseptic solutions and sterilising fluids (or at least sodium hypochloride);
- More extravagant mechanisms (e.g. portable autoclave) may be required for extended incidents.

9.3   Equipment packing
Various options exist with regard to the packing and storing of equipment. Each option has its pros and cons, and therefore the user needs to choose the option that is the most appropriate for their environment.

Storing items in their original bulk form
This is the method most commonly used in healthcare facilities, and allows for easier maintenance and turnover of stock. For mobile emergency use, however, this option can have limitations, as procedures in the field – such as initiating an intravenous line – will require a user to access multiple containers. Bulk

stock quantities do not always correlate to the associated items required for a procedure – for example, there may be 200 IV cannulae in a box but only 24 boxed fluids.

Storing items in ready-to-use packs

This option is most preferred in the pre-hospital environment as it provides the user with all the items required to perform a specific procedure in a single-pack format. However, maintenance of the stock is more intensive.

Equipment packing considerations for mobile use

Containers should ideally be:

● Reasonably secure, preferably with tamperproof seals;
● Protected from environmental factors (dust, water, insects);
● Portable – i.e. weight should not exceed 20 kg;
● Clearly marked with regard to contents and expiry date.

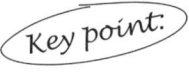 **Packaging of equipment should be of such a nature that it offers protection to the equipment while at the same time being easily portable.**

9.4   Equipment and stock maintenance

It is important that pre-packed stock is regularly checked with regard to expiry dates of consumables and medication as well as possible damage caused by environmental factors and leaking fluid containers.

Battery-operated equipment needs specific care. Items using user-removable batteries should be stored with the batteries removed to avoid damage caused by leaking batteries.

Certain installed batteries need to be kept in a charged state to avoid permanent damage to the batteries (for example, sealed lead-acid batteries). This may require equipment to be stored with trickle chargers constantly plugged in.

During major incidents and disasters, the cleaning and management of equipment is often a challenge, and it could be of value to utilise single-use items as far as possible (for example, disposable manual resuscitators, disposable splints, single-use extrication collars, disposable linen, etc.). Reusable equipment should be clearly marked with a contact number of the owning agency (preferably the 24-hour control centre number) to ease redistribution of equipment after the incident, as well as in cases where bystanders have found abandoned or lost equipment at scenes after an incident. It is the responsibility of the medical incident commander to determine a suitable equipment exchange process towards the end of the incident to ensure that agencies are able to redistribute recovered equipment to the rightful owners.

9.5   Resources

The World Health Organization – The new emergency health kit 98

US Agency for International Development – *field operations guide*, version 3.0

United Nations. Department of Peacekeeping Operations. Office of Mission Support, Logistics Support Division, Medical Support Section, *Medical Equipment Handbook for United Nations Peacekeeping Operations* (2003)

Index

Entries are listed in letter-by-letter alphabetical order. Page references in *italic* indicate where you can find a figure or table relating to the index entry term.

Multiple Choice Questions

To qualify for 9 CPD points, answer the following multiple choice questions and either fax to (021 949 7925) or email to (disastermed@emssa.org.za). Circle the correct answer on the answer sheet at the end of this section. You will receive your CPD certificate in due course.

Chapter 1

1. The ISDR has the following objectives:
   a. Increase public awareness about disaster risks and ways to reduce these risks.
   b. Obtain the commitment from public authorities to implement disaster reduction plans.
   c. Stimulate interdisciplinary and intersectoral partnership and research to address disaster reduction.
   d. All 3.

2. Ethics is:
   a. Morality or moral judgment.
   b. Right and wrong.
   c. Good behaviour.
   d. All 3.

3. The South African Disaster Management Act, 2002, provides for all of the following EXCEPT:
   a. An integrated and coordinated disaster risk management policy.
   b. An effective response to disasters.
   c. Laws to govern NGO activities in a disaster situation.
   d. The establishment of national, provincial and municipal disaster management centres.

4. With regard to ethical challenges in disaster situations, the following are true EXCEPT:
   a. They are extremely complex in nature.
   b. Controversy surrounding ethics in a disaster cannot be reduced or prevented.
   c. Medical ethics is guided by the ethical principles of beneficence, non-maleficence, autonomy and justice.
   d. Unique ethical challenges are faced by medical personnel in a disaster situation.

5. Which of the following statements is *false*? International humanitarian law:
   a. Is law set for humanitarian reasons.
   b. Is also known as the law of war or armed conflict.
   c. Regulates whether a state may actually use force.
   d. Protects persons who are not participating in the war.

6. Which of the following is a weakness of quantitative research?
    a. It provides precise, numerical data.
    b. The categories used by the researcher might not reflect local constituencies' understandings.
    c. Testing hypotheses that are constructed before the data are collected.
    d. It can study a large number of people.

7. Which of these is *not* a method of data collection?
    a. Questionnaires.
    b. Experiments.
    c. Observations.
    d. Interviews.

Chapter 2

1. The following are initial tasks that the first unit on the scene should do, EXCEPT:
    a. Make a thorough assessment of the situation.
    b. Wait for the most senior ranked officer to set up command.
    c. Assign arriving personnel to different positions with which they are familiar.
    d. Take responsibility for all functions of the Incident Command System.

2. Pick the one true statement about the tiers of command:
    a. Gold command is responsible for on-scene operational decisions.
    b. Bronze commanders are sectional heads responsible for operational teams.
    c. Silver commanders should ideally function as separate command structures.
    d. Gold command may involve international organisations.

3. Pick the one true statement about international command:
    a. Non-governmental organisations (NGOs) don't have to comply with United Nations (UN) guidelines.
    b. The World Health Organization (WHO) has no role to play on the international scene.
    c. Volunteers must register with global organisations like the UN.
    d. Volunteers not regularly involved in international major incidents might do more harm than good.

4. Which principle regarding the Incident Command System is true?
    a. A modular organisational structure only applies to major fires.
    b. A consistent basic structure should be implemented as early as possible.
    c. The most senior-ranked health services officer must immediately take over command.
    d. All key positions must be filled and appropriately identified.

5. Communication is essential for the following EXCEPT:
    a. Initial major incident activation.
    b. Inter-provider agency interaction.

c. Good command and control.

d. Giving poor staging instructions to responders.

6. The following are all electronic communications systems EXCEPT:
   a. Cellular networks.
   b. Two-way radios.
   c. Hand-held flag systems.
   d. Trunking radio networks.

7. The phonetic alphabet:
   a. Is local to South Africa.
   b. Uses words only and not numbers.
   c. Is an effective way to spell words over a radio.
   d. Cannot be used by the fire service.

8. Safety is paramount to ensure:
   a. Staff are prevented from getting infectious illness.
   b. Safety of self, scene and survivor.
   c. Biohazards are dispersed in the community.
   d. Staff are maximally utilised on the scene until they burn out.

9. The safety officer should not:
   a. Dictate to other services what to do to protect themselves.
   b. Ensure that all hazards are identified that may harm the rescuers.
   c. Let any member of staff onto the scene without appropriate PPE.
   d. Worry about the ambient temperature and weather conditions.

10. Structural stability includes all of the following, EXCEPT:
    a. Chocking the wheels of damaged vehicles.
    b. Shoring to prevent trench collapse.
    c. Removal of unstable debris when possible.
    d. Crawling into collapsed buildings without waiting for an all-clear.

11. All these statements concerning triage are true, EXCEPT:
    a. The aim of triage is to do the most for the most number of patients.
    b. Triage remains the sole responsibility of the EMS service.
    c. Triage is a dynamic process and the patient's colour code may be altered.
    d. It is important that one triage system is adopted so that all the relevant services use the same system.

12. Triage labels should have the following characteristics:
    a. Be highly visible.
    b. Be waterproof but still allow for the documentation of essential clinical notes on the label.
    c. Have a simple means whereby the label can be attached to the patient.
    d. All of the above.

13. The following are all true as regards the treatment of casualties in a major incident, EXCEPT:
    a. Much of the early treatment and first aid may be supplied by bystanders.

    b.   Patient treatment must be commenced as soon as health resources arrive at the scene.

    c.   Treatment performed at the casualty clearing station is aimed at stabilising the patients and preparing them for evacuation.

    d.   Patients classified as Green or P3 still need observation and treatment, as their condition may change.

14. Choose the one incorrect statement pertaining to transport of casualties from the scene of a major incident:

    a.   It is a critical component that requires careful planning and coordination.

    b.   Various organisations, such as a private EMS, may be able to transport patients and should take instructions only from their own control centres.

    c.   Fire and law enforcement agencies may assist with the transport of patients out of the bronze zone.

    d.   Patients triaged Green or P3 still require transportation to a health facility.

15. As regards equipment requirement for a major incident, all of the following are true, EXCEPT:

    a.   Equipment pre-planning is paramount to an effective response.

    b.   The wearing of PPE, while important, should not delay the response to getting to the patients.

    c.   Checking of safety equipment remains the responsibility of the individual who will be wearing it.

    d.   The type of equipment required may vary depending on the nature of the incident.

16. As regards training and exercising, the following are all true, EXCEPT:

    a.   It plays an important role in ensuring all role-players are comfortable in performing what is expected of them.

    b.   Exercises, when performed, need to be evaluated so as to improve on performance.

    c.   Exercises that are multi-disciplinary have proven to add no value.

    d.   Exercises may take many forms and need not be limited to expensive and time-consuming simulations.

Chapter 3

1.   The surge capacity of a hospital refers to:

    a.   Capacity to coordinate the triage of patients effectively.

    b.   The ability of a hospital to expand its normal services rapidly to meet the increase in demand.

    c.   The ability of a hospital to discharge patients to lower levels of care.

    d.   Capacity to coordinate resources through effective pre-planning.

2.   The identified triage area:

    a.   Should be in the immediate proximity to the reuniting area of the hospital to ensure logical flow of casualties.

    b.   Should be on the same floor level as the drop-off point for ambulances and Priority 1 treatment area.

    c.   Does not need effective lighting as major incidents occur during daylight hours.

    d.   Should be directly adjacent to the command centre, preferably with an interlinking door.

3.   The contact point to which the emergency services can relay a METHANE message is:

    a.   A pre-identified point staffed 24 hours per day with clear instructions on what to do.

    b.   The chief executive officer personally.

    c.   The agency staff manning casualty after hours.

    d.   The chief of security.

4.   On arrival at the hospital, lying casualties arriving by ambulance should be:

    a.   Handled on ambulance stretchers until the cervical spine has been radiological cleared.

    b.   Transferred to hospital gurneys as soon as possible to return ambulance stretchers to ambulances.

    c.   Requested to sit up and wait their turn in the waiting area.

    d.   Triaged directly as Priority 1.

5.   The purpose of Surgical Triage is to:

    a.   Identify patients that have no prognosis to receive palliative care.

    b.   Identify priority for surgical intervention.

    c.   Identify priority for resuscitation.

    d.   Re-prioritise decontaminated patients.

6.   The major incident response of the hospital should be coordinated by a hospital coordinating team (HCT), consisting of:

    a.   Chief Triage Officer; Chief Security Officer; Chief Nursing Manager; Chief Surgeon.

    b.   Chief Surgeon; Chief Physician; Chief Nursing Manager; Chief Security Officer.

    c.   Chief Executive; Chief Nursing Manager; Chief Surgeon; Chief Triage Officer.

    d.   Hospital Nursing Commander, Hospital Medical Commander and Hospital Administrative Commander.

7.   All the following are methods for the activation of staff in a major incident EXCEPT:

    a.   Human resource department calls all staff individually.

    b.   A major incident paging system can be utilised for the activation of staff (SMS).

    c.   A staff activation tree is commenced by each department.

    d.   Radio and TV can be used for the notification of staff.

8. Patient tracking in a major incident refers to:
    a. Which patient, with which condition, has been sent to which hospital and where the patient is within that hospital.
    b. Keeping track of the triage priority of the patients.
    c. Tracking patients who require urgent psychological support.
    d. Tracking the position of ambulances during a major incident to ensure optimal utilisation.

9. The rules for debriefing include:
    a. Debriefing is formal and is arranged in definite steps.
    b. Debriefing is conducted close to the incident to ensure realism.
    c. Debriefing must be conducted as soon as possible during the active phase of the major incident.
    d. Effective structured debriefing replaces counselling.

10. The discharge point (discharge lounge):
    a. Should be situated inside the emergency centre.
    b. Can be located in an open-plan restaurant facing the hospital reception area.
    c. Should be staffed by nurses and support staff such as clergy and social workers.
    d. Has psychological importance for patients involved in a major incident.

11. With regard to unidentified persons, the following are true, EXCEPT:
    a. They are not a priority for identification purposes.
    b. They may include unconscious patients, very young children and the dead.
    c. They may be identified through digital photographs as well as a coordinated effort by hospitals and the major incident enquiries centre.
    d. If paediatric, they should be allocated a specific caregiver so that secondary trauma may be avoided.

12. Major incident plans:
    a. Should be practised until stressed to detect flaws in the plan.
    b. Should be revised exclusively on an annual stipulated date.
    c. Should be made the responsibility of the emergency centre manager(s).
    d. Should include contingency plans for the hospital's evacuation.

13. Mock drills in major incident management:
    a. Are the only way of practising and testing major incident management.
    b. Benefit individuals, teams and organisations.
    c. Should always include the local emergency services.
    d. Should always be followed by counselling.

14. Tabletop exercises:
    a. Can be conducted with clinical as well as non-clinical personnel.
    b. Are a replacement for mock drills.
    c. Are particularly useful to demonstrate hospital managers' roles in major incident management.
    d. May be conducted with emergency centre staff alone.

Chapter 4

1. In pre-planning for a disruption in essential services, the standard recommended actions include:
    a. Limiting the dependence load and then assessing the remaining load.
    b. Closing the healthcare facility immediately.
    c. Contracting another company to prevent discontinuing services for maintenance.
    d. Wait and see if the disruption will have any impact.

2. When calculating a healthcare facility's emergency electrical power needs:
    a. The facility's consumption under full workload needs to be measured.
    b. The figure is not important, as any generator can supply a hospital with adequate power.
    c. Only calculate the power required in the ICU.
    d. Exercise the effectiveness by connecting a generator to the power and evaluate the effect.

3. When managing trauma patients, the limitation to determine the surge capacity is:
    a. The number of ventilators available.
    b. The number of ICU beds available.
    c. The capability of the surgical facilities.
    d. The number of resuscitation bays equipped with X-ray capabilities.

4. The components of surge capacity are:
    a. The number of theatres times the time.
    b. 5 m² per Priority 2 patient.
    c. The blood requirement per patient.
    d. Space, staff and equipment.

5. The recommended specification to calculate the surge capacity for a Priority 1 resuscitation bays is:
    a. 2m²
    b. 4m²
    c. 12m²
    d. 20m²

6. The recreation hall at the nurses' home is 120 m². Calculate the capacity of this recreation hall for nursing Priority 3 hospitalised patients:
    a. 20 patients.
    b. 40 patients.
    c. 8 patients.
    d. 12 patients.

7. The preferred minimum distance between patients in a temporary ward measured nose to nose is:
    a. 4 metres.
    b. 8 metres.
    c. 1.5 metres.
    d. Undetermined.

8. On receiving a bomb threat, a hospital should:
   a. Obtain maximum information, and use safe and accountable methods to manage the threat, without causing more harm to patients.
   b. Evacuate the total hospital, ICU and theatres immediately.
   c. Phone the fire brigade and wait.
   d. Ignore it, as such threats are often false and just seeking sensation.

9. When informed of a bomb threat, all staff members should:
   a. Not get involved, as they may blow themselves up.
   b. Immediately vacate the hospital, leaving all personal belongings behind.
   c. Immediately search their area of responsibility for any suspicious object that is out of place.
   d. Do not tell the other staff, as it may cause more panic.

10. If any suspicious object is observed after a bomb threat, staff should:
    a. Immediately remove it from the hospital to prevent injuries to patients if it explodes.
    b. Search for more objects.
    c. Not touch it, inform the command point and evacuate patients and staff from the direct surroundings.
    d. Open it to check if it is a bomb.

11. Fire prevention inspection should:
    a. Make sure that staff do not smoke in unauthorised areas, to ensure that the Tobacco Products Control Act is applied.
    b. Include all firefighting equipment, fire alarm systems and all escape routes in the facility.
    c. Ensure that hospital staff know the fire brigade staff.
    d. Not take place in hospitals due to the infection risk of firemen moving through different areas.

12. The fire alarm of the hospital should be activated:
    a. As soon as any fire is discovered in the hospital.
    b. Only if the staff with all the firefighting equipment cannot control the fire.
    c. As soon as the fire gets out of hand.
    d. When smoke cannot escape from the building in time.

13. The fire tetrahedron consists of:
    a. Fuel, oxygen, heat and the chemical reaction.
    b. Fuel, carbon dioxide, heat and the chemical reaction.
    c. Fuel, oxygen, heat and carbon dioxide.
    d. Water, dry powder and carbon dioxide.

14. Water should never be used to extinguish:
    a. A burning soiled linen basket set alight by a cigarette.
    b. Waste bags on fire in the waste collecting area.
    c. Smouldering fire in the cardiac monitor system of the ICU.
    d. Burning oily substance in the pharmacy.

15. In the absence of adequate evacuation planning, all of the following are true EXCEPT:
    a. A clear leader will emerge to assume responsibility for evacuation.
    b. Hospitals may expose themselves to lawsuits.
    c. Patients may die or suffer unnecessary complications.
    d. Unnecessary evacuations may be more likely.

16. The following correctly pair the disaster scenario with an evacuation type, EXCEPT:
    a. Noxious fumes in intensive care unit – partial horizontal evacuation.
    b. Earthquake with threat of imminent structural collapse – reverse triage complete evacuation.
    c. Approaching hurricane – reverse triage partial evacuation.
    d. Bomb threat – partial vertical evacuation of threatened floor.

17. The following correctly pair the disaster scenario with an evacuation destination, EXCEPT:
    a. Hospital fire – other local hospitals.
    b. Major earthquake with mass casualties and structural damage to most hospitals and roads – field hospital.
    c. Approaching major hurricane – other local hospitals.
    d. Credible bomb threat – staging area until further information.

18. Pick the one true statement about hospital evacuations:
    a. If hospitals have a disaster plan, they will be prepared to carry out a successful evacuation.
    b. Hospitals need to contact only fire and police departments when evacuation is needed.
    c. As world experience with hospital evacuation mounts, hospitals no longer make the same mistakes.
    d. Specialised equipment is not essential to carry out most hospital evacuations.

19. The following are core components of an evacuation plan, EXCEPT:
    a. Evacuation routes and evacuation order for all wards.
    b. A detailed approach to every possible contingency.
    c. Clear destination guidelines and/or pre-negotiated agreements.
    d. Back-up means of communication within hospital and with local authorities.

20. The following are true about the ideal evacuation drill strategy, EXCEPT:
    a. It should involve fire and police departments.
    b. Drills should occur at least once a year.
    c. The disaster scenario should always be the same.
    d. All hospital staff should be involved.

21. The management of internal major incidents in the operations suite is challenging due to:
    a. The presence of open wounds.
    b. The lack of acuity of the patient.

  c. The lack of flammable gases.
  d. Minimal electrical equipment.

22. The internal major incident is complicated by the presence of:
  a. Good communication systems.
  b. Fire in the operation room.
  c. Good access routes.
  d. Large numbers of trained staff.

23. Functional internal incidents include all of the following, EXCEPT:
  a. Logistical failure.
  b. Power failure.
  c. Flood.
  d. Water cut-off.

24. During a major incident:
  a. Surgical services must not be curtailed.
  b. Communication is unlikely to lead to effective management of the incident
  c. Ethical debates may occur relating to the relative value of the patient's life over that of the staff.
  d. Damage control surgery (life over limb) is not likely to be implemented as the standard of care is 'normal care'.

25. During an external incident, the following plans will help to prevent escalation into an internal incident:
  a. The hospital administrator is in charge of the operations suite.
  b. One team of scrub staff will be established.
  c. Hazards to staff will always be sorted out by the time the patient hits the operating room doors.
  d. Communication between the senior surgeon and the operating room nursing management will determine patient priority.

26. External incidents may lead to internal incidents because of damage to the hospital infrastructure by all of the following EXCEPT:
  a. Oversupply of pharmacy stocks.
  b. Limiting access of staff to the hospital.
  c. Breakdown in the supply of consumables.
  d. Inability to continue running back-up generators.

27. ICU management of patients during an internal incident is complicated by:
  a. Complex equipment that may be difficult to move.
  b. Patient severity making movement easy.
  c. Adequate mobile back-up gases and suction units.
  d. Many staff all trained in ICU management.

28. External incidents affect the ICU in many ways. These may include:
    a. No increase in patient surge.
    b. Ability to offer the same level of care as normal to the usual patient population.
    c. No shortage of staff.
    d. Shortage of linen during protracted incidents.

29. With regard to the evacuation of an ICU, the following are true, EXCEPT:
    a. The location of the ICU, in terms of proximity to elevators and exits, affects the ease of evacuation.
    b. Moving unstable patients on large beds adds to the difficulty of evacuation.
    c. The presence of fire or flood adds to the difficulty of evacuation.
    d. Security threats do not affect the difficulty of evacuation unless they indirectly involve the ICU ward space.

30. During protracted incidents:
    a. Generators provide completely reliable electrical backup.
    b. Support services never run out of consumables.
    c. A well-devised plan, including all role-players, is essential.
    d. Action cards are only of use in the emergency centre.

31. The management of internal major incidents is challenging due to:
    a. The ease of moving the aged.
    b. The ease of moving incubators.
    c. Cooperative psychiatric patients.
    d. Staff shortages.

32. The internal major incident is complicated by the presence of all of the following, EXCEPT:
    a. Well adults.
    b. Children.
    c. Psychiatric patients.
    d. Functional failure.

33. Functional internal incidents include the following, EXCEPT:
    a. Logistical failure.
    b. Power failure.
    c. Train crash.
    d. Water cut-off.

34. During a major incident:
    a. Action cards will assist to prepare ward staff.
    b. Command and control are optional.
    c. Safety is only an issue for staff.
    d. Communicable disease is not a threat.

Chapter 5

1. Which of the following is not a factor to be considered in mass gathering risk assessment:
    a. Presence of on-site medical facilities.
    b. Incidents occuring at previous, similar events.
    c. Presence of medically trained people among the spectators.
    d. Predicted weather conditions.

2. Which statement about mass gatherings is true?
    a. Mass gatherings are associated with a higher patient presentation rate compared to the general population.
    b. Mass gatherings of people younger than 35 years old will have relatively less patient presentations as this is an essentially healthy population.
    c. It is possible to make accurate predictions as to the number and type of medical resources necessary for a particular event based on international standards.
    d. The universally accepted definition of a mass gathering is any event with an excess of 25 000 spectators.

3. Which of the following groups would not be involved in an integrated approach to medical planning?
    a. Food vendors.
    b. Crowd control.
    c. The sports team playing at the event.
    d. The local venue management.

Chapter 6

1. The functions of a basic clinic facility in the recovery phase after a disaster includes:
    a. Providing hospitalisation capabilities for surgical interventions and amputation of septic wounds.
    b. Replacing existing health care services for the community.
    c. Providing care facilities for homeless aged inhabitants.
    d. Managing minor ailments, preventing the spreading of communicable diseases, providing medication and giving health education.

2. Environmental health intervention should be implemented as soon as possible following a major incident or disaster. These measures should include:
    a. Ensuring that safe drinking water is available and that feeding schemes adhere to hygiene requirements.
    b. Evaluating the quality of food donated and condemning all food that is not culturally acceptable to the community.
    c. Recovering all food that can be retrieved from collapsed homes and refrigerators in the area.
    d. Burying all corpses immediately.

3. In delivering psycho-social support in the post-disaster phase:
   a. Members of the clergy play no role, as survivors' religious preferences must be respected.
   b. A multi-disciplinary team of social workers, psychologists and members of the clergy is ideal.
   c. Psychological counselling is compulsory for all survivors.
   d. Financial needs should not be addressed, as this can be dealt with later.

4. In managing donations of drugs and other medicines post-disaster:
   a. All medicine donations are accepted with gratitude, as these will enable the delivery of a comprehensive health care system.
   b. They should never be accepted.
   c. Only unscheduled drugs are accepted as there is no secure storage for higher-scheduled drugs.
   d. They should be evaluated with caution, and drugs required should be accepted on specific conditions (such as understandable labelling and quality control).

5. In terms of children being affected by major incidents, all the following are true, EXCEPT:
   a. Disaster plans often include specific arrangements for dealing with children.
   b. Children are vulnerable at all phases of a disaster.
   c. The vulnerability of children is also due to health facilities not being able to deal with a large number of children in need of acute care.
   d. Treatment of children in a disaster is further complicated if the child is separated from the parents.

6. The unique needs of children include all of the following, EXCEPT:
   a. They have a limited ability to flee and seek appropriate shelter.
   b. Children are more susceptible to infections.
   c. Children have different food and pharmaceutical requirements to adults.
   d. Children tend to overcome long-term psychological problems faster than adults exposed to the same incident.

7. Select the one false statement about disaster planning:
   a. There is a need to involve paediatric trained personnel in the disaster planning process.
   b. Planning for children is further complicated by the fact that they are not a homogeneous group.
   c. Early involvement of the community is not recommended in planning, as it may cause panic.
   d. Planning should include the availability of orthopaedic equipment for children.

8. The responsibility for initial management of the deceased at a major incident in South Africa is carried by out by all of the following, EXCEPT:
   a. Police.
   b. Forensic health services.
   c. Ambulance services.
   d. Social services.

9. The process for disaster victim identification (DVI) involves all of the following, EXCEPT:
   a. Dental records.
   b. Brain matter analysis.
   c. Fingerprints.
   d. DNA comparison.

10. When selecting a suitable area for the placement of shelters for displaced populations, the following are important considerations, EXCEPT:
    a. The shelter should provide at least 3.5 square metres per person.
    b. It should be near a water source, but not in a low-lying area.
    c. As it is an emergency situation, trying to address individual cultural requirements is not important.
    d. Water provision and adequate security are important considerations.

11. With regard to surveillance of disease, the following statements are true, EXCEPT:
    a. Most common diseases include measles, diarrhoeal disease and upper respiratory tract infection.
    b. Measles vaccination is an important early intervention.
    c. Vulnerable populations include the elderly, children and immuno-compromised persons.
    d. The objective of outbreak control is to document new cases.

12. Health assessments of displaced populations are important and should include all of the points listed below, EXCEPT:
    a. Financial status, so as to determine their ability to pay for services.
    b. Size of the affected population and other demographic data.
    c. Nutritional assessment, particularly of the children.
    d. Vaccination status.

Chapter 7

1. In identifying a person to receive VIP visitors, preference should be given to:
   a. Only the CEO of the institution, as it will not be acceptable to allocate anybody else.
   b. A clinical staff member who could answer questions on the patients' diagnosis and prognosis.
   c. An identified manager senior enough to liaise effectively with the leaders but not required to make command decisions during the visit.
   d. The public relations secretary.

2. A site tour for VIPs is:
   a. Recommended if planned in advance and addresses safety and ethical issues.
   b. Not recommended, as they will be in the way of the fire-fighting teams.
   c. Should include bereaved families, so that the media can have the opportunity to film the VIP supporting the family.
   d. Should include all the ceremonial aspects, such as a guard of honour and flags, as this will lift the morale of the survivors.

3. Following a major incident, a formal media statement should be released as soon as realistic. Such a statement should include:
   a. Basic information on the event and the basic technical data that is available and confirmed.
   b. Requests for the media not to visit the hospital and that no information will be released.
   c. Deny that the incident is disrupting the routine and indicate that the hospital can cope with the situation.
   d. Decline to comment on any questions.

4. A media conference should be addressed by:
   a. Only the CEO in person.
   b. A spokesperson who has the appropriate skills and project the professional image of the institution.
   c. Any staff member that has seen the casualties.
   d. Preferably nobody from the hospital, as it will deter critical capabilities.

5. Internal information is released to all staff members to:
   a. Inform them that nobody will be allowed to go off duty.
   b. Ensure that staff are informed on the overtime payment for the disaster in time.
   c. Prevent rumours and ensure that staff have the correct facts on the incident and know what to expect.
   d. Inform staff so that they can brief family members on the situation.

6. A field treatment facility should:
   a. Always be established after any incident with more than 20 casualties as it greatly reduce mortality
   b. Contribute to the logical flow of casualties, reduce unnecessary transfers and ease the load on a already overburdened hospital.
   c. Enable surgery to be done on site and therefore reduce cost.
   d. Allow the hospital to continue functioning normally.

7. A primary health care facility can be established in a disaster area to:
   a. Replace the existing clinic service, which is often not functioning optimally.
   b. Create long-term development in the region.
   c. Provide minor ailment service to the affected population until such time as normal health and transport services are functioning normally.
   d. Provide surgical capabilities in a region where this may not be available.

8. In deploying a field hospital:
   a. A detailed appreciation must be done to identify the needs and the value of the facility.
   b. Sufficient time must be allocated to deploy the facility.
   c. There must be sufficient logistical support to move and deploy and to allow services to function.
   d. All of the above.

9. A military organisation is:
    a. Unwilling to cooperate with civilian organisations.
    b. Only used to defend the country, and not in other roles.
    c. Always strictly hierarchical, with clear lines of command.
    d. Amenable to informal liaison in civilian cooperation.

10. Various other disaster-related capabilities are embedded in the basic structures of the army, and include assets such as:
    a. Military police, mass catering capabilities, information gathering and map and photo creation capabilities.
    b. Maritime evacuation capabilities.
    c. Large aircraft for air evacuation.
    d. Only fighting elements, which are of little value in a major incident.

11. 'Rules of engagement' refer to:
    a. Rules which delineate the circumstances and limitation under which the military will initiate and continue in an engagement.
    b. Protection of military medical personnel under the Geneva Convention.
    c. Protect prisoners of war in a battle.
    d. Prohibit the use of dangerous weapons, such as phosphorus, in battle.

12. A military health or medical service often includes:
    a. Emergency care staff.
    b. Medical and nursing staff.
    c. Environmental health staff and psychologists.
    d. All of the above.

13. In assessing patients prior to mass transport, attention should be given to the following:
    a. Identify the patients with specific numbers, triaging all casualties and determining mode of transport required (sitting or lying).
    b. Triage casualties and only transport Priority 3 casualties by mass transport, as Priority 1 casualties cannot be resuscitated in transport.
    c. Only transport sitting casualties.
    d. Transport casualties for stabilisation at the receiving hospital.

14. Mass rail transport:
    a. Can be used to transport lying patients in parcel vans.
    b. Is used to evacuate critical patients only.
    c. Allows greater rapidity, as all patients can climb in and out on their own.
    d. Requires special built railway carriages.

15. In an air evacuation:
    a. All patients can be evacuated in large aircraft.
    b. Patients require specialist evaluation to determine their suitability for long-distance fixed-wing transport.
    c. It can be used as a single mode of transport from hospital to hospital.
    d. Sitting casualties can only be transported on airline seats.

Chapter 8

1. The following statements regarding the triage of burns patients are incorrect, EXCEPT:
   a. Every burns casualty needs to be referred to a specialised burns centre.
   b. Burn patients should only be triaged once all the other victims have been attended to.
   c. Total body surface area affected, age and presence of inhalational injury are important prognostic indicators.
   d. The patient needs only to be triaged once and this occurs at the site of the major incident.

2. As regards burns surge capacity, the following are incorrect, EXCEPT:
   a. It is the responsibility of the emergency centre at the receiving hospital to create burns bed capacity.
   b. Plans to create extra surge capacity can only be implemented in a major incident and not during routine daily operations.
   c. Lack of adequately trained staff is a major obstacle to the provision of extra burns and critical care surge capacity.
   d. Communication between emergency medical services and specialised burns centres is not important during a major incident.

3. Terrorism is:
   a. A relatively new phenomenon.
   b. Aimed at disrupting military targets only.
   c. Designed to cause civilian fear and panic.
   d. Of minor concern to major incident management.

4. Communication at blast scenes may be difficult due to:
   a. The risk of activating secondary devices.
   b. Noise levels that preclude use of the radio.
   c. Working cellular networks.
   d. All radio masts and repeater stations working.

5. Blast injury can be regarded as:
   a. One universal set of injuries.
   b. Limited risk for amputation.
   c. Four phases of differing injury patterns.
   d. Seldom fatal and often survivable.

6. Tertiary blast injury may lead to:
   a. Direct penetrating missile injury.
   b. Rupture of tympanic membranes
   c. Burns and respiratory distress.
   d. Crush injury and subsequent renal dysfunction.

7. Radiation incidents commonly:
   a. Are acts of terrorism at commercial facilities;
   b. Are acts of human error.
   c. Lead to surgical events rather than medical pathology.
   d. Lead to over-reaction by responding agencies.

8. In decontamination and patient evacuation:
    a. The advice of a medical physicist is useless.
    b. Special ambulances are required.
    c. Standard precautions do not apply.
    d. Water is a suitable decontaminant.

9. In hospital care of the radiation casualty:
    a. There is a high risk to hospital personnel.
    b. Internal decontamination never requires the use of chelating agents.
    c. Signs and symptoms of radiation illness are non-specific.
    d. Excision of wounds should be aggressive with limb sacrifice if involvement is suspected.

10. Bioterrorism is appealing to terrorists because:
    a. Weapons are difficult to procure.
    b. Bio-agents are more efficient than nuclear weapons.
    c. Bio-agents may take time to be detected.
    d. The effects are not well researched.

11. The common bioterrorism pathogens include:
    a. Tuberculosis.
    b. Anthrax.
    c. HIV.
    d. Beta haemolytic streps.

12. Anthrax is:
    a. Mostly not a bioterrorism episode.
    b. Found in humans rather than animals.
    c. Not known to affect the gastro-intestinal tract.
    d. Is seldom susceptible to penicillin.

13. Clues to a bioterrorism outbreak include all the following, EXCEPT:
    a. A known pathogen, but unusual resistance profile or epidemiological features.
    b. An outbreak of a rare or novel disease.
    c. An outbreak of disease in an endemic area.
    d. A seasonal disease in off-season time.

14. Viral haemorrhagic fevers include all the following, EXCEPT:
    a. Marburg.
    b. Varicella.
    c. Ebola.
    d. Congo-Crimean.

15. Post-exposure prophylaxis includes:
    a. Triple therapy for one day for all exposures.
    b. Triple therapy for 28 days for all exposures.
    c. Triple therapy for percutaneous exposure with high risk.
    d. Triple therapy for percutaneous exposure with low risk.

16. Most cases of cholera are detected in:
    a. Africa.
    b. Asia.
    c. Europe.
    d. The Americas.

17. As regards the management of a hazardous material scene, all of the following are true, EXCEPT:
    a. Incidents involving hazardous materials are managed differently, dependent on what chemical agent is present.
    b. The fire department or police service are commonly incident commander.
    c. The first responder is the first person from an emergency service to arrive on scene.
    d. Specialist services and agencies should be informed as soon as possible about the incident.

18. On approaching the scene of a hazardous material incident, all of the following statements are relevant, EXCEPT:
    a. Always approach from upwind and uphill.
    b. A safe distance from which to size up the scene is about 50 m.
    c. Air conditioners must be switched off.
    d. The presence of many dead birds in the area may be an important clue that a hazardous substance is present.

19. To control the scene, all of these actions need to be performed, EXCEPT:
    a. Safety zones need to be established.
    b. A register needs to be kept of persons entering the hot zone.
    c. The press are allowed into the hot zone, provided they are prepared to sign the required indemnity forms.
    d. Communication needs to be established early so as to update relevant control centres.

20. With respect to decontamination, which of the following statements is false?
    a. EMS should try, as far as possible, to transport only those patients that have been decontaminated.
    b. The ambulance needs to be cleaned after transporting a contaminated patient.
    c. Hospitals need to be informed of the pending arrival of casualties from a hazardous material incident.
    d. Hospitals need not worry about decontamination facilities, as the fire department will decontaminate all the patients at the scene.

21. With respect to organophosphate poisoning, the following are all true, EXCEPT:
    a. Organophosphates are commonly seen as accidental poisoning agents.
    b. Patients may present with convulsions and difficulty in breathing.
    c. Decontamination of a patient with organophosphate includes removing the clothing of the casualty.
    d. There is no specific antidote for organophosphate poisoning, and the treatment is supportive only.

Chapter 9

1. In developing an equipment plan for major incident response, the following are true, EXCEPT:
    a. The equipment supplied should be items with which the responders will be familiar.
    b. One standard equipment cache is suitable for most incidents.
    c. Planners should allow for additional stock equal to approximately 60 days' supply.
    d. The equipment plan must ensure that the responders are essentially self-sufficient.

2. Types of PPE include:
    a. Helmets specific to the hazard.
    b. Adequate eye and ear protection.
    c. Respiratory protection specific to the hazard.
    d. All of the above.

3. In terms of the packaging of equipment, the following statements are all true, EXCEPT:
    a. Battery-operated items should be stored with the batteries removed if they don't require trickle charging.
    b. Regular checks need to be made in terms of the expiry date of consumables.
    c. If equipment is to be stored in containers, then such containers need to be dust-proof.
    d. Ready-to-use packs have no role to play in the pre-hospital environment.

Answer sheet – Disaster Medicine

Name: _____   Council registration no.: _____

Email address: _____   Postal address: _____

_____

_____

Chapter 1

1.	a	b	c	d
2.	a	b	c	d
3.	a	b	c	d
4.	a	b	c	d
5.	a	b	c	d
6.	a	b	c	d
7.	a	b	c	d

Chapter 2

1.	a	b	c	d
2.	a	b	c	d
3.	a	b	c	d
4.	a	b	c	d
5.	a	b	c	d
6.	a	b	c	d
7.	a	b	c	d
8.	a	b	c	d
9.	a	b	c	d
10.	a	b	c	d
11.	a	b	c	d
12.	a	b	c	d
13.	a	b	c	d
14.	a	b	c	d
15.	a	b	c	d
16.	a	b	c	d

Chapter 3

1.	a	b	c	d
2.	a	b	c	d
3.	a	b	c	d
4.	a	b	c	d
5.	a	b	c	d
6.	a	b	c	d
7.	a	b	c	d
8.	a	b	c	d
9.	a	b	c	d
10.	a	b	c	d
11.	a	b	c	d
12.	a	b	c	d
13.	a	b	c	d
14.	a	b	c	d

Chapter 4

1.	a	b	c	d
2.	a	b	c	d
3.	a	b	c	d
4.	a	b	c	d
5.	a	b	c	d
6.	a	b	c	d
7.	a	b	c	d
8.	a	b	c	d
9.	a	b	c	d
10.	a	b	c	d
11.	a	b	c	d
12.	a	b	c	d
13.	a	b	c	d
14.	a	b	c	d
15.	a	b	c	d
16.	a	b	c	d
17.	a	b	c	d
18.	a	b	c	d
19.	a	b	c	d
20.	a	b	c	d
21.	a	b	c	d
22.	a	b	c	d
23.	a	b	c	d
24.	a	b	c	d
25.	a	b	c	d
26.	a	b	c	d
27.	a	b	c	d
28.	a	b	c	d
29.	a	b	c	d
30.	a	b	c	d
31.	a	b	c	d
32.	a	b	c	d
33.	a	b	c	d
34.	a	b	c	d

Signature: _____

Answer sheet – Disaster Medicine

Name: _____   Council registration no.: _____

Email address: _____   Postal address: _____

_____

_____

Chapter 5

1.	a	b	c	d
2.	a	b	c	d
3.	a	b	c	d

Chapter 6

1.	a	b	c	d
2.	a	b	c	d
3.	a	b	c	d
4.	a	b	c	d
5.	a	b	c	d
6.	a	b	c	d
7.	a	b	c	d
8.	a	b	c	d
9.	a	b	c	d
10.	a	b	c	d
11.	a	b	c	d
12.	a	b	c	d

Chapter 7

1.	a	b	c	d
2.	a	b	c	d
3.	a	b	c	d
4.	a	b	c	d
5.	a	b	c	d
6.	a	b	c	d
7.	a	b	c	d
8.	a	b	c	d
9.	a	b	c	d
10.	a	b	c	d
11.	a	b	c	d
12.	a	b	c	d
13.	a	b	c	d
14.	a	b	c	d
15.	a	b	c	d

Chapter 8

1.	a	b	c	d
2.	a	b	c	d
3.	a	b	c	d
4.	a	b	c	d
5.	a	b	c	d
6.	a	b	c	d
7.	a	b	c	d
8.	a	b	c	d
9.	a	b	c	d
10.	a	b	c	d
11.	a	b	c	d
12.	a	b	c	d
13.	a	b	c	d
14.	a	b	c	d
15.	a	b	c	d
16.	a	b	c	d
17.	a	b	c	d
18.	a	b	c	d
19.	a	b	c	d
20.	a	b	c	d
21.	a	b	c	d

Chapter 9

1.	a	b	c	d
2.	a	b	c	d
3.	a	b	c	d

Signature: _____